Practical Navigation; or an Introduction to the Whole art, ... By John Seller,

Lineal Maxs William James Godfrey

his Servant for Eleven years

July 28 - 1798 ye Cap. strouk me with a Stea for Vmoting

July ye 19: 1798 . I Bleded on Dross of Blood at ye nose

Practical Navigation;

OR AN

Introduction to the whole Art.

July ye 18: Thomas Shoddlworth strouk me - - - - - - -

July ye 24 he took me for - - -

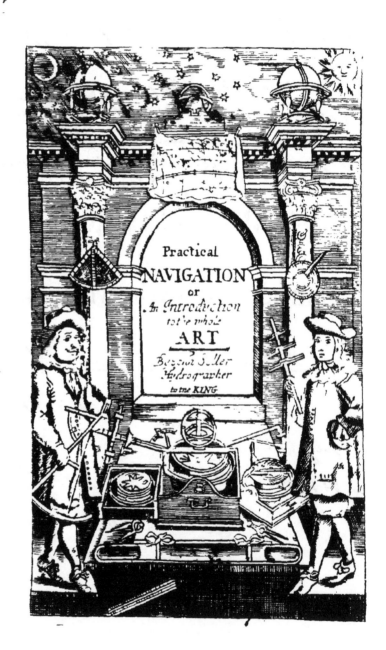

Practical

NAVIGATION

or

An Introduction
to the whole
ART

Benjamin Seller
Hydrographer
to the KING

Practical Navigation;

OR AN

Introduction to the Whole Art,

Containing many useful Geometrical Definitions and Problems, The Doctrine of Plain and Spherical Triangles, Plain Mercator, and Great-Circle-Sailing; Sundry useful Problems in Astronomy; The Use of Instruments; The Azimuth-Compass, and Ring-Dial, The Fore-Staff, Quadrant, and Nocturnal; The Plain Scale, *Gunter*'s Scale, Plain-Chart, *Mercator*'s Chart, both Globes, and Virtues of the Loadstone. Useful Tables of the Moon's Age, of the Tides, of the Sun's Place, Declination, and Right-Ascension; of the Stars Right Ascension and Declination; The Latitude and Longitude of Places, and a Table of Miridional Parts; Likewise a new Traverse-Table, and the Use thereof in keeping a Reckoning at Sea: Also a Table of 10000 Logarithms, and of the Logarithm Sines, Tangents, and Secants.

All carefully Corrected, with many useful Additions.

By *JOHN SELLER*, Hydrographer to the King.

LONDON,

Printed for R. and *W Mount* and *T. Page*, in *Postern-Row*, on *Tower-Hill*, MDCCXVIII.

BOOKS of Navigation Printed for Richard Mount.

THE Coasting Pilot for England, Scotland, Holland, &c.
The E. Pilot for the Channel. Eng. Pilot for the Straights.
The Eng. Pilot for the Northern Navigation.
The Eng. Pilot for the W. Indies. Eng. Pilot for the E. Indies.
Sea-Atlas, containing Charts of the S. Coast of the whole world
The Mariners New Kalender. By Nathaniel Colson.
The Mariners Magazine. By Capt. Samuel Sturmy, Folio.
The Seamans Kalender. By Henry Phillips.
The Seamans New Kalender. By William Leybourn.
The Seaman's Practice By Richard Norwood.
Norwood's Doctrine of Triangles, applied to Navigation.
Practical Navigation: or an Introduction to the whole Art.
The whole Art of Navigation. By Capt. Daniel Newhouse.
A Light to the Art of Gunnery, By Capt. Thomas Binning.
Theory of Navigation, By James Hodgson.
Advancement of the Art of Navigation. By Henry Phillips.
The Compleat Modelist or Art of Rigging; shewing how to raise
the Model of any Ship; and to find the Length and Bigness
of every Rope with the weight of their Anchors and Cables.
The Boatswain's Art; shewing the Art of Rigging any Ship &c.
The Compleat Shipwright; By Edmund Bushnel, Shipwright
The Ship Builders Assistance. By William Southerland.
Compleat Ship Wright and Mariner.
The Seaman's Companion. By M. Norwood.
The Seaman's Glass with the use of the Plain Scale in Navigation
Seaman's Grammer, By Capt. John Smith.
Sea-Gunners Companion, By Capt. Povey.
An Epitome of the whole Art of Navigation, containing an easie
methodical way to become a compleat Navigator. By J. Atkinson
Epitome of Navigation, the 3 kinds of Sailing, Astronomy and
Geography, with useful Tables in Navigation, By H. Gellibrand
Norwood's Epitome of Navigation, with Additions, By J. A.
Mariners Compass Rectified. By And. Wakely, much enlarged
The use of the double Scale of Proportion By Seth Partridge
An Epitome of Navigation, By William Jones.
Arithmetical Trigonometry, By Mark Fofter.
Art of Sea Fighting. By Robert Parke.
Key to Arithmetick and Algebra. By J. Parsons.
There are sold also all sorts of Mathematical and Sea Books,
Pilots and Sea-Charts for all parts of the World, Plain and Mercator; or Books of any other Subjects; Paper, or Paper Books;
the best Ink, and all other Stationary Ware.

TO THE

MARINERS

OF

Great Britain and *Ireland.*

GENTLEMEN,

THIS Book was *first Written by* Mr. John Seller, *and very much Enlarged by* Mr. John Colſon, *deceas'd, who taught Navigation for many Years in* London, *and has been much Eſteemed by the Lovers of the Art of Navigation, as has appeared by the many Impreſſions Sold off. And being informed that there were very many and conſiderable Errors in it, occaſioned by often Printing ; and that the whole wanted a Reviſe, I have therefore had it overlook'd, corrected, and amended, and added what was defective ; and renew'd the Tables, which by length of Time were worn out ; and for the Tables of* Logarithms, Sines, *and* Tangents, *there has been ſuch great Care and Pains taken in correcting and amending them, that I may juſtly Recommend them, as the moſt Correct Extant All which I hope will oblige the Ingenious Mariner, and Encourage the Learner of the Art of Navigation, into whoſe Hands it ſhall come. I am,*

Gentlemen,

Decemb. 3d.
1717.

Your moſt obliged

And humble Servant,

R. MOUNT.

On the *Practical Navigation* of my very good Friend the Author.

YOUR Book (kind Sir) I have perus'd and find
    Rich Arguments of an Ingenious Mind;
That for our good your Talent wi'l not hide,
But build a *Light House* Mariners to guide.
What others have in mighty Volumns done,
You neatly here have concluded all in one;
Yet is your Book to no great Volumn grown,
Though grac'd with large Additions of your own.
For me to praise your Work, might be my blame,
Fearing my Meaness might dispraise the same.
You want not learned Pens, in lofty Verse,
Your well-deserved Praises to Rehearse.
Mean Artists, Men Obscure (and such am I)
Ought t'wish and pray for your Prosperity.
Yet rouse for (once) my humble Muse, and let
The Country Oak Pipe drewn the Flajelet;
And 'tis but fitting (sith your pains in this
To City and to Country useful is)
That City Poetry and Country Lays
With joint Consent should eccho forth your Praise.
Who doth peruse your Work, shall surely find,
The Subject handled well, and well designed.
You much have done in little. Here we find,
What in this Art may please a curious Mind,
The *Longitude* excepted. But if we
Your Rules observe, obtained it may be
For use sufficient, but the same to get,
With certainty, is not discovered yet.
Which rare Performance, if that any can
Make plain ly out, I wish you be the Man.
But stay, my Muse, be short and not so rude;
I'll only wish you well, and so conclude.
  May these your Labours (as they profit all)
Turn to your profit, and your good withal.
May no base Plagiary arrogate
That to himself, which you by pains have got.

* Mr Wrights May never English-man be so unkind,
Charta ascribed (As famous * *Wright*, and reverend † *Ward* do find)
to Mercator. T'ascribe to Strangers, what you have set forth,
† Dr. Ward's Detracting so from their and your true Worth.
Invention of May you encourag'd be as reason is,
a Triangle .in To publish more such useful Works as this;
a Ellipsis and May you be happy ever in the End ·
applyed to A- Thus prays your humble Servant and your Friend.
tronomy, as-
cribed to Co- *Westerleigh* in
pagan.   *Glocesterfhire.*

Nathaniel Friend.

A TABLE of Contents of the following Treatise

The Contents.

𝕻𝖗𝖆𝖈𝖙𝖎𝖈𝖆𝖑

𝕻𝖗𝖆𝖈𝖙𝖎𝖈𝖆𝖑 𝕹𝖆𝖛𝖎𝖌𝖆𝖙𝖎𝖔𝖓.

CHAP. I.

A Preliminary Discourse of Navigation and Arithmetick.

SECT. I. *Of the Preliminary Discourse of Navigation.*

NAVIGATION (that useful part of the *Mathematicks*) is a Science which has been highly valued by the Ancients, especially by our Ancestors of this Island; it being indeed the Beauty and Bulwark of *England*, the Wall and Wealth of *Britain*, and the Bridge that joins it to the Universe.

It consists of two general Parts.

First, That which may be called the *Domestick*, or more *common Navigation*, (I mean Coasting or Sailing along the Shore.) This Part employs the Mariners *Compass* and *Lead*, as the chief Instruments, and for an Introduction of this kind, I refer you to the Books, entituled, *The English Pilot*, describing the Sea-Coast, Capes, Soundings, Sands, Rocks, and Dangers, the Bays, Roads, Harbours, Rivers, and Ports, in most of the known Parts of the World *Being furnished* with New and Exact *Draughts* and *Descriptions* collected from the Experience of divers of our *Able Navigators*; Sold by Mr. *Mount* on *Tower-Hill*.

Secondly, That which may more properly bear the Name and principally deserves to be entituled the *Art of Navigation*, is that Part which guides the Ship in her Course through the Immense Ocean, to any Part of the known World, which cannot be done unless it be determined in what place the Ship is at all times, both in respect of *Latitude* and *Longitude* : this being the principal Care of a *Navigator*, and the *Masterpiece* of *Nautical Science*.

To the Commendable Accomplishment of which knowledge, these four things are subordinate Requisites:

Viz. {
  Arithmetick,
  Geometry,
  Trigonometry and
  Astronomy.

B

Of

Of the firſt of which (namely *Arithmetick*) I ſhall give you a brief Specimen

Arithmetick is the Art of Numbering, from the Greek Word *Arithmos*, which ſignifies Number, and in it there are five eſpecial Parts, *viz. Numeration, Addition, Subtraction, Multiplication,* and *Diviſion.* Of which in order.

Sect. II. *Of NUMERATION.*

NUmeration teaches how to ſet down any Number ſpoken or propoſed; and to read it truly when written.

To which purpoſe you are to obſerve, That Numbers are commonly expreſſed by theſe Nine Figures

$$1 \quad 2 \quad 3 \quad 4 \quad 5 \quad 6 \quad 7 \quad 8 \quad 9$$

One, Two, Three, Four, Five, Six, Seven, Eight, Nine.

And o which is called a Cypher (and by ſome a Nought) becauſe of it ſelf it ſignifies nothing, yet encreaſes the Value of other Figures that ſtand behind it; for every Figure augments its proper Value according to the place it happens in, except the firſt: And are reckoned from the right hand unto the left (and the reaſon is, becauſe this Art of Numbering was firſt taught by the Oriental Nations, whoſe Languages are read that way) ſo that the Figure that ſtands fartheſt to the right hand, is ſaid to be in the firſt place, the next to that to be in the ſecond place, and ſo of the reſt.

Any of the nine Figures in the firſt place ſignifies only its ſingle Value; in the ſecond place, as many Tens as its own ſimple Value; in the third place, ſo many Hundreds; in the fourth place, ſo many Thouſands; in the fifth place, ſo many ten Thouſands, in the ſixth place, ſo many Hundred Thouſands; and in the ſeventh place, ſo many Millions; as may appear in this following Table.

Units	1	2	3	4	5	6	7	8	9
Tens		1	2	3	4	5	6	7	8
Hundreds			1	2	3	4	5	6	7
Thouſands				1	2	3	4	5	6
Ten Thouſands					1	2	3	4	5
Hundred Thouſands						1	2	3	4
Millions							1	2	3
Ten Millions								1	2
Hundred Millions									1

To be read this way.

The laſt Line of this Table is thus read, *One hundred twenty three Millions, four hundred fifty ſix thouſand, ſeven hundred eighty nine.*

SECT.

SECT. III. *Of ADDITION·*

A Ddition is the putting together of two or more Numbers into one Sum, so that the total Value of them all may be discovered.

Example 1. *In whole Numbers.*

Suppose here were a Squadron of Men of War of five Ships I demand (according to the quantity of Men in each Ship) how many Men there is in the whole Squadron?

Aboard of the biggest Ship there are ————————————	500
Aboard another, ————————————————	450
Aboard another, ————————————————	362
Aboard another, ————————————————	278
Aboard the last, ————————————————	110
There are in the Squadron ———————————	1700

To add these together, begin at the first Row on the Right-hand, and say 8 and 2 is 10, set down 0 under the first; then I carry the 1 (which stands for 10) to the next Row, and say 1 and 1 is 2, and 7 is 9, and 6 is 15, and 5 is 20, then set down 0 under the second Row, and carry the 2, which is 20, to the next Row; and say 2 and 1 is 3, and 2 is 5, and 3 is 8, and 4 is 12, and 5 is 17; which 17 set down under the third Row, and the Sum is 1700, the Number of Men in the whole Squadron.

Example 2. *Of Pounds, Shillings, Pence.*

Now if you would know how much Money all the Captains Pay comes to for one Month

	l.	*s.*	*d.*
Supposing that the Captain of the greatest Ship hath *per Month* ————————————	10	00	00
The Captain of the other—————————	08	10	00
The Captain of the other—————————	07	10	00
The Captain of the other—————————	06	10	00
The Captain of the last —————————	05	00	00
	37	10	00

	l.	*s.*	*d.*
The Question is *How much Mony it amounts to for 1 Month?* Answer ———————————	37	16	00

To effect which you must begin at the Row of Pence, and seeing there is no Pence in the whole Row, you must set down 00 under the Row of Pence Then proceed to the Row of Shillings, and add up the Shillings in that Row, which amounts to 30 Shillings, set down the 10 Shillings under the Row of Shillings, and carry the 20 Shillings, or 1 Pound, to the Row of Pounds, and say 1 and 5 is 6, and 6 is 12 and 7 is 19, and 8 is 27, and 10 is 37, which 37 set down under the Row of Pounds; and the whole Sum amounts to *Thirty seven Pounds, Ten Shillings,* the Sum of all the Captains Pay for one Month.   B 2   SECT

SECT. IV. *Of SUBTRACTION.*

SUbtraction (commonly called *Subftraction*) is a Rule that teaches how to take any leffer Number out of a greater, fo as to know how much remains.

1. Set down your greater Number, and under that your fmaller, Units under Units, Tens under Tens, &c and in Mony each Denomination anfwering to its kind, as Pence under Pence, and Shillings under Shillings, and Pounds under Pounds.

2. Draw a Line under them, and begin at the Right-hand, and take the leffer Number out of the greater, and fet down what remains under the Line

3. If any Figure of the fmaller Number happen to be bigger than that over it, then you muft borrow a Unite from the next Place, or higher Denomination, to be added to the leffer Figure, fubtracting from that Sum, and fubfcribe the Remainder ; which Unite muft be added to the next Place, or Denomination to be Subtracted.; as will appear in the Example following.

Example.	l.	s.	d
Suppofe I borrow ———————————	296	15	06
And I paid at feveral Times———————	125	17	04
There remains due ————————————	170	18	02

The Work is thus performed: Begin with the Row of Pence, and fay 4 from 6 and there remains 2 ; then go to the Row of Shillings, and fay 17 from 15 I cannot take, then you muft borrow 20 Shillings from the Row of Pounds; and fay 17 from 35, and there remains 18, which 18 fet under the Row of Shillings. Then proceed to the Row of Pounds, and fay 1 that I borrowed and 5 is 6, 6 from 6 there remains 0, which 0 fet under the firft Row of Pounds; and proceed to the next, and fay, 2 from 9 and there remains 7, which 7 fet under the fecond Row, and proceed to the third Row, and fay 1 from 2 and there remains 1 ; then is the Queftion finifhed and there remains 170*l.* 18*s.* 2*d.* unpaid.

And the Queftion ftands thus,

	l.	s.	d.
Now to prove whether the Queftion is truly wrought, add the Remainder and the lower Number together; and if the total of that Addition be the fame with the upper Number then is the Work right.	296	15	06
	125	17	04
	170	18	02
	296	15	06

Sect. V. *Of* MULTIPLICATION.

1. **M**Ultiplication teaches how to increase the greater of two Numbers given, as often as there are Units in the lesser; and serves instead of many Additions.

2. In Multiplication there are three Parts.
  1. The Multiplicand, or Number to be Multiplied.
  2. The Multiplier, or Number by which it is Multiplied
  3. The Product made by the Multiplication.

792	Multiplicand
32	Multiplier.
1584	
2376	
25344	Product.

Example

Before you can make any Progress in this Rule you must perfectly get the following Table by Heart.

Multiplication Table.

	1	2	3	4	5	6	7	8	9
1	1	2	3	4	5	6	7	8	9
2	2	4	6	8	10	12	14	16	18
3	3	6	9	12	15	18	21	24	27
4	4	8	12	16	20	24	28	32	36
5	5	10	15	20	25	30	35	40	45
6	6	12	18	24	30	36	42	48	54
7	7	14	21	28	35	42	49	56	63
8	8	16	24	32	40	48	56	64	72
9	9	18	27	36	45	54	63	72	81

The Use of the foregoing Table.

Note; That on the Top and left Side are placed the 9 Digits, which are to be multiplied one by another, and in the common Angle of meeting you will have the Product.

Example. Suppose I would multiply 7 times 9; look on the left side of the Table for 7, and on the Top of the Table for 9, and in the Angle of meeting (in the Column next the right Hand) you will find 63, the Answer of the Question.

Question 1.

Suppose there are 1700 private Seamen in a Squadron of Ships, and they have 33 Shillings *per* Month; How much Money will pay them

for

for one Month ? Set your Numbers thus, the greater Number uppermoſt.

     1700 Multiplicand.
       23 Multiplier.

     5100

    3400

   39100   Shillings ; the Anſwer of the Queſtion.

The Numbers being placed, as is before directed, begin thus, and ſay, 3 times 0 is 0, ſet that under the 3, and proceed to the next Figure in the Multiplicand, and ſay again 3 times 0 is 0 ; then ſet that 0 under the 2, and proceed to the next, and ſay, 3 times 7 is 21 ; ſet down 1 under the 7, and bear 2 in mind, and proceed to the next Figure in the Multiplicand, and ſay, 3 times 1 is 3, and 2 that I carry is 5, ſet that down under the 1, then have you done with the firſt Product : Then go to the next Figure in the Multiplier, and proceed as you did before, and the ſecond Product will be 3400, which muſt be ſet down under the other, only with this Caution, to move it one place more to the left Hand, as you may ſee in the Work ; then add thoſe two Numbers together, and the Product will be 39100, which are Shillings, the whole Sum of Wages for 1700 Men for one Month.

               Example 2.   235
In 235 Degrees, how many Minutes ?   60
   Multiply the Degrees by 60, the   ────────
   Number of Minutes in one Degree.   14100 Minutes.

Note, For a Contraction in this Rule, if any Number is given to be multiplyed by 10, 100, or 1000, it is but adding ſo many Cyphers to the Number given, and that will be the Product. As thus,

If 232 be multiplied by 10, it will produce 2320, by 100, 23200; by 1000, it will be 232000, &c:

Or, If any Number be given to be multiplied by 20, 30, 600, 5000, &c. multiply only by the Figures, and add as many Cyphers to your Product on the Right-hand as there is in the Multiplier, the Sum is the Product. Thus 257 multiplied by 700, the Product is 179900, &c.

Sect. VI. *Of DIVISION.*

Diviſion teacheth to find how many times a leſſer Number is contained in a greater, and ſheweth what remains, ſupplying the uſe of many Subtractions, it conſiſts of three Parts, Dividend, Diviſor and Quotient. The Dividend is the Number to be divided. The Diviſor is the Number to divide by, which is always leſſer than the Dividend : The Quotient is the Sum produced, by ſhewing how many times the Diviſor is contained in the Dividend. And if any thing happen to remain, it is called the Remainder.   *Example 1.*

Example 1.

To divide 250 by 4, how much is the Quotient?

First, Set down the Dividend 250, at each end
of which make a Scratch, as you see in the Margin. Then on the Left-hand set the Divisor 4 (the
Scratch on the right-hand being for the Quotient)
then (because I cannot have the Divisor 4 in the
first Figure of the Dividend 2) say how oft 4 in

```
4)250(62
  24
  ──
  10
   8
   ──
   2
```

25, which because there is 6 times, set 6 in the Quotient, and say 6
times 4 is 24, which set down under the 25 in the Dividend, and by
the common Rules of Subtraction take 24 from 25, there rests 1, which
set down under the 4, and to that 1 bring down the 0 in the Dividend
it makes 10, then say how oft 4 in 10, which because I can have 2
times, I set 2 in the Quotient, and (as before) say 2 times 4 is 8,
which set under the 10, and subtracted from it, the last Remainder is 2, so
that 250 being divided by 4, the Quotient is 62 and 2 remaining, &c.

Examp. 2. Suppose 4684 Pounds be to be divided among 54 Men,
How much is each Man's Share?

```
54)4684(86
   432
   ───
   364
   324
   ───
    40
    20  The Shillings in one Pound.
   ────
54)800(14 Shillings.
   54
   ──
  260
  216
  ───
   44
   12  The Pence in one Shilling.
   ──
   88

   44
  ────
54) 528(9 Pence.
    486
    ───
     42

      4 Farthings in one Penny.
   ─────
54)168( 3 Farthings.
   162
   ───
     6  ;4/4 or 1/9 of one Farthing.
```

Having

Having diſpoſed of your Numbers as directed *Example* 1. they will ſtand as you ſee them ; becauſe I cannot have 54 (the Diviſor) in 46 (the two firſt Figures of the Dividend) I ſay how oft 54 in 468, or (for the more Eaſe in working) how oft 5 in 46, which though I can have 9 times and 1 remaining, yet becauſe I foreſee that I cannot have 9 times 4 in 16, I take but 8 times, which I ſet in the Quotient, then ſay 8 times 4 is 32, ſet down 2 under the 8 in the Dividend, and carry 3, then ſay 8 times 5 is 40 and 3 is 43, which ſet down beſides the 2, as you ſee, then ſay 2 from 8 there reſts 6, which ſet down under 2, and then 3 from 6 there reſts 3 , then to the 36 ſo found, bring down 4 the laſt Figure in the Dividend, and begin a ſecond Operation, ſaying How oft 5 in 36, which you can have 6 times, ſet 6 in the Quotient, and ſay 6 times 4 is 24, ſet down 4 and carry 2, and 6 times 5 is 30 and 2 I carry is 32, then 4 from 4 there reſts 0, and 2 from 6 there reſts 4, and thus you have 40 remaining at laſt, ſo that each Man's ſhare is 86 Pounds and 40 remaining : Now to know the Value of this 40 that remains (which in Fractions is $\frac{40}{54}$ of a Pound) multiply 40 by 20 (the Shillings in a Pound) the Product is 800, which divided by 54 (the former Diviſor) the Quotient is 14 Shillings and 44 remains ; then multiply 44 by 12, the Pence in one Shilling, the Product 528 divided by 54, the Quotient is 3 pence and 42 remains, which 42 being multiplied by 4, the Farthings in one penny, and the Product 168 divided by 54 the Quotient is 3 Farthings and 6 remains, which is only $\frac{6}{54}$ of a Farthing.

Note, In finding the Value of any Fraction or Remainder in Diviſion, you always multiply the Remainder by ſuch a Number as the next leſs Denomination is contained in the greater (as in this Example, the firſt Remainder is 40, which becauſe the firſt Operation is Pounds, and I deſire to know the Value of that Fraction in Shillings, you multiply by 20 the Shillings in one Pound, &c and always divide the Product by the firſt Diviſor which here is 54, as you ſee above

If your Queſtion had been in Hundreds, Quarters and Pounds, you muſt have multiplied your firſt Remainder by 4, the Quarters in one Hundred, and your next by 28 the Pounds in one Quarter, and ſo in any other Denomination

Thus, if 4684 Pounds be divided amongſt 54 Men, each Man's ſhare appears to be 86 *l.* 14 *s* 9 *d*. 3 *q*.

Note, That the beſt Proof of Diviſion is by Multiplication thus : multiply the Quotient by the Diviſor, and add the Remainder (if any be) and if the Product be the ſame with the Dividend, then is the Work right, otherwiſe there is ſome miſtake.

Sect.

THE *Rule of Three,* for its excellent Ufe is called the *Golden Rule,* which teaches from three Numbers given, to find a fourth in Proportion thereunto, which is done by multiplying the fecond and third Numbers together, and dividing the Product by the firft, and the Quotient of the faid Divifion is the Anfwer of the Queftion.

As if 25 Tuns of Wine coft 800*l.* What fhall 35 coft?

Here *Note,* That the firft Number and the third muft always be of the fame Denomination. As if one be Pounds, Pence, Yards, Tuns, Hours, Men, &c. fo refpectively muft the other be: And the like is to be underftood by the fecond and the fourth, as in the following Numbers, which are thus difpofed   *Tuns*   *Pounds.*   *Tuns.*

25————————800————————35

This Rule is performed (after an apt difpofal of the Terms) by *Multiplication* and *Divifion* But note, that this Rule hath two Varieties, *viz.* Direct and *Reverfe* Now for the proper difpofing the Terms in any Queftion propounded, it is neceffary to give a General Rule to know whether the Queftion muft be wrought by the Direct Rule, or the Reverfe; which is this: When in the Queftion more requires more, or lefs requires lefs · As in this Queftion.

If 25 Tuns of Wine coft 800*l.* What will 35 Tuns coft? Here it is evident that the third Term is more than the firft, and therefore requires more. So in this Queftion ·

If 750*l.* give 45*l.* Intereft for a Year, What fhall 50*l.* give? Here it's plain that 50*l.* is lefs than 750*l.* and requires lefs Intereft. Therefore both thefe and all fuch like Queftions, muft be wrought by the Rule of Three Direct, wherein the Rule is plainly thus: Multiply the fecond Number by the third, and divide by the firft, the Quotient fhall be the fourth Number fought. As in the firft of thefe Examples, multiply 800 by 35, and the Product is 28000 : which being divided by 25, the Quotient is 1120 *l.* which fhews that 35 Tuns will coft 1120 *l.*

The Operation.

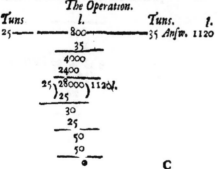

Tuns.   *l.*   *Tuns.*   *l.*
25————————800————————35 *Anfw.* 1120
                              35
                          ————
                          4000
                          2400
                  25) 28000 (1120*l.*
                       25
                      ————
                        30
                        25
                      ————
                        50
                        50
                      ————
                         0

          C   And

And ſo in the ſecond *Example* : Multiply 50 by 45, it makes 2250, which divided by 750, the Quotient is 3 , which ſhews that the Intereſt of 50l. for a Year is 3l.   *The Operation.*

l.	*l.*	*l.*
750————	45———	50
	50	

75|0)   225|0   (3l.

The Rule of Three Reverſe, is to be uſed when the third Number more requires leſs, or leſs requires more ; and then the Rule is thus :

Multiply the firſt Number by the ſecond, and divide the Product by the third, the Quotient ſhall be the fourth Number ſought, which always (as in the Direct Rule) ſhall be of the ſame Denomination with the ſecond Number. For Inſtance :

If 24 Pioneers require 16 Months to dig a Retrenchment about a Town, How many Pioneers muſt there be employed to dig the like Trench in 4 Months ?

In ſtating this Queſtion you muſt note, That 24, tho' it be the firſt named, is not to be the firſt Number in the Work, becauſe the middle Term muſt always be of the ſame Denomination with that which is ſought. And the three Numbers put in order ſtand thus,

Months.	*Pioneers.*	*Months.*
16————	24———	4

Here 'tis plain leſs requires more, that is, leſs Time more Hands : Therefore it muſt be wrought by the Rule Reverſe, and accordingly you may multiply 24 by 16, and divide the Product by 4, the Quotient is 96, as doth appear by the Work : which is, that 96 Pioneers muſt be employed to finiſh the Trench in 4 Months.

The Operation.

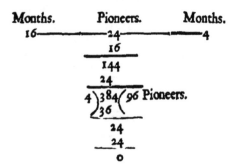

Months.	Pioneers.	Months.
16————	24———	4
	16	
	144	
	24	

4)384(96 Pioneers.
36
24
24
0

SECT. VIII.

Some Questions answered, and the Way of working them directed, serving to illustrate the foregoing Rule.

In ADDITION.

Quest. An ancient Lady being demanded how old she was: To avoid a direct Answer, said thus, I have 9 Children, and there were three Years between the Birth of every one of them, my Eldest was born when I was 19 Years old, which is now exactly the Age of my Youngest, How old now, is the Lady?

Answ. It is resolved by *Addition* thus First, Set down her Age when her first Child was born, which was 19, then the difference between that and the Birth of her Youngest which is 24, and then the Age of the Youngest 19, which being added together, shews the Lady to be 62 Years of Age.

```
19 Her Age.
24 Difference between the Children.
19 Age of her Youngest.
62 Lady's Age.
```

In SUBTRACTION.

Quest. In the Year of our Lord 1588, was the Spanish Invasion; In the Year 1715, I demand how long it is since?

Answ. Subtract 1588 out of 1715, there remains 127, the Time since, to the Year 1715.

In MULTIPLICATION.

Quest. How many Statute Miles are there in the Circumference of the Body of the Earth, whose Circuit is 360 degrees, and each degree contains (according to Vulgar Computation) 60 Miles.

Answ. Multiply 360, by 60, (the Miles contained in one degree) and the Product is 21600 Statute Miles.

The Operation.

```
  360
   60
-----
21600
```

In DIVISION.

Quest. If the Circuit of the Terrestrial Globe is 21600 Miles. Suppose a Man travel continually in a direct Line (under one of the Greater Circles of the Sphere) 15 Miles a day: In how many days can he compass it?

C 2 *Answ*

Anſw. Divide 21600 by 15, your Quotient will be 1440, which ſhews that in ſo many days he may effect it, that is, in ſomewhat leſs than 4 Years.

The Operation.

$$15)\,21600\,(1440$$
$$\underline{15}$$
$$66$$
$$\underline{60}$$
$$60$$
$$\underline{60}$$
$$0$$

In the Rule of THREE.

Queſt. A Man lent me 400*l.* for 7 Months, without Intereſt: How much muſt I lend for 12 Months to retaliate his Kindneſs?

Anſw. This muſt be ſolved by the Reverſe Rule of *Three*, and muſt be thus ſtated.

Months.	*l.*	*Months.*
7————————	400————————	12

Where 'tis plain that more requires leſs; that is, tho' the third Number be more than the firſt, yet it requires a leſſer Number to anſwer unto it than the ſecond: Therefore you muſt multiply 400 by 7, and it makes 2800, which I divide by 12 (the third Number) the Quotient is 233*l.* and 4*l.* remaining, the 12th part of which is 6*s.* 8*d.* So the Anſwer to the Queſtion is, That I muſt lend him 233 *l.* 6*s.* 8*d.* for 12 Months.

The Operation.

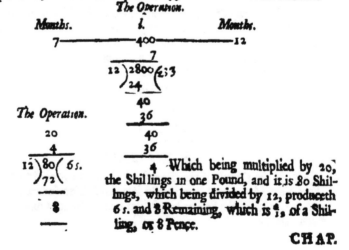

Months.	*l.*	*Months.*
7————————	400————————	12

The Operation.

4 Which being multiplied by 20, the Shillings in one Pound, and it is 80 Shillings, which being divided by 12, produceth 6*s.* and 8 Remaining, which is $\frac{8}{12}$ of a Shilling, or 8 Pence.

CHAP.

CHAP. II.

Containing sundry useful Definitions and Problems of GEOMETRY.

SECT. I. *Geometrical Definitions.*

A *Point* is that which cannot be divided, having neither Part nor Quantity, and therefore void of Length, Breadth or Depth; and is represented in the Margin, by the Letter A;

A *Line* is Length, without Breadth or Thickness, and is Right, as A; Or Curved, as B.

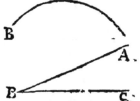

An *Angle* is the Inclination of two Lines one to another, the one touching the other yet not so as to make one Line, as the Lines BA and BC.

A *Right-lined Angle*, is that which is contained by Right Lines, as the Angle ABC.

A *Right-lined Angle*, is either Right-Angle or Oblique.

A *Right-Angle* is when a Right Line standing upon a Right Line, makes the Angles on each side equal to each other; as the Right-Angles ACD, and BCD.

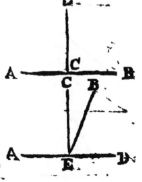

An *Oblique-Angle* is either Acute or Obtuse.

An *Acute-Angle* is less than a Right, as the Angle DEB.

An *Obtuse-Angle* is greater than a Right-Angle, as AEB.

A *Plain Figure* is contained under one Term, or many.

A

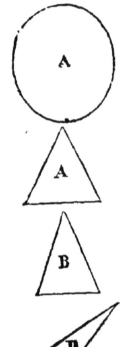

A *Circle* is a Plain Figure contained under one Term or Line called the *Circumference*, unto which all Lines drawn from a certain Point within the Figure are equal, and that Point is called the Center, as A.

A *Right-lined Figure* is contained by Right-Lines, and is either three-sided, four-sided, or many-sided.

A *Triangle* is a three sided Figure, and is considered either in respect of its Sides, or Angles.

In respect of its Sides, 'tis either,

Equilateral, having three equal Sides: as A.

Or *Equicrural,* having two equal Sides; as B.

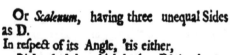

Or *Scalenum,* having three unequal Sides as D.

In respect of its Angle, 'tis either,

Right-Angled, which hath a Right-Angle; as E.

Or *Oblique-Angled,* which hath no Right-Angle, but hath two Acute-Angles, and one Obtuse-Angle; as C.

Or three *Acute-Angles;* as G.

Of

Of four-sided Figures.

A *Square* is that which hath four equal Sides, and four Right-Angles ; as A.

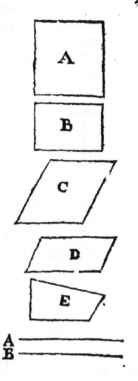

An *Oblong* hath four Right-Angles, and the oppofite Sides equal ; as B.

Rhombus hath four equal Sides, but is not Right-angled ; as C.

A *Rhomboides* hath the oppofite Sides and Angles equal, but is neither equal-fided nor Right-angled ; as D.

All other four-sided Figures are called *Trapezia's*, as E:

Parallel, or equi-diftant Right-Lines are fuch, which being in the fame Superficies, if infinitely produced, would never meet, as A and B.

Sect. II. *Geometrical Problems.*

Prob. 1. *How to raife a Perpendicular on the middle of a given Line.*

LET the given Line be AB, and C be a Point therein, whereon it is required to raife a Perpendicular. Firft, open the Compaffes to any convenient diftance, and fetting one foot in the Point C, with the other fet off on either fide thereof the equal diftances, CA and CB : Then opening the Compaffes to any convenient (wider) diftance, fetting one foot in the Point A, with the other ftrike the occult Arch at E, then with the fame same diſtance, ſet one foot in the Point B, and with the other ſtrike the Arch F, croſſing E in the Point D, from whence draw the Line DC, which Line is a Perpendicular unto the given Line AB, as was required.

Prob. 2. *To let fall a Perpendicular from a Point aſſigned, to the Middle of a given Line*

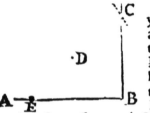

Let BCD be the given Line, and A the Point aſſigned, from whence you would have a Perpendicular let fall. Firſt, ſet one foot of your Compaſſes in the Point A, and opening them to any convenient diſtance, deſcribe an Arch of a Circle that may cut the Line BCD at E and F; then find the middle between theſe, which will be the Point C, from which Point draw the Line AC, which is the Perpendicular Line required.

Prob. 3. *To raiſe a Perpendicular upon the End of a Line given.*

Let the given Line be AB, Firſt, open your Compaſſes to a convenient diſtance, and ſet one Foot in the Point B, and let the other point fall any where above the Line, as at the point D, and in that point let one foot of your Compaſſes remain, turning the other about, until it cut the Line AB in the point E; then turn the foot of the Compaſſes towards C, and draw an occult Arch, and lay the edge of a Ruler to thoſe points E and D; and where the ſame edge of the Ruler doth cut the Arch C, from that point draw the Line CB, which ſhall be a Perpendicular at the end of the Line AB, as was required.

Prob. 4. *To let fall a Perpendicular from a Point aſſigned, unto the End of a given Line.*

Let the Line AB be given, unto which it is required to let fall a Perpendicular from the Point D, to the end A: Firſt, from the Point D draw a Line unto any part of the given Line AB, which may be the Line DCE; find the Middle of the Line, which is at C, place one foot of your Compaſſes in that Point, and extend the other unto D or E, with which Diſtance deſcribe the Semi-Circle DAE, which ſhall cut the given Line AB in the Point A, and DCE in D, from which Point draw the Line DA, which is the Perpendicular on the End of the given Line AB, as was required.

To

Prob. 5. *To draw a Line Parallel to a Line given.*

Let AB be a given Line, whereunto
it is required to draw a Parallel. First,
set o e foot of your Compasses in the
Point C, and opening the other at pleasure, describe the Arch E; then with

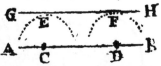

the same Distance set one foot in the Point D, describe the other Arch F;
Lastly, lay a Ruler to the Convexities of both those Arches, and draw
the Line GH, which shall be a Parallel to AB, as was required.

Prob. 6. *How to make an Angle equal to an Angle given.*

Let ABC be the given Angle, draw the Line DE, and upon B, as a
Center, describe the Arch GH, between the Sides BA and BC, and upon
the Point D, with the same Extent describe the Arch KL, and place
the Extent GH from K to L, then through the Point L, draw DF: So
is the Angle EDF equal to ABC, which was required.

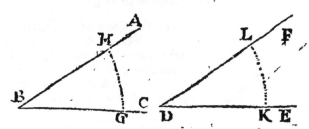

Prob. 7. *To divide a given Line into two equal Parts, properly called Bisecting a Line.*

Let the given Line be AB, open
your Compasses to any convenient Extent more than half the Line, and
with one foot in A describe the *Arch*
C and D, then with the same Extent,
and one foot in B, cross the aforesaid
Arches in C and D, a Ruler laid
from the crossing at C, to that at D,
cuts AB in E, the middle of the Line
required.

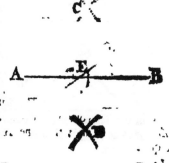

D   Prob.

Prob: 8. *To bring three Points (not scituate in a Right Line) into the Circumference of a Circle.*

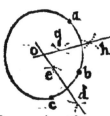

Suppose it be required to draw a Circle thro' the Points a b c ; First, with any Extent of the Compasses, and more than half a b, and one foot in a, draw the occult *Arches* g and h, and with the same Extent and one foot in b, cross the aforesaid *Arches* in g and h , then with any Extent more than half b c, and one foot in b, draw the *Arches* d and e, and with the same Extent and one foot in e, cross the said *Arches* in d and e, then through the d and e draw the Line d e o ; also through h and g, draw the Line h g o ; where these Lines cross each other as at o, is the Center required, then with the Extent o a draw a Circle, it shall pass through the three given Points.

Prob 9 *With a given Line AB to make any given Angle. Suppose an Angle of 36 Degrees.*

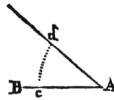

With the Chord of 60 Degrees, and one foot in A draw the *Arch* c d, upon which set off the Chord of the given *Angle* 36 from c to d, and through d draw the Line A d, which shall make an *Angle* at A of 36 Degrees, with the Line AB as was required.

Prob. 10. *With three given Sides to make a Triangle.*

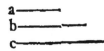

Suppose the given Sides be a b and c with them to constitute the Triangle ABC.

Take the longest Side c in your Compasses, and set from A to B, then with the Length of the Side b in your Compasses, and one foot in B sweep the small *Arch* at c, and with the length of the Side a in your Compasses and one foot in A cross the aforesaid *Arch* at c, then draw the Lines A c and B C, so have you the Triangle required.

By

By thefe Problems you may project any Plain Triangle, or lay down any Queftion in *Plain* or *Mercator's* Sailing, as fup-pofe in the Triangle ABC the Angle at A, and the *Hypothenufe* AC be given. Firft (as in all Cafes) draw the Line AB and by Prob. 9. make the given Angle at A, and from a Scale of Equal parts fet off the given *Hypothenufe* from A to C, and let fall the Perpen-dicular CB to cut AB in B, fo is your Triangle fini-fhed.

Likewife, if the Side AB had been given (which if in a Queftion of Navigation had been the Differ-ence of Latitude) you muft make the Angle as before, and fet off the Side AB from A to B, and at B Erect a Perpendicular to cut AC in C, and 'tis done; and this with a little Application is fufficent for Project-ing all Cafes in Plain Trigonometry and Navigation, as a little Practice will make Evident.

CHAP. III.

Treateth of the Doctrine of Plain or Right-lined Triangles.

Sect. I. *Containing fome Things neceffary to be underftood rela-ting to the* Science of PLAIN TRIGONOMETRY.

THE *Doctrine of Triangles* is converfant in the *Menfuration* of *Triangles, Plain* or *Spherical,* comparing the Sides and Angles to-gether, according to known Analogies, whereby three things being gi-ven, either Sides, Angles, or both, a fourth Side or Angle may be found.

But becaufe the Angles, of both Plain and Spherical-Triangles are meafured by Arches of Circles, and the Sides likewife of Spherical Tri-angles are themfelves Arches of great Circles, therefore thefe Arches, are in a manner *reduced into the Right-lines applied thereunto.*

The Right-Lines applied to Circles, are *Chords, Sines, Tangents,* and *Secants.*

A *Chord* is a Right-line drawn in a Circle, from one part of the Cir-cumference to the other; as in the annexed Figure.

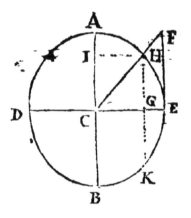

HK is the Chord of the Arches HEK, and HDK; also DE the diameter, is the Chord of the Semi-Circles DAE and DBE.

The right Sine of an Arch is half the Chord of twice that Arch, as HG being half the Chord HK, is the right Sine of the Arch HE, also of the Arch HAD, the Arch HE being the half of HEK, and the Arch HAD being half the Arch HDK. The Sine Complement of the Arch HE is HI, equal to CG.

The Versed Sine of an Arch, is that part of the Diameter which lies between the right Sine of that Arch and the *Circumference*, so that GE is the Versed Sine of the Arch HE, and GD the Versed Sine of the Arch HAD

The *Tangent* of an Arch, is a right-line touching the Arch, being Perpendicular to the Radius drawn to the Point of Contact, and concurring with a line drawn from the *Center*, through the Term or End of that Arch: so EF is a *Tangent* of the Arch EH.

A *Secant* is that Right-line drawn from the *Center* of the Arch, until it meet with the *Tangent*, so CF is a *Secant* of the Arch EH.

It is to be understood that every *Circle* is divided into 360 equal Parts, called Degrees · every Degree into 60 Parts, called Minutes; and every Minute into 60 Parts, called Seconds, &c.

The Complement of an Arch or Angle, is commonly the Complement thereof, to (or that which makes it up) 90 degrees. But if it be meant the Complement thereof to a Semi-Circle, it is expressed by saying the Complement to 180 deg.

A Plain-Triangle is contained under three Right-lines, and is either Right-Angled or Oblique.

In all Plain Triangles, two Angles being given, the third is also given; And one Angle being given, the Sum of the other two is also given; because the three Angles together are equal to two right Angles.

Therefore in a Plain Right-angled Triangle, one of the accute Angles is the Complement of the other, to 90 deg.

In the Solution of Plain Triangles, the Angles being only given, the Sides cannot be found, but only the Ratio of the Sides: It is therefore necessary that one of the Sides be known: As

In

In a Right-angled Triangle two things (befides the Right-angle) will ferve to find the third, fo one of them be a Side:

In Oblique-angled Triangles, there muft be three things given (one of them being a Side) to find a Fourth.

Some Symbols ufed in the Doctrine of Triangles for Brevety's fake.

= Equal to.

-┼ Móre.

— Lefs

x Multiply by, or drawn into.

° Over a Number ftands for **Degrees**, as 12° fignifies 12 deg.

' Signifies Minutes, as 12' is 12 Minutes.

ct. a Side. crs. Sides.

∠ An Angle, ∠s Angles.

Z The Sum.

X The Difference.

S. Sine.

Sc. Co-Sine, or Sine Complement.

Co. Ar. Complement Arithmetical.

t. Tangent.

tc. Co-Tangent, or Tangent Complement.

2 R Ang. two Right-Angles.

Q. Square.

In Right-angled Plain Triangles, the Sides comprehending the Right-Angle are called the *Legs*; and the Side fubtending (or oppofite to) the Right-Angle, is called the *Hypothenufe.*

In the Doctrine of Triangles; three Letters denote an Angle, as BAC fignifies the Angle at A ; ACB the Angle at C. Two Letters fhew a Side, as Side AB, or AC.

In the Doctrine of Triangles, the given Sides or Angles are noted with a Dafh, thus (')

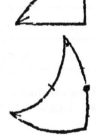

The required Sides or Angles with a Cypher, thus, (o)

In Right-angled Plain Triangles, there are feven Cafes, and in Oblique Triangles fix; For the Solution of which, thefe Four *Axioms* are fufficent.

AXIOM 1 *Of Right-angled Triangles*

In all Plain Right-angled Triangles, any of the Sides may be made Radius, and the other Sides will be Sines, Tangents or Secants: and what Proportion the Side put for Radius, hath to Radius, the fame Proportion hath the other Sides, to the Sines, Tangents, and Secants by them reprefented

AXIOM 2 *Of Oblique Triangles.*

In all Plain *Triangles*, the Sides are in fuch proportion one to another as the Sines of their oppofite Angles.

AXIOM 3.

In all Plain *Triangles*, As the Sum of two Sides is to their Difference; fo is the *Tangent* of the half Sum of their two oppofite Angles, to the *Tang* of the Diff. of either of them, above or under the half Sum

AXIOM 4.

In all Plain *Triangles*; as the Bafe is in Proportion to the Sum of the other Sides, fo is the Difference of thefe Sides, to the Difference of the Segments of the Bafe.

SECT. II. *Of Right-Angled Plain Triangles.*

Cafe I.

THE *Angles*, and one of the Legs given, to find the other Leg.

Example.

In the Triangles ABC
There is given
BAC 33° 45' ⎱
AB 90 parts. ⎰ BC required.

The Operation by the Logarithms

As S. ACB 56° 15' Log———————————	9.919846
To AB 90 parts———————————————	1.954242
So is S. BAC 33° 45'—————————	9.744739
	11.698981
To BC required, 60, 13 parts———————	1.779135

The General Rule for working Proportions by the Logarithms.

Add the Logarithms of the fecond and third Numbers together, from

from that Sum subtract the Logarithm of the first, and the Remainder is the Logarithm of the fourth Number sought, as is apparent by the precedent Operation.

Note, That the Work may be abreviated in this and the following *Cases* · When Radius is not put in the Proportion, then take the *Complement Arithmetical* of the first Logarithm ; and then adding the Logarithms of the second and third, and the *Complement Arithmetical* of the first into one Sum, from which bating Radius, or an Unite (towards the left-hand) the Remainder is the Logarithm of the fourth Number.

The Operation by the Compl. Arith.	*Co. Ar.*
As S. ACB 56° 15′ Log.———————————	0 080154
To AB 90 parts ———————————	1.954242
So is S BAC, 33° 45′———————————	9 744739
To AC required, 60, 13 parts ———————————	11.779135

The *Compl. Arith* of a Log. is the Remainder thereof, being subtracted from Radius.

So the Compl. Arith. of S 59° 15′	10.000000
is 0080154, as here appears:	9.919846
	0 080154

But a readier way is hinted by Mr. *Norwood*, thus : By taking the Compl. or Residue of the first Figure towards the left-hand unto 9, and so of the rest, until you come to the last Figure towards the right-hand thereof, set down the Residue to 10, thus, To take the Compl. Arith. of 9.91984. For 9 I write this Residue unto 9, which is 0 ; for 9, 0 ; for 1, 8 ; for 9, 0 ; for 8, 1 ; for 4, the Compl. to 10 ; which is 6. And so I have 008016, which is the Compl. Arith. of 9.91984.

How to work this and the following Cases by *Gunter's Scale*, shall be shewn in the Use of that Instrument.

Case II.

The Angles, and one of the Legs given, to find the *Hypothenuse*.

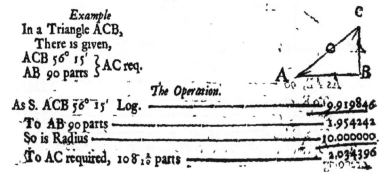

Example
In a Triangle ACB,
   There is given,
   ACB 56° 15′ } AC req.
   AB 90 parts }

The Operation.

As S. ACB 56° 15′ Log. ———————————	9.919846
To AB 90 parts ———————————	1.954242
So is Radius ———————————	10.000000
To AC required, 108 10/13 parts ———————————	2.034396

In the Operation of this Cafe there is no need to take the Compl. Arith: becaufe Radius is one of the four Terms in Proportion; nor of adding the Log. of the fecond and third together, according to the general Rule aforegoing, only fubtract the former Figures of the firft Log. from the fecond Logs. And in fubtracting the laft Figure of the firft Log. add 10 to the correfponding Figure of the fecond Log. *viz.*

Say 9 from 11, there remains 2; This Remainder 2.034396 gives the Log of the fourth Number required.

But if the Compl. Arith of the Log. of the firft Term be taken, the Labour of Subtraction may be faved.

Cafe III.

The Angles and *Hypotenufe* given, to find either of the Legs.

Example.

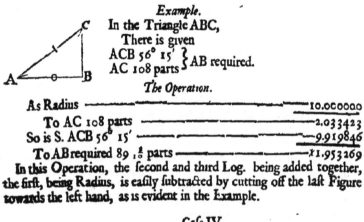

In the Triangle ABC,
There is given
ACB 56° 15' } AB required.
AC 108 parts }

The Operation.

As Radius —————————————————— 10.000000
    To AC 108 parts ————————— 2.033423
So is S. ACB 56° 15' ——————————— 9.919846
    To AB required 89 $\frac{4}{10}$ parts ————— *1*1.953269

In this Operation, the fecond and third Log. being added together, the firft, being Radius, is eafily fubtracted by cutting off the laft Figure towards the left hand, as is evident in the Example.

Cafe IV.

The Legs given to find an *Angle*.

Example.

In the Triangle ABC,
There is given
AB 90 } BAC required.
BC 60 }

The Operation.

As AB, 90 ——————————————— 1.954242
    To Radius ————————————— 10.000000
So is BC 60 ——————————————— 1.778151
    To t. BAC required, 33° 41' ————— 9.823909

This Operation is performed as the Example in the fecond Cafe be-oregoing.

    Cafe

Cafe V.

The *Hypotenufe*, and one of the Legs given to find the Angles.

Example.

In the Triangle ABC
    There is give
      AC 108 ⎰
      AB 90 ⎱ ACB required.

The Operation.

As AC 108 ———————————————————— 2.033423

  To Radius——————————————————— 10.000000

So is AB 90 ————————————————— 1.954242

    To S. ACB required, 56° 26' —————— 9.920819

This is performed as the precedent Operation in the fourth Cafe.

Cafe VI.

The Legs given to find the *Hypotenufe.*
  In the Triangle ABC
    There is given

AB 90 ⎰
BC 60 ⎱ AC required.

This Cafe requires a double Operation
  1. By the 4*th* Cafe to find the Angles.
  2. By the 2*d* Cafe to find the *Hypotenufe.*

The firft Operation.

As AB, 90 ———————————————— 1.954242

  To Radius ———————————————— 10.000000

So is BC 60————————————————— 1.778151

    To t. BAC, 33° 41' ——————————— 9.823909

The fecond Operation.

As S. BAC 33° 41'——————————————— 9.743981

  To BC 60 ——————————————————— 1.778151

So is Radius ————————————————— 10.000000

    To AC required 108 ——————————— 2.034170

Cafe VII.

The *Hypotenufe*, and one of the Legs given, to find the other Leg.

Example.

In the Triangle ABC
    There is given

AC 108 ⎰
AB 90 ⎱ BC required.

E   This

This Cafe likewife requires a double Operation.
1. By the 5th Cafe to find the *Angles.*
2 By the 1st or 3d Cafe to find the Leg required.

The first Operation.

As AC 108 ————————————————— 2.033428
To Radius ————————————————— 10.000000
So is AB 90 ————————————————— 1.954242
To S. ACB 56° 26' ————————————————— 9.920814

The second Operation.

As Radius ————————————————— 10.000000
To AC 108 ————————————————— 2.033428
So is S. BAC 33° 34' ————————————————— 9.742652
To BC required 60 ————————————————— 11.776080

The fixth and feventh Cafes before-going, may be performed without the Cannon of Sines and Tangents, by the 47 Prop. 1. *Euclid viz.* that in plain Right-angled Triangles, the Square of the *Hypothenufe* is equal to the Sum of the Squares of the two Legs.

Example of the fixth Cafe.
In the Triangle ABC
There is given
AB 90 ⎫
BC 60 ⎭ AC required.

Square the given Legs feverally, add their Squares together, the Square-Root of that Sum is the *Hypothenufe* required.

In multiplying 90 by 90, you need not regard the Cyphers, but 9 times 9 is 81, to which fet the two Cyphers, the Sum 8100 is the Product required, &c.

The Operation.

AB 90   Square of AB, 8100
   90   Square of BC, 3600
————————
 8100   Their Sum 11700(108 AC required.
BC 60   1
   60   20)17
————————   00
 3600   1700
                 1664
                ————
                  36

Otherwife by the Logarithms

From the double Log. of the greater Leg fubtract the Log. of the lefs, and

and to the abfolute Number anfwering to the Difference of the Logs, add the lefs Leg; half the Sum of the Logs. of the faid Sum and lefs Leg, is the Log. of the *Hypothenufe* required.

The Operation.

The greater Leg AB, 90 Log.	1.954242
The fame again	1.954242
The double Log.	3.908484
The Lefs Leg BC 60 Log. fubtr.	1.778151
The abfolute Number 135	2.130333
The Sum — 195 Log.	2.290034
Lefs Leg BC 60 Log.	1.778151
Sum	4.068185
The *Hypothenufe* AC 108 ½ Sum	2.034092

Example of the Sixth Cafe.

In the Triangle ABC,
There is given

AC 108
AB 90 } BC required.

From the Square of the *Hypothenufe*, fubtract the Square of the given Leg, the Square Root of the Remainder is the Leg required.

The Operation.

	AB 90	the Square of AC 11664
AC 108	90	the Square of AB 8100
108	00	Remainder 3564 59
864	810	25
1080	Square 8100	109) 1064
Squ. 11664		981
		83

Otherwife by the Logarithms.

Half the Sum of the Logs. of the Sum, and of the Difference of the *Hypothenufe* and given Leg, is the Log. of the Leg required.

The Operation.

The *Hypothenufe* AC	108		
The given Leg AB	90		
The Sum	198	Log.	2.296665
The Diff.	18	Log.	1.255272
		Sum	3.551937
The Leg. BC 59 required,	½ Sum	1.775988	E 2 SECT.

SECT. III. *Of* Oblique-angled Plain Triangles.
Cafe I.

THe Angles, and one of the Sides given, to find one of the other Sides.

Example.
In the Triangle ABC.
There is given,
BAC 33° 45' ⎫
ABC 45 00 ⎬ BC required
AC 40 parts ⎭

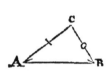

The Operation of this and the following Cafe, depends upon the fecond *Axiom* aforegoing.

The Operation.	Co. Ar.
As S ABC 45° 00'	0 150515
To Side AC 40	1 602060
So is S BAC 33° 45'	9 744739
To Side BC required, 31	11.497314

After the fame manner you might find the Side AB if it were required.

Cafe II.

Two Sides, and an Angle oppofite to one of them, being given, to find the other oppofite Angle.

Example.
In the Triangle ABC;
There is given,
ABC, 45° 00' ⎫ ACB required,
AB 100 ⎬ being Obtufe.
AC 80 ⎭

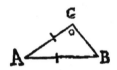

1 In this cafe, If the given Angle be Obtufe, the Angle required is Acute

2. If the given Angle be Acute, and oppofite to the greater of the given Sides, the required Angle is Acute

3 If the given Angle be Acute and oppofite to the leaft of the given Sides, it's doubtful whether the Angle fought be Acute or Obtufe, and ought to be determined before the Operation, as in this *Example.*

The Operation.	Co. Ar.
As Side AC 80	8.096919
To S ABC 45° 00'	9.849485
So is Side AB 100	2.000000
To S. ACB required, 117° 54'	19.946404

This

This Operation produces the Log. Sine of 62° 06' for the Angle sought, but because it is Obtuse, you must take its Complement to 180° *viz* 117° 54'.

Case III.

Two Sides, and an Angle opposite to one of them, being given, to find the third Side.   *Example.*

In the Triangle ABC.

There is given,

ABC 45° 00'
AB 100 } BC required.
AC 80

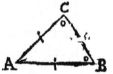

First find the Angle at C, by case the second   **Co. Ar.**

As Side AC ————————— 80 ————— 8.096919
     To Sine of *ABC* ————— 45° 00' ————— 9.849485
     So Side *AB* ————————— 100 ————— 2.000000

     To Sine of *ACB* Obtuse, ——— 117° 54' ——— 19.946404
Angle *ABC* ———————————— 45° 00'
Angle *ACB* found ————————— 117° 54'

     Sum ——————————————— 162° 54' Subtracted from 180
there Rests the Angle *CAB* 17° 6'. Then by case the first,

As Sine of *ABC* ——————————— 45° 00' ——— 0.150515
     To Side *AC* ———————————— 80 ——— 1.903090
     So Sine of *BAC* ——————— 17° 06' ——— 9.468407

To Side *BC* required ————— 33 ————— 11.522012

Case IV

Two Sides, and their contained Angles given, to find the other Angles.   *Example*

In the Triangle *ABC*,

There is given,

AB 25
AC 20 } *ACB* and *ABC* required.
C.AB 33° 45'

The Operation of this case depends upon the third *Axiom.*

The Operation.

The Side   *AB* 25   180° 00'
The Side   *AC* 20   BAC -33 45
The Sum of the Sides 45   Sum   146 15
Their Difference   05

       half Sum 73   07 of the unknown Angles.
                        Co. Ar.

		Co. Ar.
As the Sum of the Sides *AB* and *AC* 45 Log.	——	8.346788
To their Difference 05	——	0.698970
So is t. half Sum of the opposite Angles 73 07′	——	10.517833
To t. of their half Difference —— 20 06	——	19.563591

The half Difference added to the half Sum, gives the greater An- and subtracted leaves the less.

	° ′
The half Sum of the Angles	73 07
The half Difference	20 06
Added, gives *ACB*	93 13
Subtracted, *ABC*	53 1

Case V.

Two Sides, and their contained Angle given, to find the third Side

Example.

In The Triangle *ABC*,
There is, given,

$\left.\begin{array}{l} AB\ 335 \\ AC\ 271 \\ BAC\ 14°\ 40' \end{array}\right\}$ *BC* required.

This Case requires a double Operation.
1. By the 3d Case to find the Angles
2. By the 1st Case to find the Side required.

The first Operation

		Co. Ar.
As the Sum of the Sides *AB* and *AC* 606 Log.	——	7.217528
To their Difference —— —— 64	——	1.806180
So is t. half Sum Angles ——— 82° 40′	——	10.890440
To t. half their Difference —— 39 22	——	19.914148

By which you will find the Angle *ABC*, to be 43° 18′

The second Operation.

		Co Ar.
As S. *BAC* 34° 18′ Log	——	0.163791
To Side *AC* 271	——	2.432969
So is S. *BAC* 14° 40′	——	9.403455
To Side *BC* required, 100	——	12.000215

· *Case*

Cafe VI.

Three Sides given to find an *Angle.*
Example.

In the Triangle ABC
  There is given
    AB 64 ⎫
    AC 47 ⎬ BAC required.
    BC 34 ⎭

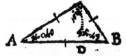

The Refolution of this *Cafe* depends upon the *4th Axiom,* reducinng the Oblique-angled Triangle into two Right-angled Triangles, by letting fall the Perpendicular CD, upon the *Bafe* or greater fide AB, and requires a double Operation.

The *Bafe* is that fide upon which the Perpendicular falls,
  1 To find the Segment of the *Bafe* AD.
  2. To find (by the 5*th Cafe* of Rectangular) the *Angles* required

The firft Operation.

				Co. Ar.
AC 47	As the *Bafe* AB		64 Log.	8.193820
BC 34	To the Sum of the fides AC and BC		81	1.908485
Sum 81	So is the Difference of the fides AC & BC		13	1.113943
Diff. 13	To the Differ. of the Segments of the *Bafe*		16	1.216248

          The *Bafe* is   64
        The Difference of the Segments 16
                    Sum 80
          $\frac{1}{2}$ Sum 40 is AD the greater Segment of the *Bafe,* becaufe adjacent to the greater fide AC.

The fecond Operation.
In the Triangle ACD, Right-angled at D.
  There is given AD and AC, to find CAD.

As AC 47 ———————————————	Log.	1.672097
To Radius———————————————		10.000000
So is AD, 40 ———————————————		1.602060
To fc. CAD 31° 40' ———————————		9.929963

CHAP.

CHAP. IV.
The Doctrine of Spherical TRIANGLES.

SECT. L. *Containing the Affections of Spherical Triangles, and their Axioms.*

1. A Spherical Triangle is that which is described on the Surface of the Sphere

2 The sides of a Spherical *Triangle* are the *Arches* of three great *Circles* of the Sphere mutually interfecting each other.

3 Spherical *Angles* are measured by the *Arch* of a great *Circle*, intercepted between the sides containing the *Angle*, the *Pole* of that *Circle* being the *Angular Punct*

4. Those are said to be great *Circles* which divide the Sphere into two equal Parts.

5. Those *Circles* which cut each other at Right-angles, pass through the Poles of each other, and the contrary.

6 In every Spherical Triangle, each side is less than a Semi-circle.

7 In every Spherical Triangle, any two sides together are greater than the third.

8 The Sum of the sides of a Spherical Triangle is less than two Semicircles.

9. If two sides of a Spherical Triangle be equal to a Semi-circle, the two *Angles* at the Base shall be equal to two Right angles; if they be less than a Semi-circle, the two *Angles* shall be less; but if greater than a Semi-circle, the two *Angles* shall be greater than two Right-angles

10. The Sum of the three *Angles* of a Spherical Triangle are greater than two Right-angles, and less than six.

11 Two *Angles* of any Spherical Triangle are greater than the Difference between the third *Angle* and a Semi-circle, therefore,

12 Any side being continued, the Exterior *Angle* is less than the two Interior opposite ones.

13. In any Spherical Triangles the Difference of the Sum of two *Angles* and a whole *Circle*, is greater than the Difference of a third *Angle* and a Semi-circle.

14. In any Spherical Triangle, one side being produced, if the other two sides be equal to a Semi-circle, the outward *Angle* shall be equal to the inward opposite *Angle* upon the side produced: If they be less
than

than a Semi-circle, the outward *Angle* shall be greater than the inward oppofite *Angle*, if they be greater than a Semi-circle the outward *Angle* shall be lefs than the inward oppofite *Angle*.

15. A Spherical Triangle is either Right, or Oblique-angled.

16 A Right-angled Spherical Triangle, is that which hath one Right Angle at the leaft.

17 The Legs of a Right-angled Spherical Triangle are of the fame Affection with their oppofite *Angles*.

18. In a Right-angled Spherical Triangle, if either Leg be a Quadrant, the *Hypothenufe* shall be alfo a Quadrant : but if both the Legs be of the fame Affection (that is, be both greater or both lefs than a Quadrant) the *Hypothenufe* is lefs than a Quadrant, or if of different Affections, then greater, and the contrary

19 In a *Right-angled Spherical Triangle*, if either of the *Angles* at the *Hypothenufe* be a Right Angle, the *Hypothenufe* shall be a Quadrant ; but if both shall be of the fame Affection, it shall be lefs ; if of different, it shall be greater, and the contrary.

20. In a *Right-angled Spherical Triangle*, the Sum of the *Oblique-Angles* are lefs than three *Right-Angles*

21. An *Oblique Spherical Triangle* is either acute or obtufe.

22 An *Acute-angled Spherical Triangle* hath all its *Angles Acute*

23 An *Obtufe-angled Spherical Triangle* hath all its *Angles* either Obtufe or Mixt, viz. fome *Acute* and fome *Obtufe*.

24 In any *Spherical Triangle* whofe *Angles* are all *Acute*, each fide is lefs than a Quadrant.

In *Spherical Triangles* there are 28 Cafes, 16 in *Rectangular*, and 12 in *Oblique Angular*. The 16 Cafes of Rectangular are refolved by thefe two *Axioms* following.

AXIOM 1.

In all *Spherical Rectangular Triangles*, having the fame *Acute Angle* at the *Bafe*, the Sines of the *Hypothenufa's* are proportional to the Sines of their Perpendicular.

AXIOM 2.

In all *Spherical Rectangular Triangles*, having the fame *Acute Angle* at the *Bafe*, the Sines of the *Bafes*, and the *Tangents* of the *Perpendiculars* are proportional.

That all the Cafes of a *Right-angled Spherical Triangle*, may be refolved by thefe two *Axioms*.

The feveral parts of the *Spherical Triangle* propofed, muft fometimes be continued to Quadrants, that fo the *Angles* may be turned into Sides,

F　　　　　　　　　　the

the *Hypothenufa*'s into Bafes and Perpendiculars, and the contrary. By which means the Proportions, as to the Parts of the *Triangle* given, inftead of Sines do fometimes fall in Co-fines, and fometimes in Co-tangents inftead of *Tangents.* Such Parts as do change their Proportion, are noted with their Complements, *viz.* the *Hypothenufe*, and both the *Oblique Angles*, but the Sides containing the *Right Angles* do not fo change.

These are called the five circular Parts of a *Triangle*, amongft which the *Right Angle* is not reckoned, and therefore the two Sides which do contain it, are fuppofed to be joined together.

Each of thefe circular Parts, may by fuppofition be made the middle Part, and then the two circular Parts, which are next to that middle Part, are the Extreams Conjunct ; the other remote from the Part affumed, are the Extreams Disjunct.

As in the *Triangle* ABC, if *Comp.* AC be made the middle Part *Comp* A and *Comp.* C are the Extreams Conjunct, and the Side, AB and BC are the Extreams Disjunct : and fo of the reft, as in the Table following.

Mid. Part.	Extr. Conj.	Extr. Disj.
Leg. AB	Comp. A Leg. BC	Comp. AC Comp. C
Comp. A	Comp. AC Leg. AB	Comp. C Leg. BC
Comp. AC	Comp. A Comp. C	Leg AB Leg BC
Comp C	Comp. AC Leg. BC	Comp. A Leg. AB
Leg BC	Comp. C Leg. AB	Comp. A Comp. AC

The Parts of a Right-angled Spherical Triangle, being thus diftinguifhed into 5 circular Parts, for the more eafe in refolving all Spherical Triangles, obferve this Catholick and Univerfal Proportion invented by the Lord *Napier.*

The *Sine* of the Middle Part and Radius, are reciprocally proportional to the Tangents of the Extreams Conjunct, and the Co-fines of the Extreams Disjunct.

That is ; As Radius to the Tangent of fone of the Exreams Conjunct ;

fo is the Tangent of the other Extream Conjunct, to the Sine of the Middle part.

And alfo, as Radius, to the Co-fine of one of the Extreams Disjunct; fo is the Co-fine of the other Extream Disjunct to the Sine of the Middle part.

Therefore if the Middle part be fought, the Radius muft be in the firft place; if either of the Extreams, the other Extream muft be in the firft place.

Only Note, that if the Middle part, or either of the Extreams Conjunct, be noted with its Complement in the Circular Parts of the Triangle inftead of the Sine or Tangent, you muft ufe the Co-fine or Co-tangent.

If either of the Extreams Disjunct be noted by its Complement in the Circular parts of the Triangle, inftead of the Co-fine you muft ufe the Sine of fuch Extream Disjunct.

That the Directions may be the better underftood, there is in the Table following the Circular parts of a Triangle under their refpective Titles, whether they be taken for the Middle part, or for the Extreams, whether Conjunct or Disjunct; and unto thofe Parts there is prefixed the *Sine* and *Co-fine*, the *Tangent* or *Co-Tangent*, as it ought to be by the Catholick Proportion.

Mid. Part.	*Extr. Conj.*	*Extr. Disj.*
Sine. AB	Co.-tang. A *Tang.* BC	*Sine* AC *Sine* C
Co-fine A	Co-tang. AC *Tang.* AB	*Sine* C Co-fine BC
Co-fine AC	Co-tang. A Co-tang. C	Co-fine AB Co-fine BC
Co-fine C	Co-tang. AC *Tang.* BC	*Sine* A Co-fine AB
Sine BC	Co-tang. C *Tang.* AB	*Sine* A *Sine* AC

AXIOM 3.

In all Spherical Triangles, the Sines of the Sides are in direct proportion to the Sines of their oppofite Angles, and the contrary.

AXIOM

F 2

AXIOM 4.

In all Oblique angled Spherical Triangles, in which two **Sides are less** than a Semi-circle:

As the Sine of half the Sum of the two sides,
To the Sine of half their Difference;
So is the Co-tangent of half the contained Angle,
To the Tangent of half the Difference of the opposite Angles.
And, As the Co-sine of half the Sum of the Sides,
To the Co-sine of half their Difference;
So is the Co-tangent of half the contained Angle,
To the Tangent of half the Sum of the opposite Angles.

AXIOM 5.

In all Oblique angled Spherical Triangles, in which two Angles are less
than two Right-angles.
As the Sine of half the Sum of two Angles,
To the Sine of half their Difference;
So is the Tangent of half the interjacent Side,
To the Tangent of half the Difference of the opposite Sides.
And, As the Co-sine of half the Sum of the Angles,
To the Co-sine of half their Difference;
So is the Tangent of half the interjacent Side,
To the Tangent of half the Sum of the opposite Sides.

AXIOM 6.

As the Rectangle of the Sines of the containing Sides,
To the Square of Radius;
So is the Rectangle of the Sines of half the Sum of the three Sides,
and of the Difference of the opposite Side therefrom,
To the Square of the Co-sine of half the Angle sought.

This being premised, the several Cases shall be set down, with their
Anologies, and resolved by the Logarithms.
First, Of *Right-angled Triangles*
Then Of *Oblique.*

SECT. II. Of *Right-angled* Spherical Triangles.

Case I.

A Leg, and an Angle opposite thereto, being given to find the other
Leg; if it be known, whether the *Hypothenuse,* or other Angle,
be greater or lesser than a Quadrant. *Example*

Example.

In the *Triangle* ABC,
  There is given,
BAC 23° 30' } AB required.
BC, 17 43 }

The Operation.

As Radius ———————————————— Log. 10.000000
  To tc. BAC 23° 30' ——————————— 10.361698
  So is t. BC 17 43 ———————————— 9.504418
  To S. AB required, 47° 17' ———————— 19.866116

Cafe II. A Leg and an adjacent Angle given, to find the other Leg.
Example.

In the Triangle ABC
  There is given,
BAC 23° 30' } BC required.
AB 47 19 }

The Operation.

As tc. BAC 23° 30' ————————————— Log. 10.361698
To Radius ————————————————— 10.000000
So is S. AB 47° 19' ————————————— 9.866353
To t BC required, 17° 43' ———————— 9.504655

Cafe III. The Legs given to find an Angle.
Example.

In the Triangle ABC,
  there is given,
AB 47° 19' } BAC req.
BC 17 43 }

The Operation.

As t. BC, 17° 43' ————————————— Log. 9.504418
  To Radius ———————————————— 10.000000
  So is S. AB 47° 19' ——————————— 9.866353
  To tc. BAC required, 23° 30' ———————— 10.361935

Cafe IV. The *Hypothenufe* and a Leg given, to find the contained Angle.
Example.   In the *Triangle ABC*,
  There is given,
AC 49° 48' } ACB required.
BC 17 43 }

The

The Operation.

As Radius ———————————————————————— Log. 10.000000
   To t. AC 49° 48' ————————————————— 9.926890
   So is tc. BC 17° 43' ————————————————— 9.504418
  , To fc. ACB required, 74° 21' ———————————— 19.431308

Cafe V. A Leg and the adjacent Angle given to find the *Hypothenuse.*

                Example. In the Triangle ABC,
                    There is given,
                BAC 23° 30' } AC required.
                AB 47 19 }

The Operation.

As t. AB 47° 19' ————————————————— Log. 10.035158
To Radius ————————————————————————— 10.000000
So is fc. BAC 23° 30' ———————————————— 9.962397
To tc. AC required, 49° 47' ————————————— 9.927239

Cafe VI. The *Hypothenuse* and an Angle given, to find the Leg adjacent to the given Angle.

              Example. In the Triangle ABC
                There is given
              ACB 74° 19' } BC required.
              AC 49 48 }

The Operation.

As tc. AC 49° 48' ————————————————— Log. 9.926890
   To Radius ——————————————————————— 10.000000
   So is fc. ACB 74° 19' ——————————————— 9.431878
To t. BC required, 17° 44' ———————————— 9.504988

Cafe VII. The Oblique Angles given to find the *Hypothenuse.*

            Example. In a Triangle ABC
              There is given,
           ACB 74° 19' } AC required.
           BAC 23 30 }

The Operation.

As Radius ——————————————————— Log. 10.000000
   To tc. ACB 74° 19' —————————————————— 9.448356
   So is tc. BAC 23 30 —————————————————— 10.361698
   To fc. AC required, 49° 47' ————————————— 19.810054

Cafe VIII. The *Hypothenuse* and one of the Angles given, to find the other Angle.

                                      Example

Example.

In the Triangle ACB
  There is given
ACB 74° 19' } BAC required.
AC 49 48

The Operation.

As tc ACB 74° 19' ———————————— Log. 9.448356
To Radius —————————————— 10.000000
So fc. AC 49° 48' ————————————— 9.809867
To tc. BAC required, 23° 31'———————— 10.361511

Cafe IX. The *Hypothenuse* and an Angle given, to find the Leg oppofite to the given Angle.

Example.

In the Triangle ABC,
  There is given
BAC 23° 30' } BC required.
AC 49 48

The Operation.

As Radius ————————————————— 10.000000
To f. BAC 23° 30' ———————————— 9.600699
So is f. AC 49° 48' ———————————— 9.882977
   To f. BC required 17° 43'———————— 19.483676

Cafe X. A Leg and an *Angle* oppofite thereto being given, to find the
Hypothenuse, if it be known, whether it or the other Leg, or unknown
Angle be greater or lefs than a Quadrant.
    Example.

In the Triangle ABC,
  There is given
BAC 23° 30' } AC required.
BC 17 43

The Operation.

As f. BAC, 23° 30' ———————————— Log. 9.600699
To Radius — ————————————— 10.000000
So is f. BC 17° 43' ———————————— 9.483316
To f. AC required, 49° 45' ——————— 9: 882617

Cafe XI. The *Hypothenuse* and a Leg given, to find the *Angle* oppofite
to the given Leg.   Example

Of Spherical Triangles.

Example.

In the Triangle ABC
There is given
AC 49° 48' ⎱
BC 17 43 ⎰ BAC required.

The Operation

As f. *AC* 49° 48' ——————————————— Log. 9.882977

To Radius ——————————————————10.000000

So is f *BC* 17° 43' ——————————————9.483316

To f. *BAC* required, 23° 28' —————————9.600339

Case XII. A Leg, and an *Angle* adjacent thereunto being given, to find the other *Angle*.

Example.   In the Triangle ABC
There is given,
BC 17° 43' ⎱
ACB 74 19 ⎰ BAC required.

The Operation

As Radius ——————————————————Log. 10.000000

To f *ACB* 74° 19' ——————————————9.983522

So is fc *BC* 17 43 ——————————————9.978898

To fc. BAC required, 23° 30' —————————19.962420

Case XIII. A Leg and an *Angle* opposite thereto, being given, to find the other *Angle*, If it be known whether it, the other Leg, or the *Hypothenuse*, be greater or less than a Quadrant

Example.   In the Triangle ABC,
There is given
BAC 23° 30' ⎱
BC 17 43 ⎰ ACB required.

The Operation

As fc. BC 17° 43' ——————————————— Log. 9.978898

To Radius ——————————————————10.000000

So is fc. BAC, 23° 30' —————————————9.962397

To f. ACB required, 74° 19' —————————9.983499

Case XIV. The Oblique-angles given, to find either Leg.

Example.

In the Triangle ABC,
There is given,
ACB 74° 19' ⎱
BAG 23 30 ⎰ BC required.

The Operation.

As ſ ACB 74° 19' ——————————————— Log. 9.983522
  To Radius ——————————————————— 10.000000
  So is ſc. BAC 23° 30' ————————————— 9.962397
  To ſc. BC required, 17° 43' ——————— 9.978875

Caſe XV. The Legs given, to find the *Hypothenuſe.*
Example.
In the Triangle ABC
  There is given
  AB 47° 19' } AC required.
  BC 17   43 }

The Operation.

As Radius ——————————————————— Log. 10.000000
  To ſc. AB 47° 19' —————————————— 9.831195
  So is ſc. BC 17   43 ——————————— 9.978898
  To ſc. AC required 49° 47' —————— 19.810093

Caſe XVI. The *Hypothenuſe* and a Leg given, to find the other Leg.
Example.
In the Triangle ABC,
  There is given
  AC 49° 48' } AB required.
  BC 17 43 }

The Operation.

As ſc. BC 17° 43' ——————————————— Log. 9.978898
  To Radius ——————————————————— 10.000000
  So is ſc. AC 49° 48' ————————————— 9.809867
  To ſc. AB required, 47° 21' —————— 9.830969

SECT. III. *Of Oblique-angled Spherical Trianlges.*

Caſe I.

TWO Sides, and an *Angle* oppoſite to one of them being given, to
  find the other oppoſite *Angle*; if it be known, whether the *Angle*
ſought be greater or leſs than a *Right-Angle.*

G

Example

Example.
In the Triangle ADE,
There is given
AE 69° 47 ⎱ ADE required,
DE   38 28 ⎰ being Obtuſe.
DAE 37 03

The Operation.   Co. Ar:

As ſ. DE 38° 28' ─────────────────── Log. 0.206169
To ſ. DAE 37 03 ─────────────────── 9.779965
So is ſ. AE 69 47 ─────────────────── 9.972384
To ſ. ADE required 114° 39' ──────────── 19.958518

Caſe II. Two *Angles* and a Side oppoſite to one of them, being given, to find the other oppoſite Side ; if it be known whether it be greater or leſs than a Quadrant

Example.
In the Triangle ADE,
There is given
ADE 114° 38' ⎱ AD required,
AED 45 00 ⎰ being leſs than
AE   69 47   a Quadrant.

The Operation.   Co. Ar.

As ſ. ADE—114° 38' ─────────────── Log. 0.041439
To ſ. AE—69   47 ─────────────────── 9.972384
So is ſ. AED 45 00 ─────────────────── 9.849485
To ſ. AD required, 46° 53' ──────────── 19.863308

The Reſolution of this and the former Caſe depends upon the third *Axiom.*

Caſe III. Two Sides and their contained *Angles* being given, to find the other *Angles.*

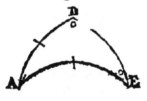

Example.
In the Triangle ADE,
There is given
DAE 37° 03' ⎰ ADE⎰
AE 69 47 ⎰ and ⎰ required.
AD 46 53 ⎰ AED⎰

The

The Operation,

AE 69° 47'
AD 46 53
Sum, 116 40 ½ Sum ; 58° 20'
Diff. 22 54 ½ Diff. 11 27
DAE 37 03 half thereof is 18° 31'

As f. ½ Z cr². AE and AD 58 20 ——————————————Log. 0.070011
   To f. ½ X cra. ——————— 11 27 —————————————9.297788
   So is tc. ½ DAE ————18 31 —————————— 10.475060
   To t. ½ X ∠s D and E—34 51——————————— 19.842859

As fc. ½ Z cra. AE and AD 58 20———————————Log. 0 279861
   To fc. ½ X cra. ————11 27 ——————————9.991269
   So is tc. ½ DAE ————18 31 —————————— 10.475060
   To t. ½ Z ∠s D and E—79 49—— ——————10.746190
    ½ Z ∠s D and E ——79 49
    ½ X ∠s ————34 51

Sum, 114 40 ADE ⎱ required.
Rem. 44 58 AED ⎰

Having by the fourth *Axiom* found the half Sum, and half Difference, of the *Angles*; if to that half Sum you add the half Difference, the Total is the greater *Angle* ; and if from the half Sum, you subtract the half Difference, the Remainder is the lesser *Angle* sought.

Note ;] If the Sum of the two containing Sides exceed a Semi-Circle then subtract each Side severally from 180, and proceed with those Complements as with the Sides given in the Example aforegoing. The Operation produces the Complements of the *Angles* sought to a Semi-circle.

Cafe IV. Two *Angles*, and the interjacent Side being given, to find the other Sides.

Example.
In the Triangle ADE,
There is given,

DAE 26 23 ⎱ AE ⎱
ADE 137 55 ⎰ and ⎰ required;
AD 81 50 ∠ DE ⎰

The Operation.

```
              °   ′
ADE    137 55
DAE     26 23
Sum    164 18    ½ Sum——82° 09′
Diff.  111 32    ½ Diff. ——55 46
AD      81 50    half thereof 40 55                    Co. Ar.
As ſ ½ Z ∠s A and D——82° 09′————————————Log. 0 004889 0
  To ſ. ½ X ∠s————55 46    ————————————9 917376
  So is t ½ AD ————40 55    ————————————9 937887
  To t. ½ X cri. AE & DE 35 52 ————————————19.859352

As ſc ½ Z ∠s A and D ——82 09    ———————— Log 0 864613
  To ſc ½ X ∠s————55 46    ————————————9.750172
  So is t. ½ AD————40 55    ————————————9.937887
  To t. ½ ZAE and DE——74 21    ————————————10.552672
½ Z cri. AE and DE——74 21
½ X cri. ————35 52
         Sum,  110 13 AE ⎫ required.
         Rem.   38 29 DE ⎭
```

This Caſe is wrought by the *5th Axiom*, and the half Sum of the Sides added to the half Difference, gives a greater Side ; and the half Difference ſubtracted, leaves the leſs.

Note ;] If the Sum of the given *Angles* exceed 180°, ſubtract each *Angle* from 180° and proceed with the Reſidues, the Operation will produce each ſides Compl to a Semi-circle.

Caſe V. Two Sides and an *Angle* oppoſite to one of them, being given, to find the third Side, if it be known whether the other oppoſite *Angle* of the required ſide, be greater or leſs than a Quadrant.

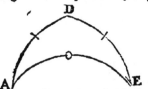

Example.

In the Triangle ADE,
There is given
AD 46° 53′ ⎫ And AE required,
DE 38   28 ⎬ being leſs than
AED 45   00 ⎭ a Quadrant.

The Operation of this Caſe depends upon the *3d* and *5th Axioms*.

Firſt, By the *3d Axiom* find the *Angle* oppoſite to the other given *Side.*

Secondly, Having two ſides, and their oppoſite *Angles*, you may find the third ſide by the former part of the *5th Axiom* inverted.

The

The Operation.

	°	'		Co. Ar.
As f. AD	46	53	Log.	0.136699
To f AED	45	00		9.849485
So is f. DE	38	28		9.793831
To f DAE	37	03		19.780015
AED	45	00		
DAE	37	03		

Sum 82 03 half Sum, 41° 01'

Diff. 07 57 half Diff. 03 58

AD 46 53

DE 38 28

Diff. 08 25 half Diff. 04 12

	°	'		Co. Ar.
As S. ½ X ∠s A and E	03	58	Log.	1.160044
To f. ½ Z 7s	41	01		9.817088
So is t. ½ Xcrª. AD and DE	04	12		8.865905
To t. ½ AE required.	34	52		19.843037

34 52

34 52

AE 69 44 required.

Cafe VI. Two Angles and a Side oppofite to one of them, being given, to find the third *Angle,* if it be known, whether the oppofite Side, or *Angle* required, be greater or lefs than a Quadrant.

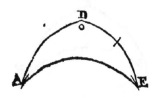

Example.

In the Triangle ADE,
There is given,
DAE 37° 03' ⎫ ADE required,
AED 45 00 ⎬ being Obtufe.
ED 38 28 ⎭

The Refolution of this Cafe depends upon the third and fourth *Axioms.* *Firft,* By the third *Axiom* find the Side oppofite to the other *Angle.* *Secondly,* Having the two *Angles,* and their oppofite Sides, the third *Angle* may be found by the former part of the fourth *Axiom* inverted.

The

The Operation.   Co. Ar.

As ſ. DAE——37 03 ——————————————Log. 0.220035
   To ſ. DE 38 28 ————————————————9.793831
   So is ſ. AED 45 00 ——————————————9.849485
      To ſ. AD 46 53 ————————————————19.863351
         AD 46 53
         DE 38 28

         Sum 85 21 ½ Sum, 42° 40′
         Diff 08 25 ½ Diff. 04 12

         AED 45 00
         DAE 37 03
         Diff. 07 57 ½ Diff. 03 58

                        °   ′   Co. Ar.
As ſ. ½ X crs. AD and DE 04 12 ——————— Log. 1.135263
   To ſ. ½ Zcrs.   42 40 ————————————9.831058
   So is t. ½ X ∠s A and E 03 58 ————————————8.840997
      To tc. ½ AD required, 57 19—————————19.807318
                           57 19
                          114 38 required.

Caſe VII. Two Sides, and an *Angle* oppoſite to one of them being given, to find the contained *Angle*; if it be known, whether the other
oppoſite, or the *Angle* required be *Acute* or *Obtuſe*.
       Example.

In the *Triangle* ADE,
   There is given
   AED 45° 00′ ⎫ DAE required,
   AE 110 13 ⎬ being *Acute.*
   AD 81 50 ⎭

This Caſe is wrought by the help of the third and fourth *Axioms.*
Firſt, By the third *Axiom* to find the other oppoſite *Angle*.
Secondly, By the fourth *Axiom* to find the contained *Angle*.
                        The Operation.   Co. Ar.
As ſ. AD   81 50 ——————————— Log. 0.004427
   To ſ. AED 45 00 ————————————————9.849485
   So is ſ. AE 110 13 ——————————————9.972384
      To ſ. ADE 137 55 required, ——————19.826296
                                            A

ADE 137 55
AED 45 00

Diff 92 55 half Diff. 46° 27'
AE 110 13
AD 81 50

Sum, 192 03 half Sum, 96 01
Diff. 28 23 half Diff. 14 11

As ſ. ½ X cra. AE and AD   14° 11' ——————————Log. 0.610789
To ſ. ½ Zcra.   96 01 —————————————9.997601
So is t. ½ X ∠s D and E   46 27——————————————10.021991
To tc. ½ DAE required,   13 11 ——————————————10.630381
                             13 11

DAE 26 22 required.

Caſe VIII. Two Angles and a Side oppoſite to one of them. being given, to find the interjacent Side, if it be known, whether the other oppoſite Side, or Side ſought; be greater or leſſer than a Quadrant.

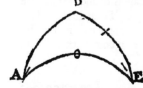

Example.

In the Triangle ADE,
     There is given,
     AED 45° 00' ⎱ AE required, being
     DAE 37 03 ⎰ leſs than a Quadrant.
     DE 38 28

This Caſe is reſolved by the third and fifth *Axioms.*
   Firſt, By the third *Axiom,* to find the other oppoſite Side.
   Secondly, by the fifth *Axiom,* to find the interjacent Side.

                  °   '   *The Operation.*   Co. Ar.

As ſ. DAE   37 03 ———————————— Log. 0.220034
To ſ. DE   38 28 ——————————————9.793831
So is ſ. AED 45 00 ——————————————9.849485

To ſ. AD   46 53 ——————————————19.863350
     AED 45° 00'
     DAE 37 03

Sum 82 03 ½ Sum 41° 01'

Diff. 07 57 ½ Diff. 03 58
AD 46 53
DE 38 28
Diff. 08 25 ½ Diff. 04 12

                                       Co

				Co. Ar.
As ſ ½ X ∠s A and E	03 58		Log. 1.160044	
To ſ ½ Z ∠s	41 01			9.817088
So is t ½ Xcr: AD and DE	04 12			8.865905
To t.½ AE required	34 52			19.843037

$$34 \quad 52$$
$$\overline{69 \quad 44 \text{ required.}}$$

Caſe IX. Two Sides and their contained *Angle* being given, to find the third Side

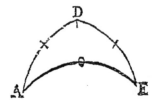

Example

In the Triangle ADE,
There is given
ADE 137° 55'
AD   81   50 } AE required
DE   38   28

The Reſolution of this and the following Caſe is deduced from the Lord *Napier's* *Catholick Propoſition* (the Oblique Triangle by a ſuppoſed Perpendicular being reduced into two Rectangulars) by the Ingenious [Mr. *Cclure*, in his *Sector on a Quadrant*, whom in this I ſhall imitate

The Operation

As Radius		Log 10.000000	
To ſc ADE the contained *Angle* 137° 55'			9.870503
So is t DE the leſſer Side	38 28		9.900086
To t. of a fourth *Arch*	30 31		19.770589

If the contained *Angle* be leſs than 90°, ſubtract the fourth *Arch* from the greater Side; but if it be greater than 90°, from its Complement to 180°, the Remainder is the Reſidual *Arch*.

				Co. Ar.
As ſc. of the fourth *Arch*	30 31		Log. 0.064755	
To ſc. of the Reſidual	67 39			9.580084
So is ſc. of the leſſer Side DE	38 28			9.893745
To ſc of the Side required, AE	110 13			19.538584

Caſe X. Two *Angles*, and the interjacent Side being given, to find the third *Angle*.

Ex-

The Bearings of the Ships are N.eafterly 75° 31', and S.wefterly 75° 31', or *E N. E* ¼ *E.* and *W. S W.* ¼ *W.* nearly.

To find their Diftance, by Cafe 1.   Co Ar·

As f. AED	53° 01'	Log.	0.097556
To AD	20		1.301030
So is f. DAE	33 45		9.744739
To DE	14		11.143325

PROB. IV.   A Ship fails from a certain Port *S S E* 68 Min. and then 72 min.more *Eafterly,* but is forced back, by foul Weather 82 min. to the Port from whence fhe firft fet fail, I demand what Courfe fhe fteered from the fecond Place to the third, and how fhe failed back to the firft Port   *Plate* 1. *Fig.* 11.

Let A reprefent the Port,
E the fecond Place,
D the third Place.

The Operation

To find the Courfe from the fecond Place to the third, by Cafe 6.

AD 82
AE 68
Sum, 150
Diff. 14   Co. Ar·

As DE the Bafe	72'	Log.	8.142668
To Z cra. AE and AD	150		2.176091
So is their Difference	14		1.146128
To X Segments of the Bafe	29		11.464887

DE	72'	DE	72
Segment	29	Segment	29
Diff.	43	Sum	101
½ Diff.	21 ½, or 21 1/10 EB.	½ Sum,	50½ DB 50 5/10

As *AE*	68'	Log	1.832508
To Radius			10.000000
So is EB 21' 1/10			1.332440
To fc. AEB, or AED 71° 34'			9.499932

The Courfe from the fecond Place to the third, is *N. E.* 49° 04', or *N. E.* ¼ *E.* almoft.

L
. . . . uiftance of the Po. . . .
portion . . . . AB and BC, *viz.* as
                                 I 2

To find the Course back to the Port.   Co. Ar.
As AD 82 min ───────────────────────── Log. 8.086186
  To f. AED, 71° 34' ──────────────────────── 9977125
  So is AE 68 min. ──────────────────────── 1832509
  To f ADE 51° 53' ──────────────────────── 29895820
The Course to the Port is N. W 79° 03', or W. by N. a little W.erly.

Of CURRENTS.

When a Ship fails in a Current her Motion is compounded of two Motions, *viz.* the apparent Motion of the Ship, which is known by the Compass, Log, &c and the Motion of the Current, which if known before-hand, you may eafily find the true compound Motion of the Ship; or if the Currents Motion be not known, you may find it if you do but know how far you are deceived, *viz* how far, and which way, you are unexpectedly carried As for Inftance,

Queft. I

A Ship fails 5 Miles an hour, *S* by *W* for 16 hours, in a Current that fets 3 Miles an hour, *W* by *S* I demand the Courfe and Dift made good.

In the Triangle ABC, there is given, AB the Diftance failed 80 Miles, *S* by *W* and BC the Currents Motion 48 Miles *W* by *S* and the Angle ABC ten Points, or 112° 30', to find AC the Diftance made good, and the Angle BAC the true Courfe ───── *Plate* 1 *Fig* 12

And firft for the Angle BAC, the Courfe by Cafe the fourth, of Oblique Plain Triangles

Side AB—80 ⎫   From ──── ── ── 180° 00'
Side BC—48 ⎰   Subtr. Angle ABC ── 112 30
Sum   128 ⎰   Refts Sum of the Angle 67 30
Diff   32 ⎱   half Sum 33 45

			Co. Ar.
As Sum of the Sides AB and BC,	128	──── ── ──	7892790
To their Difference	32	──── ── ──	1.505150
So t half Sum of unknown Angles	33° 45'	──── ── ──	9824893
To t half their Difference	9 29	──── ── ──	9.222833
To the half Sum	33° 45'		
Add the half Difference	9 29		
The Sum is ACB	43 14	the greater Angle.	
Subt. the Diff. is BAC	24 16	the lesser Angle.	

Secondly

Secondly, to find the Side AC, by Cafe the fift.

                      °   ′   *Co Ar.*

As Sine of the Angle BAC   24 16 ———————————— 0.386175
To Side oppofite BC   48 ————————————— 1.681241
So Sine of the Ang. ABC 112 30 —————————————9.965615
To Side oppofite AC   108 ————————————— 2.033031

              To AB South by Weft,   11° 15′
              Add the Angle BAC   24 16
              The Sum is the Courfe 35 31

The way made good is 108′ S. 35° 31′ W. or S. W. by S 1° 46′ W.erly.

Queftion 2.   *Plate* 1 *Fig.* 12.

Suppofe three Ports, A, B, and C, a Ship at A, fteers South by Weft 80 Miles, and expecting to arrive at B, he finds himfelf at C, a Port diftant from A 108 Miles, South 35° 31′ Weft, being deceived by a Current. I demand which way the Current fets, and how faft, fuppofing the Ship fails five Miles an hour

In the Triangle ABC you have given, the Side AB, the diftance failed by the Log 80 Miles, South by Weft, and AC the diftance made good 108 Miles South 35° 31′ Weft, and then contained Angle CAB, 24° 16′, to find the Angle ABC, the Courfe of the Current, and BC its Race, which becaufe it is found by *Cafe the fourth* and *firft*, of Oblique Plain Triangles, and performed exactly in the fame manner as the foregoing *Queftion* is, I fhall leave the *Operation* for the Readers practice.

The Angle ABC will be found to be 112° 30′ or ten points, which reckoned from North by Eaft, the Courfe from B to A, it will be found Weft by South and the Side BC 48, the Currents Race in the time that the Ship fails 80 Miles, which at five Miles an hour, is 16 hours; fo that the Current fets 3 Miles an hour.

But fuppofe you know, or have formerly found the Currents Courfe and Race, and know the true bearing and diftance between the Ports given, and defire to know what Courfe you muft fteer, and how many Miles you muft fail by the Log, to arrive at the defired Port.

Queftion 3

A Ship at A Bound for C, which bears from A South 35° 31′ Weft, 108 Miles off, but knowing there is a Current that fets Weft by South 3 Miles an hour. I demand what Courfe he muft fteer by the Compafs, and how far he muft fail by the Log, to arrive at his Port at C, the the Ship failing 5 Miles an hour   *Plate* 1. *Fig.* 12.

Here is given, AC the diftance of the Ports 108 Miles, and the proportion of the Sides AB and BC, *viz.* as 5 to 3, becaufe the Ship fails

I 2

5 Miles an hour, from A to B, while the Current sets 3 Miles an hour from B to C; you have also given, the Anlge ACB 43° 14'. Therefore by *Cafe* 2,

			Co Ar
As Side AB	5	———	9.301030
To its opposite Angle ACB	43° 14'	———	9.835672
So Side BC	3	———	0.477121
To its opposite Angle BAC	24° 16'	———	19.613823

Angle ACB	43° 14	From 180° 00'
Angle BAC	24 16	Subtr 67 30
Sum	67 30	Rest ABC 112 30

Then l, Cafe the fi.st of Oblique   Co. Ar.

As Sine of the Angle ABC	112° 30'	———	0.034385
To Side opposite AC	108	———	2.033424
So Sine of the Angle ACB	43 14	———	9.835672
To Side opposite AB	80	———	11.903481

The Distance sailed AB is 80 Miles, the Rate of sailing, is 5 Miles an hour, Divide 80 by 5, the Quotient is 16, the time the Ship should sail from B to A.

Likewise, Multiply 16, the hours that the Ship is sailing by 3, the Miles the Current sets in an hour, the product 48 is the Side, BC the Currents Race, the truth of which may be proved by a Canon,

As Sine ACB, To Side AB; So S. BAC, To Side BC.

Then from the whole Angle, that the line AC makes with the Meridian ——————————————————— 35° 31'

Subtr the Angle BAC ———————————— 24 16

Rests DAB the Course steered *S.* by *W* ———— 11 15

The Distance by the Log, AB 80 Miles

There are other Curiosities in Current sailing, but these being the most useful, we forbear to Enlarge

CHAP. VI

The Doctrine of Plain Right-angled Triangles applied in PROBLEMS *of* Mercators Sailing.

THE true Sea Chart, commonly called *Mercator's Chart*, (which is the useful Invention of our Country-man Mr. *Edward Wright*, although this Stranger hath got the Name thereof) performs the like Conclusions, and almost in the same manner for ease, and yet

most

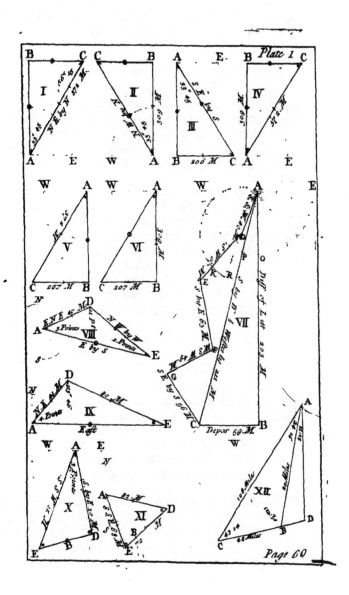

Plate 1

moſt exactly ; becauſe all Places may be laid down upon this Chart, with the ſame Truth as upon the Globe, both as to the Latitude and Longitude, Bearing and Diſtance from each other.

PROB I. To find the Meridional Difference of Latitude, or the Difference of Latitude in Meridional Parts

Firſt, If one Place be under Equinoctial, and the other in North or South Latitude, the Meridional Parts (in the Table of Meridional Parts) anſwering to the Degrees and Minutes of the Place's Latitude is the Meridional Diff. of Latitude.

Example. One Place in the Latitude 37° 27′ North, the other under the Equinoctial · I demand the difference of Latitude in Meridional Parts.

Lat 37° 27′————————2426
2426 is the Meridional Diſt. Latitude.

· *Secondly,* If two Places be both in North, or both in South Latitude, ſubtract the Meridional Parts of the leſs Latitude from thoſe of the greater, the Remainder is the Meridional Diff. Lat.

Example 1.	*M. Pts.*
One Place in the Latitude 37° 20′ N. -	2418
The other in the Latitude 17 10 N.	1046
The Meridional Diff Latitude,	1372
Example 2.	*M Pts.*
One Place in the Latitude 45° 56′ S.	3110
The other in the Latitude 29 17 S.	1839
The Meridional Diff Latitude,	1271

Thirdly, If of the two Places the one have North Latitude, the other South, add the Meridional Parts of each Latitude together, the Sum is the Difference of Latitude in Meridional Parts.

Example.	*M. Pts.*
One Place in the Latitude 42° 17′ S.	2805
The other in the Latitude 27 19 N.	1705
The Meridional Diff. Latitude,	4510

PROB. II. One Latitude, Courſe and Diſtance given, to find the other Latitude, Departure and Difference of Longitude.
Example. A Ship in Latitude 42° 12′ N. ſails S. E. by S 397 Miles ; I demand the other Latitude, Departure and Difference of Longitude
In the Triangle ABC, *Plate* 2. *Fig.* 1.
Ac repreſents the Diſtance,

A b

AD the difference of Latitude,
bc the Departure, as in *Plain Sailing,*
AB the Meridional Difference of Latitude,
BC the difference of Longitude, according to the true Chart, commonly called *Mercator's-Chart*

The Operation. To find the Departure.

As Radius ———————————————90° 0'   10 000000
To the Distance Ac ——————————397   2 598790
So Sine bAc the Course ——————33° 45'   9 744739
To bc the Departure————————22c 6   12.343529

To find the Difference of Latitude

As Radius ———————————————90° 00' 10 000000
To the Distance Ac ——————————397   2 598790
So Sine Acb Comp Course——————56 15   9 919846
To difference of Lat. Ab——————330   12.518636

To find the Difference of Longitude

Lat failed from————42° 12' Merid Parts ————2798
Dif Lat ——————— 5 3c
Lat come to————36 42 Merid Parts ————2370
Meridional difference of Latitude——————— 428
As Radius ————————————90° 0' ——— 10 000000
To AB to Merid dift Lat,————— 428 ——— 2.631444
So Tang. BAC the Course———— 33° 45' ——— 9.824894
To BC the difference of Longitude ——286 ——— 12.456338
Which reduced is——— 4° 46'

PROB. III. Both Latitudes and Course given, to find the Distance, Departure and Difference of Longitude.
A Ship sails N. W by N from Lat 36° 42' N. to Latitude 42° 12' N. I demand the Distance, Departure, and Difference of Longitude.

Latitude 42° 12' Merid. Parts,   2798
Latitude 36 42 Merid Parts,   2370   Plate 2. Fig 2.
Merid. Diff. Latitude   428

The Operation, to find the Distance.

As Radius————————————90° 0' ——— 10 000000
To AB Dif. Latitude————————— 330 ——— 2 518514
So Secant of bAc the Course———— 33° 45' ——— 10.080154
To Ac the Distance——————— 396 9 ——— 2.598668
                                              To

To find the Departure.

As Radius ———————————————90° 0' ———— 10.000000
To the diftance A c ——————— 396 9 ——— 2 598681
So Sine b A c the Courfe ————— 33 45 ——— 9 744739
To b c the Departure———————— 220 5 ——— 2 343420

To find the Difference of Longitude.

As Radius ————————————90° 0' ——— 10.000000
To AB Merid. Diff Lat. ————— 428 ——— 2.631444
So tang. BAC the Courfe———— 33° 45' — 9 824893
To BC Diff. Longitude———— 286———— 12 456337

PROB. IV. Both Latitudes and Diftance given, to find the Courfe, Departure, and Difference of Longitude.

A Ship fails in the S. E Quarter 397 miles, from Lat. 42° 12' N to Lat 36° 42' N I demand the Courfe, Departure, and Difference of Longitude.

Lat. 42° 12' merid. parts   2798
Lat. 36 42 merid parts   2370   *Plate 2. Fig. 3*
Merid. Diff. Lat.   428

The Operation, to find the Courfe:

As A c the Diftance——————————397 —— 2.598790
To Radius——————————90° 0' —— 10 000000
So Ab the Diff. Latitude————— 33° —— 2.518514
To Sine of A c b Comp Courfe———56° 15' — 9 919724

To find the Departure

As Radius ——————————— 90° 0' ——— 10 000000
To the Diftance Ac—————— 397 — 2.598790
So Sine b A c, the Courfe ——— 33° 45' ——— 9 744739
To b c the Departure ———— 220 6 —— 12.343529

To find the Difference of Longitude.

As Radius———————————90° 0' — 10.000000
To merid. Diff Lat AB ——— 428 — 2.631444
So tang. of BAC the Courfe —— 33° 45' — 9.824893
To BC Diff. Longitude ———— 286 — 12.456387

PROB

PROB. V. Both Latitudes and Difference of Longitude given, to find the Course, Distance, and Departure

A Ship sails from Latitude 63° 55′ North; and sails into Latitude 59° 12′ North, her Difference of Longitude 4° 7′, I demand her Course Distance and Departure. *Plate. 2. Fig. 4.*

Lat 63° 55′ Merid. parts 5028
Lat 59 12 Merid parts 4433

Diff Lat 04 43 Merid Diff. Lat. 595
60

Diff Lat in miles 283
Diff. Long 4° 7′
60

Diff. Long. in Minutes 247

The Operation To find the Course.

As AB Merid. Diff. Lat	595	2.774517
To Radius	90° 0′	10.000000
So BC Diff. Longitude	247	2.392697
To Tang. BAC, the Course	22 32	9.618180

To find the Distance

As Radius	90° 0′	10.000000
To Ab the Diff. Latitude	283	2.451786
So the Sec. of BAC the Course	22 32	10.034489
To Ac the Distance	306 4	12.486275

To find the Departure

As Radius	90° 0′	10.000000
To Ac the distance	306 4	2.486289
So Sine bAc the Course	22 32	9.583449
To bc the Departure	117 4	12.069738

Or,

As Radius	90° 0′	10.000000
To Ab the Diff. Lat.	283	2.451786
So Tang. bAc the Course	22° 32′	9.617939
To bc the Departure	117.4	12.069725

PROB. VI One Latitude, Course, and Difference of Longitude given, to find the other Latitude, Distance, and Departure.

A

Mercator's Sailing. 73

A Ship in Latitude 35° 56' North, fail *S. E.* by *E.* half *E.* and makes Difference of Longitude 7° 42'. I demand the other Latitude, Diftance, and Departure.

$$\begin{array}{r} 7^\circ \ 42' \\ 60 \\ \hline 462' \ \text{Diff. Long.} \end{array}$$

Plate. 2. Fig. 5.

The Operation, to find the other Latitude.

As Tang. BAC the Courfe —— 61° 53' —————— 10:2721952

To BC Diff. Long. ———— 462 ———— 2 6646420

So Radius ———— 90° 0' ———— 10.0000000

To the Merid. Diff. Lat. AB —— 247 ———— 2 3924468

Lat. failed from 35° 56' Merid. parts ———— 2313

Merid. Diff. Lat. fubtract ———— 247

Refts Merid. parts for Lat. come to 32 32 ———— 2066

To find the Diftance.

As Radius ———— 90° 0' ———— 10.0000000

To Ab the Diff. Lat. ———— 204 ———— 2.3096301

So fecant bAc the Courfe —— 61 53 ———— 10 3267316

To Ac the Diftance ———— 432 9 ———— 2.6363617

To find the Departure.

As Radius ———— 90° 0' ———— 10 0000000

To Ab the Diftance ———— 432.9 ———— 2.6363875

So S. bAc the Courfe— —— 61° 53' ———— 9.9454636

To the Departure bc —— — 381 8 ———— 2 5818511

PROB. VII Both Latitudes and Departure given, to find the Courfe, Diftance, and Difference of Longitude.

There are two Ports, one in Latitude 57° 3' North, and the other Latitude 61° 10' North, and by a true Reckoning, according to Plain Sailing, the Wefting made good in failing from the Southermoft, to the Weftermoft, is 200 miles. I demand the Courfe, Diftance, and Difference of Longitude between them.

Lat. 61° 10' Merid. parts   4670

Lat 57 03 Merid parts   4188

Diff. Lat. 4: 7 Mer. Diff. Lat.   482

$$\begin{array}{r} 60 \\ \hline 247 \end{array}$$

• Plate 2. Fig. 6.

K

The

The Operation To find the Courſe.

As Diff. Lat Ab ———————— 247 ——— — ———— 2 3926969

  To Radius ———— — — — — — ———— 10 0000000

So Departure bc — — - — - — 200 ——— ———— 2 3010400

  To Tang. bAc, the Courſe — — 39° 0′ ——— —— 9.9083431

               To find the D ſtance

As S Acb Comp Courſe ———— 51° 0′ ——— 9.8905026

  To Diff Latitude Ab ——— — 247 ——— — 2.3926969

So Radius —— — — — — — — - — 10 0000000

  To the Diſtance Ac — — —— — 317 8 ——— 2 5021943

         To find the D ference of Longitvde.

As Radius ——— — — — — ———— 10 0000000

  To the Merid Diff Lat AB ——— 482 —— ———— 2.6830470

So Tang of BAC the Courſe——— 39° 0′ —— - - — 9 9083692

  To Diff. Longitude BC——— —— 390 ——— ——— 12 5914162

There are other Problems, that are frequently and indeed properly Rank'd amongſt the Queſtions in _Mercator's Sailing_, Nevertheleſs becauſe theſe relate only to Sailing in the ſame Latitude, viz upon an Eaſt or Weſt Courſe, we ſhall here diſtinguiſh them by the Name of,

Parallel Sailing.

A Ship in Latitude 60° 0′ North, ſails due Weſt till her Difference of Longitude be 7° 17′, I demand how many Miles ſhe hath ſailed.

             7 17

             60

Diff. Long.   437

        The Operation.   _Plate 2 Fig 7._

As AB Radius——— —— 90° 0′ ———— 10 0000000

  To BC Diff Long ——— 437 — —— ———— 2 6404814

So Ab S Comp Lat ——— 30 0 —— ——— — 9 6989700

  To bc the Diſtance- —— 218 5 ——— — ——— 12.3394514

See the Demonſtrations of the Proportions uſed in this and the two following Problems, in the uſe of the Plain Scale, Chap 11. in the latter part of this Book.

PROB. II The Parallel of Latitude, and Diſtance between two places given, to find the Diff of Long.   _Plate 2 Fig 8._

A Ship in Lat 42° 10′ ſails Weſt 397 Miles, I demand the Difference of Longitude.

As Sine Comp Lat, Ab ———— 42° 10' ——————————— 9 8699326

   To the Diftance bc ———————— 397 ——————————— 2.5987905

   So Radius AB————————————90 0 ——————————— 10 0000000

   To Diff. Long. BC———————535 6——————————— 2.7288579

PROB III The Diftance, and Difference of Long. between two Places in the fame Lat. given, to find the Lat   *Plate.* 2. *Fig.* 9.

   There are two places in the fame Latitude, their Diftance 597, and Difference of Longitude 769, I demand the Parallel or Latitude.

As BC the Diff. Long.————————— 769————————— 2.8859263

   To Radius AB ——————————90.0—————————— 10.0000000

   So bc the Diftance—————— ———597——————————— 2 7759743

   To Ab Sine Comp. Lat —————39.4——————————— 9 8900430

The foregoing Prob. in Mercat Sailing, Illuftrated by a Practical Examp.

   There are two Ports, one in Lat 40° 00' North, the other in Lat. 43° 25' North, the Difference of Longitude 4° 52' the Southermoft Port being the Wefteimoft. A Ship at the Northeimoft fails S. W by S. 47' then S. S. W half W 51, then S by E a quarter E 62, then W N. W three quarters W 61, then W. S. W. a quarter W. 51. I demand,

  1   The Courfe and Diftance between the two Ports,

  2   What Latitude the Ship is in,

  3.   What Difference of Longitude fhe hath made,

  4.   What Courfe and Diftance fhe hath made good, from the firft Port failed fiom,

  5.   What is the Courfe and Dift to the 2d. Port, the Port bound for.

    The Operation To find the Courfe between the two Ports.

Lat ————43.25 Merid parts 2897⎫

Lat ————40 0 Merid parts 2623⎬   *Plate* 2 *Fig* 10.

Diff Lat - —3 25 Mer Diff. Lat. 274⎭

As Merid· Diff. Lat AD——————274——————— 2 4377505

   To Radius ———————————90 0——————— 10 0000000

   So Diff Long ED————————292——————— 2 4653828

   To Tang Courfe—————————46·49 ——— 10.0276323

    To find the Diftance.

As Sine Comp. Courfe s c——— 46.49——————— 9 8352688

   To Diff Lat. A d——————205——————— 2.3117538

   So Radius————————90 °.0'——————— 10 0000000

   To the Diftance A e ————299 5——————— 2.4764850

The Courfe from the Northermoft Port, to the Southermoft, is South 46° 49' Weft, or South Weft 1° 49' W. the Diftance 299.5 Miles.

         Then

Then for the first Course South West by South, 47ʳ,
To find the other Latitude.

As Radius —————————90° 0′—————————— 10 0000000
  To the Distance————47————————— 1 6720978
So Sine Comp. Course sc—33 45————————9 9193464

  To the diff Latitude ——— 39 1 ———————— 11.5919442
Latit sailed from   43° 25′ Merid. parts, ——— 2897
Diff. Lat. Subtr   0 39
Lat come to   42 46   Merid parts 2844
                Merid. Diff Lat.   53

As Radius ———————————90° 0′——————— 10 0000000
  To Merid Diff Lat————53————————— 1 7242758
So Tang. Course————33 45—————————9 8248926

  To Diff. Longitude ————35 4—————————11 5491684
The second Course S S. W. half W. 51 min.
To find the Difference of Latitude, and Latitude come to.

As Radius———————————90° 0′——————— 10 0000000
  To the Distance————51————————— 1.7075701
So Sine Comp. Course sc.—28.7————————9.9454636

  To the Diff Lat ————45—————————11.6530337
Lat. sailed from——42° 46′ Merid parts————2844
Diff. Lat. subtr.——0 45
     Lat. come to——42 1 Merid parts————2783
            Merid Diff. Lat   61

As Radius ———————————90° 0′————— 10 0000000
  To the Mer. differ. Latitude — 61———————— 1 7853298
So Tang. Course ————28 7————————9.7278048

  To Diff Long.————32 6—————————11 5131346
The third Course S by E. ¼ E 62 Miles.
To find Diff Lat. and Lat. come to.
          —90° 0′———— 10 0000000

As Radius —————————62———— 1 7923916
  To the Distance——————14° 4′——9 9867778
So Sine Comp. Course sc. ————— 60 1——11.7791694

To Diff Lat. —————————
Lat. fail'd from———42° 1′ merid. parts 2783
Diff. Lat. subt.————1 0
     Lat come to ———— 41 1 merid parts 2703
         merid. Diff. Lat. 80

                                As

As Radius	90° 0'	10.00000C0
To Merid. Dif. *Lat*	80	1 9030900
So tang Courfe	14° 4'	9 3989191
To Dif. Longitude	20	11.3020091

The fouth Courfe W NW. ¼ W 61.
To find Dif. *Lat* and *Lat* come to.

As Radius	90° 0'	10.0000000
To the Diftance	61	1 7853298
So Sine Comp Courfe fc.	75° 56'	9 3856969
To Diff *Lat*.	14 8	11.1710267
Lat. fail'd from	41° 01' merid. parts	2703
Dif. *Lat*. add.	0 15	
Lat. come to	41 16 merid. parts	2723
	Merid. Dif *Lat*	20

As Radius	90° 0'	10 0000000
To merid Dif *Lat*.	20	1 3010300
So tang Courfe	75° 56'	10 6010809
To Dif. *Long*	78 8	11.9021109

The fifth Courfe W S W. ¼ W. 51,
To find Dif *Lat*. and *Lat*. come to

As Radius	90° 0'	10 0000000
To the diftance	51	1 7075702
So Sine Comp. Courfe fc.	70 19	9 5273997
To Dif. *Lat*	17 2	11 2349699
Lat. fail'd from	41° 16' merid. parts	2723
Dif *Lat*. fubt	0 17	
Lat. come to	40° 59' merid parts	2700
	Merid Dif. *Lat*	23

As Radius	90° 0'	10.00000C0
To merid Dif. *Lat*	23	1 3617278
So tang Courfe	7° 19	10 4464523
To Dif Longitude	64 3	11.8081801

To find the Courfe and Diftance made good from the Port firft failed from.

Make a fmall Table, as you are taught in the Ufe of the Tables of the difference of Latitude and Departure in the latter part of this Book, only this confifts of feven Columns, as below.

Courfes

Course	Dist.	Lat	Diff.	Lat	Diff.	Long.
	M D	M	N	S.	E.	W.
S W b, S	47	42.46		39 1		35 4
S S W ½ W	51	42. 1		45 0		32 6
S. b. E. ½ E.	62	41. 1		60.1	20 0	
W N W ½ W	61	41 16	14 8			78 8
W S W ½ W	51	40 59		17 2		64 3
				161 4		211 1
				14 8		20 0
				146 6		191 1

The first Column contains the Courses, the second the Distances t e third the *Latitude* come to, the fourth the Difference of *Latitude* Northerly, the fifth the Difference of *Latitude* Southerly, the sixth the Difference of *Longitude* Easterly, and the seventh the Difference of *Longitude* Westerly, which is thus found,

Observe the *Latitude* and *Longitude* of the Place sailed from, and the Course and Distance sailed, and then by *Case* 1 of *Plain Sailing*, find the Difference of *Latitude*, and by *Prob* 2 of *Mercator*, find the Difference of *Longitude* as you see in the Operation for the first Course, where you find the Difference of *Latitude* 39 min and Difference of *Longitude* 35 4 and because the Course is between the South and West, I set the Difference of *Latitude* 39 1 in the South Column, and the *Difference* of *Longitude* 35 4 in the West Column as you see in the Table, also subtracting the *Difference* of *Latitude* 39' from 43° 25' the *Latitude* sailed from, the Remainder 42° 46' is the *Latitude* come to, which I place in the third Column under *Lat* and so proceed to the second and third Courses, &c and having found the *Difference* of *Latitude* and *Longitude* and placed them all in their proper Columns in the Table add up each Column alone, as you see in this Example, where the North Column is only 14 8, the South Column 161 4, which being the greatest, I subtract the Northing 14 8, from it, and the Remainder 146.6 I set in the South Column for the South *Latitude* made good, do the same by the East and West Columns, and you have the *Longitude* made good, which in this Example is 191 1 West *Longitude*, which divided by 60, gives 3° 11' Also the *Difference* of *Latitude* 146 6, or rather 147 divided by 60 gives 2° 27' which subtracted from the *Latitude* sail'd from, gives 40° 58' the *Lat* the Ship is in. And thus you have both *Latitudes*
and

and *Difference* of *Longitude* to find the *Courfe* and *Diftance* failed from the firft Port, by *Prob. 2* of *Mercator's Sailing.*

As merid. Dif. *Lat.* AB ———— 198 ——— 2.2966652

   To Radius ——————————— 90° 0'   10.0000000

   So *Diff Longitude* BC ———————— 191 —— 2 2810334

   To tang. Courfe ————————— 43° 58' 9 9843682

To find the Diftance failed.

As Sine Comp. Courfe ———————— 43° 58' 9 8571779

   To *Diff Lat* A b ———————— 147 —— 2.1673173

   So Radius ————————— 90° 0' 10 0000000

   To the Diftance Ac ———————— 204.2 2.3101394

Then to find the Courfe and Diftance from the Ship to the Port bound for, you have given the *Latitude* and *Longitude* the Ship is in, *viz.* Lat. 40° 58' and *Latitude* of the Port 40° 0', the *Difference* of Longitude between the Ports is 4° 52', or 292' the *Diff. Longitude* made by the Ship is 191', which fubtracted from 292', reft 101, the *Diff. Longitude* from the Ship to the Port reprefented by the Line *E M*.

   Lat 40° 58' merid parts ———— 2699

   Lat. 40 0 merid. parts ———— 2623

Diff. Lat 0 58 merid. *Diff. Lat.* ——— 76

As merid. *Diff Lat* CM ———— 76 ——— 1 8808136

   To Radius ————— 90° 0' ——— 10.0000000

   So *Diff. Longit.* E M ——— 101 ——— 2 0043214

   To tang Courfe ———— 53° 2 ——— 10.1235078

To find the Diftance.

As Sine Comp Courfe fc ————— 53° 2' —— 9 7791275

   To *Diff Lat.* C L ———— 58 —— 1.7634280

   So Radius ———— 90° 0' ——— 10 0000000

   To the Diftance CR ———— 96 5 ——— 1 9843005

From the Ship to the Port bound for, is South 53° 2' Weft, or South Weft almoft ¼ South, the Diftance 96.5 miles, or 96 miles and a half, reprefented by the prick'd Line C R.

This method of working by a Canon, is the moft exact, and the Foundation of all other Methods of Working. Neverthelefs, a Traverfe may be wrought, and an Account of a Ship's Way kept with fufficient Exactnefs, both in Latitude and Longitude, only by the Tables of Difference of Latitude and Departure, as will be plainly taught when we come to fhew the Ufe of thefe Tables towards the latter end of the Book, and the true Projection thereof you will have in the Ufe of the *Plain Scale,* &c.   *How*

How to work any Question in Mercator's Sailing, without a Table of Meridional Parts.

BUT for the Learner's Instruction, and (if possible) to invite all Mariners to the frequent use of *Mercator's* Sailing, I shall incert one Proportion which may well be called the *Catholick Proportion*, in Mercator, because by it all Neceflary Cases in *Mercator* may be refolved, and it is thus performed without a Table of Meridional Parts,

As Log. Tangent 51° 38′ 9″ (*viz* 10.101510) To Tangent Courfe, So is the Difference between the Log. Tangent of half the Complement of the two Latitudes, to the Difference of Longitude.

You need not regard the degree, *viz* 51° 38′ 9″ becaufe the Tang. of it is always a stared Number, to work with, and is easie to remember, for if you set it down by two figures together 'tis, 10, 10, 15, 10, the firft 10 being the Characterifick, the reft ftand as you fee above.

Now if one Latitude, Courfe, and Diftance be given to find the Difference of Longitude, the Terms ftand as above.

Example

A Ship in Latitude 50° 10′ fails South South West half West, 1650 Miles, I demand the Latitude come to, and Difference of Longitude.

Firft, find the Diff. of Lat. by Cafe the firft of Plain Sailing.

As Radius	90° 0		10.0000000
To the Diftance	1650		3.2174839
So Sine Comp. Courfe &c.	28 7		9.9454636
To Difference Latitude	1455		13.1629475

The Difference of Latitude 1455′ or 24° 15′ fubtracted from 50° 10′ gives 25° 55′ the Latitude come to

50° 10′ Comp. 39° 50′ half Comp 19° 55′ Tangent			9.559097
25° 55′ Comp. 64 5 half Comp. 32 2½ Tang.			9.796491
		Diff.	2373.94

From the Difference 237394, cut off two figures to the Right-hand, and you have 2373 94 but the firft figure of the Decimal being 9, I add 1 to the laft figure of the Number, and make it 2374, and proceed by the foregoing Proportion.

As the Common Tangent			10.101510
To Tangent Courfe	28° 7′		9.727805
So is Diff. of the Tangents	2374		3.375480
			13.103285
To Diff. Longitude	1004		3.001775

Or

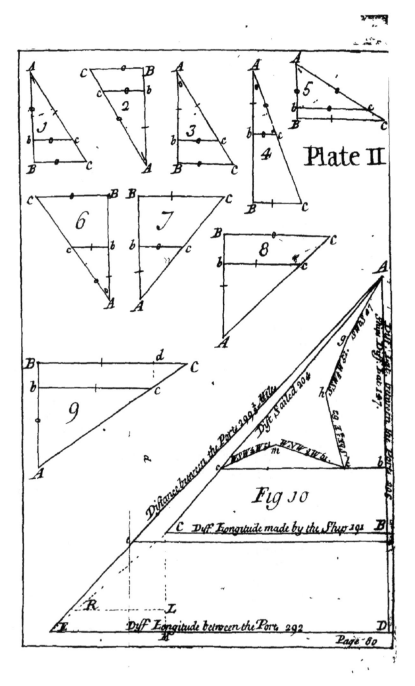

Plate II

Fig 10

Distance between the Ports 299 3/4 Miles

Diff Sailed 204

Diff Longitude made by the Ship 191

Diff Longitude between the Ports 292

Or the Proportion may be altered, and fuited to any other Cafe in Mercator's Sailing; as if both Latitudes, and Dift. of Longitude were given, to find the Courfe it would be,

As the Dif of the Tang. of half Complement of the two Latitudes, To Dif. Longitude, So is the common Tangent 10.101510, To Tang of the Courfe.

Or If both Latitudes, and Courfe were given, to find Difference of Longitude it will be,

As common Tang 10 101510, To Diff Tang ½ Comp. of the two Lat So Tang Courfe, To Diff Long &c. But thefe Varieties we fhall leave to the Reader's Practice.

Middle Latitude Sailing, commonly called Mercator's Sailing by Middle Latitude.

THIS, as well as *Mercator's Sailing*, fuppofeth the Earth and Sea to make one entire Globe, and is grounded upon this manifeft Truth derived from thence, that the Semidiameter of any Parallel of Latit. is in Proportion to the Semidiameter of the Equinoctial, as the Sine Complement of that Parallel is to Radius, and becaufe the Circumference of all Circles are Proportionable to their Semidiameters, the Circumference of any Parallel bears alfo the fame Proportion to the Circumference of the Equinoctial; and becaufe there are the fame Number of *Degrees* of *Longitude* in any Parallel that there are in the Equinoctial, it will follow, that the miles in one *Degree* of *Longitude* in the Equinoctial, *viz.* 60, are in Proportion to the Miles in one *Degree* of *Longitude* in any other Parallel, as Radius to the Sine Complement of that Parallel; and hence to reduce miles Eafting or Wefting in any Parallel to *Difference* of *Longitude*, or miles Eafting or Wefting in the Equinoctial, the Proportion is, As Sine Complement of *Latitude* to Radius, fo the Eafting or Wefting (commonly called *Departure*) to *Difference* of *Longitude*

This is abfolutely exact if you fail Eaft or Weft (as hath been fhew'd in *Parallel Sailing*) and fufficiently fo, if you fail upon an ObliqueCourfe, provided you take the *Middle Latitude* between the two extream *Latitudes* (from whence it is called *Middle Latitude Sailing*) which is found by adding both *Latitudes* together, and if they are both *North* or both *South*, half their Sum is the *Middle Latitude*, &c.

Note; If there be an odd Minute in the fum of the two *Latitudes*, take always the greater half of the fum for *Middle Latitude*.

L   Example

Example. One Latitude, Course and Distance given, to find the other Latitude, Departure and Difference of Longitude.

A Ship in *Latitude* 50° 0′, sails *S W* by *S.* 88 miles ; I demand the *Latitude come to, with the Departure and Difference of Longitude?*

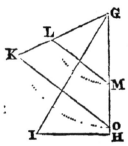

Lay down the Triangle GHI, as you are taught in the use of the *Plain Scale* in *Plain Sailing* with the *Sine* of the Comp of *Middle Lat* in your Compasses, and one Foot in G, draw the Arch LM, till the line LM be equal to IH, and through L draw *GLK* ; with the *Sine* of 90 in your Compasses, and one Foot in G, describe the Arch *KO*, the Line *K O* measured on the same equal Parts from which you projected the Question, gives the *Difference of Longitude* required.

To find Arithmetically what is required.

First, by Case the first of Plain Sailing.

As Radius	90° 0′	10 0000000
To the distance GI	88	1.9444827
So Sine of the Course IGH	33 45	9 7447390
To the Departure IH	49	11.6892217

As Radius	90° 0′	10 0000000
To the Distance G I	88	1 9444827
So S. Comp. Course GIH	56 15	9.9198464
To Diff. Latitude GH	73	11.8643291

Diff. Lat. 73′ or 1° 13′ Lat. come to	48° 47′
Latitude sailed from	50 00
Sum	98 47
Half Sum or Middle Latit.	49 24

To find the Difference of Longitude.

As Sine Comp. Middle Lat.	49° 24′	9 8134303
To Radius	90 00	10 0000000
So Departure	49	1.6901961
To Diff. Long.	75	1.8767658

Or

Or the Diff of Long. may be thus found,

Firſt, as in Caſe the firſt of Plain Sailing, with the given Courſe and Diſtance, lay down the Triangle GHI, and having found the Middle Lat which in this Example is 49° 24′ draw the Line I R to make an Angle of 49° 24′ with the Line I H continue GH till it cut I R in R, then is G I the Diſtance, the Angle IGH the Courſe, G H the Diff of Lat I H the Departure, and the Angle HIR the Middle Lat. HRI the Complement of Middle Latitude. Hence is Demonſtrated the proportion by which we have found the Longitude, for As Sine of the Complement of Middle Latitude HRI, To Departure I H, So is Radius, or the Right Angle IHR, To Difference of Longitude IR.

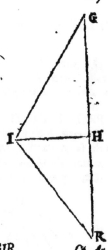

And in the Oblique Triangle GIR, &c. Ar.

As Sine Compl Middle Latitude IRH — 40° 36′ ———— 0.1865697
To Side oppoſite GI the Diſtance — 88 ——.—— 1.9444826
So Sine Courſe IGR ——— 33 45 ——— 9.7447390
To Side oppoſite IR Diff. Long———75 ——.—— 11.8757823

By this Method you may project and anſwer all the uſeful Caſes in Middle Latitude Sailing, as ſuppoſe both Latitudes, and Difference of Longitude were given, in *Fig.* 2. draw the line GR, and at R make the Angle GRI, equal to the Complement of Middle Latitude, and ſet the Difference of Longitude from R to I, and let fall the Perpendicular IH, Then ſet the Difference of Latitude, from H to G, and draw I G and then is the Projection finiſhed. The Angle IGH is the Courſe, G I the Diſt. and IH the Dep. And by Arithmetical Calculation it is,

As Radius, to RI Diff. Longitude, So Sine of HRI the Complement of Middle Latitude, to HI the Departure.

And as GH the Difference of Latitude, To Radius; So HI the Departure, To Tangent of HGI the Courſe.

And, As Sine of HGI the Courſe, To IH the Departure, So is Radius, to IG the Diſtance.

But for the Operations, in this and other Varieties of this kind, I ſhall leave them to the Reader's Practice, ſuppoſing that what hath been ſaid may be ſufficent to Introduce the Learner into the further knowledge of Middle Latitude Sailing; and is as much as our intended Brevity in theſe new Additions to this Treatiſe will permit.

L 2

CHAP.

CHAP. VII

The Doctrine of Spherical Triangles, applied in PROBLEMS of
Great Circle Sailing.

Although it be hardly possible for a Ship exactly to trace out the
Arch of a Great Circle, yet it may be of Advantage to keep
conveniently near it, especially in a Parallel (or East and West)
Course.

PROB I. Two Places differing only in Longitude.

Example. A Ship being in the Latitude 50° North, is bound to a Port
in the same Parallel, whose Difference of Longitude Westerly is 47°;
I demand the Angles of Position, the Distance in the Arch of a Great
Circle, by what Latitudes and Longitudes the Arch shall pass, likewise

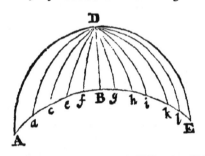

the Course and Distance
from Place to Place, ac-
cording to *Mercator.*

Let A represent the first
Place, E the second.

The Operation.

To find the Angles of
Position, BAD and BED.

The Oblique-angled Tri-
angle ADE is reduced in-
to two equal Right-an-

gled Triangles ABD and EBD, the Sides and Angles being equal;
therefore in either of them there is given the *Hypothenuse,* and the Angle
at D, to find the Angle at A or E.

In the Triangle ABD.

As tc. ADB———23° 30'———	Log.	10.3616981
To Radius ———		10 0000000
So is sc. A D——40 00		9.8842540
To tc. BAD —— 71 35———		9.5225559

2. To find the Distance AE.
In the Triangle ABD.

As Radius	Log.	10 0000000
To s. DA———40° 00' ———		9 8080675
So is s. ADB —— 23 30———		9 6006997
To s. AB ——14 51———		19.4087672
AB —— 14 51 being doubled, produces		
AE——29 42, or 1782'.		3. To

3. To find the Latitudes by which the Arch shall pass at every five Degrees of Longitude from A; representing the first Port.

First, You must find the greatest Latitude by which the Arch passesDB.

In the Triangle ABD.

As tc. AD————————40° 00'——————————Log 10.0761865

To Radius ——————————————————— 10.0000000

So is sc ADB ———23 30——— ·——————————9.9623978

To t. BD——— 37 35 ——————————•——— 9.8862113

The Compl. of BD (to 90°) 5e° 25' is the greatest.

Secondly, To find the Latitude by which the Arch passes at every five Degrees of Longitude from A, you must resolve the several Right-angled Triangles, BDa, BDc, BDe, &c

Subtracting 5° from ADB 23 30
There remains ——aDB 18 30
Subtracting 5° from aDB 18 30
Remains ——— BDc 13 30

And so for the rest, as follows in the Table.

a D B   18° 30'   In the Triangle aBD,
B D c   13   30
B D e   o8   30   To find by what Latitude the Point (a) passes.
B D f   03   30
B D g   01   30   As Radius —— —— ——————Log. 10.0000000·
B D h   06   30   To tc. BD————————37° 35'———10.1137122
B D i   11   30   So is sc aDB ——— 18   30 ——— 9.9769566
B D k   16   30   To tc. Da——— 39   04——— 10.0906688
B D l   21   30

The Complement of Da 50° 56' North, is the Latitude of the Point (a) After the same manner are found the Latitudes for the Points c, e, &c. in the subsequent *Table.*

Long		Lat.	
A 00°	00'	50°	00'
a 05	00	50	56
c 10	00	51	38
e 15	00	52	06
f 20	00	52	22
g 25	00	52	24
h 30	00	52	14
i 35	00	51	51
k 40	00	51	14
l 45	00	50	24
E 47	00	50	00

Thirdly, Having the Latitudes and Longitudes by which the Arch passes, you may find the Course and Distance from Place to Place by *Mercator.*

So to find the Course and Distance Aa, there is given both Latitudes, 50° North, and 50° 56' North.

And the difference of Longitude 5° West.

The

The Meridional Difference of Latitude is 87 Minutes.

For the Course

As Merid. Diff Lat ———————— 87' ————————Log 1 9395192

To Radius ———————————————— 10 0000000

So is the Diff of Long ——————300 ————————2.4771212

To t. Course———————————73° 49' ————————10.5376020

For the Distance.

As Sc. Course ——————— 73° 49 ————————— Log. 9.4451553

To theDiff of Lat ——————— 56 ——————— 1.7481880

So is Radius ——————————————————— 10 0000000

To the Distance ——————— 200 ————————— 2 3030327

After the same manner you will find the Courses and Distances a c, c e, &c as they follow in the Table.

Places	Courses.	Distances
From A to a	N W 73° 49'	200
From a to c	N W 77 13	189
From c to e	N W 81 28	188
From e to f	N W 85 02	184
From f to g	N W 89 22	180
From g to h	S W 86 45	179
From h to i	S W 82 58	187
From i to k	S W 78 41	188
From k to l	S W 75 14	196
From l to E	S W 72 51	081

But in regard most of the Courses afore-found are so near the West, you may sail W. N.W. 917', until you are in theLatitude 55° 51' N. and then W. S. W. 917' further, you will arrive at your Port. By this means you will alter your Latitude almost 6°, and theDistance is but 52 more than that of a Great Circle, and not above 22' more than the Parallel or West Distance.

PROB. II. Two Places differing both in Latitude and Longitude.

Example. Suppose the two Places to be, one in Latitude 36° North, the other in the Latitude 50° North, the Difference of Longitude between them 68° Easterly. I demand the Angles of Position, the Distance in the Arch, the Latitudes and Longitudes by which the Arch passes, and the Course and Distance from Place to Place, through those Latitudes and Longitudes, according to the true Chart.

Let

Let A reprefent the firft place, in the Lat. 36°.
E the fecond, in the Lat. 50°.

The Operation.

1ft, To find the Ang of Pofition
In the Triangle ADE.

AD 54 00	ADE 68 00
DE 40 00	half ADE 34 00
Sum, 94 00	half Sum, 47 00
Diff. 14 00	half Diff. 07 00

As f ½ Zcrᵃ AD and DE 47 00 ——— Log. 0.1358725
To f ½ Xcrᵃ ———— 07 00 ——— 9.0858945
So is tc ½ ADE ——— 34 00 ——— 10.1710126
To t ½ X ∠s A and E 13 52 ——— 19.3927796

As fc ½Zcrᵃ. AD and AE 47 00 ——— Log. 0.1662167
To fc ½ X crᵃ. —— 07 00 ——— 9.9967507
So is tc ½ ADE—— 34 00 ——— 10.1710126
To t ½ Z ∠s A and E—65 08 ——— 10.3339800

½ Z ∠s 65° 08'
½ X ∠s 13 52

Sum 79 00 AED ⎱ The Angles of Pofition.
Diff. 51 16 DAE ⎰

Secondly, To find the Diftance. In the Triangle ADE.

As f. AED ——— 79 00 ——— Log.0.0080534
To f. AD ——— 54 00 ——— 9.9079576
So is f. ADE ——— 68 00 ——— 9.9671659
To f. AE ——— 49 50 ——— 19.8831769

The Diftance is 49° 50', which reduced into Minutes, makes 2990'.
Thirdly, To find the Latit. and Longit. by which the Arch paffes.
Firft, Find the greateft Latitude by which the Arch paffes.
In the Right angled Triangle ABD.

As Radius ——— Log.10.0000000
To f. AD ——— 54° 00' ——— 9.9079576
So is f. DAB ——— 51 16 ——— 9.8921316
To f. DB ——— 39 07 ——— 19.8000892

DB

DB is 39° 07′, whofe Comp 50° 53′ is the greateſt Latitude.
Secondly, To find the Vertical Angles ADB, and BDE.

In the Right angled Triangle ABD.

As tc BAD ———————————— 51° 16′ ——————— Log. 9 9042321
To Radius ——————————————————— 10.0000000
So is ſc. AD ——————— 54 00 ——————— 9 7692187
To tc ADB ——— ———— 53 46 ——————— 9.8649866
From ————— ADE 68° 00′
Subtract ——— ADB 53 46
Remains — BDE 14 14

Thirdly, To find the Latitudes by which the Arch paſſes at every 5
Degrees of Longitude from A, you muſt reſolve the ſeveral Right-angled
Triangles BDa, BDb, BDc, &c

Subtracting five deg. from ADB 53° 46′
There remains   ADb 48 46
Subtracting five deg. from   48 46
Remains ————————— bDB 43 46
So of the reſt, in the follwing Table.

BDa 48 46	BDh 13 46
BDb 43 46	BDi 08 46
BDc 38 46	BDk 03 46
BDd 33 46	BDl 01 14
BDe 28 46	BDm 06 14
BDf 23 46	BDn 11 14
BDg 18 46	

In the Triangle aDB, to find by what Latitude the Arch paſſes at the Point a.

As t. DB —————————— 39° 07′ ——————— Log. 9 9101766
To Radius —————————————————— 10 0000000
So is ſc. aDB ————— 48 46 ——————— 9.8189692
To tc aD ————————— 50 59 ——————— 9.9087926

Whoſe Complement 39° 01′ is the Latitude at *a*.

After the ſame manner are found the Latitudes of ſeveral Points
b, c, d, e, &c. as in the ſubſequent Table.

Fourthly

Latitude.		Longit.
A 36°	00'	00°
a 39	01	05
b 41	36	10
c 43	47	15
d 45	37	20
e 47	09	25
f 48	22	30
g 49	20	35
h 50	33	40
i 50	40	45
k 50	49	50
l 50	53	55
m 50	43	60
n 50	20	65
E 50	00	68

Fourthly, Having thus the Latitudes and Longitudes of the Arch, you may find the Courses and Distances from Place to Place, according to *Mercator.*

So to find the Course and Distance *A a.*

Both Latitudes are 36 degrees and 39 degrees 01 minute.

The Difference of Long. 5 deg.

The proper Difference of Latitude 181 minutes.

The Merid. Difference of Latitude 228 minutes.

For the Course.

As Merid. Diff. Lat. —————— 228' —————— Log. 2.3579348
To Radius —————————————————— 10.0000000
So is the Diff. Longitude ——— 300 ——— 2.4771212
To t. Course ————— 52° 45' ————— 10.1191864

For the Distance.

As Sc. Course ————— 52° 45' ————— Log. 9.7819664
To the Diff. of Latitude, 181 ——— 2.2576786
So is Radius ———————————————— 10.0000000
To the Distance ——— 299 ——— 2.4757122

After the same manner you may find the Courses and Distances *a b, bc, c d,* &c. as they follow in the Table.

Places.	Courses.			Distances
From *A* to *a*	N E	52°	45'	299'
From *a* to *b*	N E	55	54	276
From *b* to *c*	N E	59	10	255
From *c* to *d*	N E	62	40	239
From *d* to *e*	N E	66	05	226
From *e* to *f*	N E	70	01	212
From *f* to *g*	N E	73	39	202
From *g* to *h*	N E	77	35	199
From *h* to *i*	N E	81	05	193
From *i* to *k*	N E	85	14	192
From *k* to *l*	N E	89	02	177
From *l* to *m*	S E	87	19	192
From *m* to *n*	S E	83	09	193
From *n* to *E*	S E	80	13	117

M

CHAP.

CHAP. VIII.

The Doctrine of the Sphere ; containing sundry Astronomical *Definitions and* Problems *useful in the* Art of Navigation.

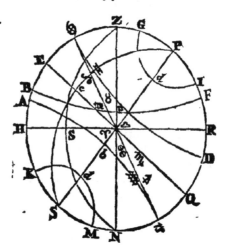

Sect I. *Astronomical Definitions.*

THE *Poles of the World* are two fixed Points in the Heavens diametrically oppofite to one another, the one vifible in our Hemifphere, called the North, or *Artick Pole,* noted with the Letter P.

The other not feen of us, being in the lower Hemifphere, ealled the South or *Antartick Pole,* noted with S.

The *Axis of the World* is an *imaginary Line* drawn from Pole to Pole, about which the *Diurnal Motion* is performed from Eaft to Weft.

The *Meridians* are great Circles concurring and interfecting one another in the Poles of the World; as P E S, and P c S.

The *Equinoctial,* or *Equator,* is a *Great Circle* 90° diftant from the Poles of the World, cutting the *Meridians* at Right-Angles, and dividing the World into two *Parts,* called the *North* and *South Hemifpheres* ; as E ♎ Q.

The *Ecliptick* is a *Great Circle,* croffing the *Equinoctial* in the two oppofite Points *Aries* and *Libra,* and making an Angle therewith (called its *Obliquity*) of 23 deg. 30 min. reprefented by ♋ ♎ ♑.

This Circle is divided into 12 Signs, each containing 30 deg. whofe Names and Characters follow.

Aries,

Aries	♈		Libra	♎	
Taurus	♉		Scorpio	♏	
Gemini	♊	Which are *Nor-*	Sagittarius	♐	These are *Sou-*
Cancer	♋	*thern* Signs.	Capricornus	♑	*thern* Signs.
Leo	♌		Aquarius	♒	
Virgo	♍		Pisces	♓	

The *Zodiack* is a Zone or Girdle, having eight degrees of Latitude on either side of the *Ecliptick*, in which space the Planets make thier Revolutions. 'Tis divided and distinguished by the twelve Signs.

The *Colures* are two *Meridians*, dividing the *Equinoctial* and the *Ecliptick* into four equal parts ; one of these passes by the *Equinoctial* Points *Aries* and *Libra*, and is called the *Equinoctial Colure*, as P ♎ S.

The other by the beginning of *Cancer* and *Capricorn*, called the *Solstitial Colure*, as P ♋, S ♑.

The *Poles of the Ecliptick* are two Points, 23° 30' distant from the Poles of the World, as I and K.

The *Tropicks* are two small Circles, parallel to the *Equinoctial*, and distant therefrom 23° 30', limiting the Sun's greatest *Declination*.

The *Northern Tropick* passes by the Beginning of *Cancer*, and is called the *Tropick of Cancer* ; as ♋ a D.

The *Southern Tropick* passes by the Beginning of *Capricorn*, and is called the *Tropick of Capricorn*; as A b ♑.

The *Polar Circles* are two small Circles parallel to the *Equinoctial*, and distant therefrom 66° 30', and from the Poles of the World, 23° 30'.

That which is adjacent to the N. Pole, is called the *Artick Circle*, as G d I. And the other the *Antartick Circle*, as K d M.

The *Zenith* and *Nadir* are two Points diametrically opposite.

The *Zenith* is the *Vertical Point*, or the Point right over our Heads, as Z. The *Nadir* is directly opposite thereto, as N.

The *Azimuth* or *Vertical Circles*, are great Circles of the Sphere, concurring and intersecting each other in the *Zenith* and *Nadir*, as Z S N.

The *Horizon* is a great Circle 90° distant from the *Zenith* and *Nadir*, cutting all *Azimuths* at Right-angles, and dividing the World into two equal Parts, the *Upper* and visible *Hemisphere*, and the *Lower* and invisible. This Circle is represented by H ♎ R.

The *Meridian* of a Place, is that *Meridian* which passes by the *Zenith* and *Nadir* of the Place, as PZSN.

The *Almicanthers*, or *Parallels of Altitude*, are small Circles parallel to the *Horizon*, imagined to pass through every Degree and Minute of the *Meridian*, between the *Zenith* and *Horizon* ; as B a F.

Parallels of Latitude, or *Declination*, are small Circles parallel to the *Equinoctial* : They are called *Parallels of Declination*, in respect of the

M 2

Sun or Stars in the Heavens ; and *Parallels of Latitude,* in reſpect to any Place upon the Earth.

The *Latitude of a Place,* is the Heighth of the *Pole* above the *Horizon* or the Diſtance between the *Zenith* and the *Equinoctial*

The *Latitude of a Star,* is the Arch of a Circle contained between the Center of a Star, and the *Ecliptick* Line ; this Circle making Right-Angles with the *Ecliptick,* and counted either Northward or Southward, according to the Situation of the Star.

Longitude on the Earth is meaſured by an Arch of the *Equinoctial,* contained between the primary *Meridian* (or *Meridian* of that Place where Longitude is aſſigned to begin) and the Meridian of any other Place counted either Eaſterly or Weſterly.

The *Longitude* of a Star is that Part of the *Ecliptick* which is contained between the Star's Place in the *Ecliptick,* and the beginning of *Aries,* counting them according to the Succeſſion of the Signs.

Altitude of the Sun or Stars, is the Arch of an *Azimuth* contained betwixt the Center of the Sun or Star and the Horizon.

Aſcenſion is the riſing of any Star, or any part of the *Equinoctial* above the *Horizon,* and *Deſcenſion* is the ſetting thereof.

Right-Aſcenſion is the Number of Degrees and Minutes of the *Equinoctial* (counted from the beginning of *Aries*) which cometh to the *Meridian* with the Sun or Star, or with any Portion of the *Ecliptick.*

Oblique Aſcenſion is an Arch of the *Equinoctial* between the beginning of *Aries* and that part of the *Equinoctial* that riſeth with the Center of a Star, or with any Portion of the *Ecliptick,* in an *Oblique Sphere.*

Oblique Deſcenſion is that part of the *Equinoctial* which ſets therewith.

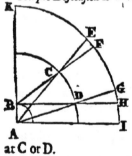

Aſcenſional Difference is an Arch of the *Equinoctial,* being the Difference between the *Right* and *Oblique Aſcenſion.*

The *Amplitude* of the Sun or Star, is the Diſtance of the riſing or ſetting thereof, from the Eaſt or Weſt Points of the *Horizon.*

The *Parallax* is the Difference between the true and apparent Place of the Sun or Star ; ſo that the true Place in reſpect of Altitude is in the Line ACE or ADG the Sun or Star being at C or D.

And the apparent Place in the Line BCF, or BDH.

So the Angles of *Parallax* are ACB or ECF ; and ADB, or GDH. In this Scheme, ABK repreſents a Quadrant of the Earth's Superficies. A the Center of the Earth. B any Point of the Earth's Surface.

Re-

Refraction of the Stars, Observed by Tycho,	
Alt.	Refract.
0°	30′ 30″
1	21 30
2	15 30
3	12 30
4	11 00
5	10 00
6	9 00
7	8 15
8	6 45
9	6 00
10	5 30
11	5 00
12	4 30
13	4 00
14	3 30
15	3 00
16	2 30
17	2 00
18	1 15
19	0 30
20	0 00

The *Refraction* is caused by the *Atmosphere*, or Vaporous Thickness of the Air near the Earth's Superficies, whereby the *Sun* and *Stars* seem always to rise sooner and set later than really they do.

In the Latitude of 55 degrees, and thereabouts, it is allowed to be as follows in the *Table*, altho' it varies by the Weather.

And in the more Northern Parts it hath been observed to be greater.

The Use whereof is this:

Suppose the Altitude observed were 10 degrees; the correspondent Refraction is 5 min. 30 seconds, which subtracted from 10 degrees, the Remainder 9 degrees 54 minutes 30 seconds, is the true Altitude.

SECT. II. *Astronomical Problems.*

PROB. I. THE Sun's Place in the *Ecliptick*, and greatest Declination being given, to find his present Declination.

Example 1. The Sun's Place being in 26° 41′ of *Taurus*, and his greatest Declination, or the Angle of the *Ecliptick* with the *Equinoctial*, 23° 30′, to find his present Declination ⸺ *Plate 3. Fig. 1.*

In the Right-angle Spherical Triangle ♈ BC there is given ♈ C the *Hypothenuse* 56° 41′ the Sun's Distance from *Aries*, and the *Angle* B ♈ C, the greatest Declination (by the *9th* Case) to find the opposite Leg BC, the Sun's present Declination.

Therefore the Proportion and Operation is;

As Radius ⸻⸻⸻⸻⸻⸻ Log. 10.0000000
To f. B ♈ C 23° 30′, the Sun's greatest Declinat. ⸺9.6007000
So is f. ♈ C 56 41, the Sun's distance from ♈ ⸺9.9220232
To f. BC ⸺ 19 28, the present Declination N. ⸺19.5227232

Note, That the Sun's distance is always accounted from the nearest of the Equinoctial Points *Aries* or *Libra*. Therefore if the Sun be in the Northern Signs, *Aries, Taurus*, or *Gemini*; or in the *Southern Signs, Capricornus, Aquarius*, or *Pisces*, his Distance is computed from *Aries*.

But if his Place be in the *Northern Signs, Cancer, Leo* or *Virgo*, or in the

the *Southern Signs*, *Libra*, *Scorpio* or *Sagittarius*, 'tis reckoned from *Libra*,

If the *Sun* be in the *Northern Signs*, his Declination is *Northerly*; if in the Southern Signs, *Southerly*.

Example 2. The Sun's Place is 22° 12' of *Aquarius*, his greatest Declination (as before) 23° 30'; to find his present Declination.

The Sun's distance from *Aries* is 37° 48'.　　　*Plate 3. Fig. 1.*

The Operation.　In the Right-angled Triangle ♈ DF.

As Radius ———————————————— Log. 10.0000000

To f. D ♈ F 23° 30, the greatest Declination——————9.6007000

So is f. ♈ F 37 48 the distance from *Aries* ————— 9.7873946

To f. DF— 14 08 the present *Declination* S ———————19.3880946

You may find the Sun's Place by the *Tables* in *Astronomia Carolina.*

PROB. II. The Sun's Place given, to find his Right-Ascension.

Note; the *Sun's* greatest *Declination* is concluded by Mr. *Street*, in his *Caroline Tables*, to be 23° 30', therefore it is always given.

Example 1. The *Sun's* Place is 26° 41' of *Taurus.*

To find the Right-Ascension.　　　　　　　　*Plate 3. Fig. 1*

In the Right-angled Triangle ♈ BC, there is given the *Hypothenuse* ♈ C 56° 41', the Sun's place from *Aries.*

The Angle B ♈ C 23° 30' the greatest *Declination*, (by the *6th* Case) to find the adjacent Leg ♈ B, the Right-Ascension.

The Operation.

As Radius ——————————————————— Log 10.0000000

To t. ♈ C — 56° 41' the *Sun's* Long. from ♈ ———— 10 1822405

So is fc. B ♈ C 23 30, the greatest Declination——————9.9623978

To t. ♈ B — 54 22, the Right-Ascen. from ♈ —— 10.1446383

Example 2. The *Sun's* Place is 22° 12' of *Aquarius.*

To find the Right-Ascension.　　　　　　　*Plate 3. Fig. 1.*

The Operation.

In the Right-angled Triangle ♈ DF.

As Radius ———————————————————— Log 10.0000000

To t. ♈F————37° 48', the *Sun's* Long. from ♈ ——— 9.8896823

So is fc. D ♈F— 23 30, the greatest Declination —— 9.9623978

To t. ♈D — 35 25, the Right Ascension from the ⟩

next Equinoctial Point. ⟩ 19.8520801

This Proportion finds the Right-Ascension from the nearest Equinoctial Point, as you account the Longitude in the Operation. But the Right-Ascension is to be reckoned from *Aries*, according to the Succession of the Signs.

Therefore in this last *Example*, the Complement of 35° 25' to 360, which is 324° 35', is the Right Ascension sought.　　　**PROB.**

PROB. III. The Sun's Declination given, to find his Place or Longitude from *Aries*.

Example 1. The Sun's Declination is 19° 30' North, encreasing. To find his Place.

Plate. 3. Fig. 1.

In the Right-angled Triangle ♈ B C.
There is given the Leg BC 19° 30', the Sun's present Declination.
The opposite Angle B ♈ C 23° 30', the greatest Declination.
And the *Hypothenuse* ♈ C required by (the tenth Case) being the Sun's Distance from *Aries* or *Libra*.

The Operation.

As ſ B♈C ———————23° 30', the greateſt Declinat. Log. —— 9.6007000
To Radius ——————————————————— 10.0000000
So is ſ. BC ‑‑19 30, the preſent Declination——— 9.5234953
To ſ. ♈ C——56 50 ————————————— 9.9227953
  Which ———56 50 reduced into Signs, is 1 Sign 26° 50',
  or ———26 50 of *Taurus.*

If the Sun's Declination be North, and encreasing, this Proportion finds the Sun's Distance from *Aries*; if decreasing, from *Libra* in the Northern Signs.

If the Sun's Declination be South, and encreasing, from *Libra*; if decreasing, from *Aries*, among the Southern Signs.

Example 2. The Sun's Declination is 14° 10' South decreasing. To find the Longitude from *Aries*. Plate 3. Fig. 1.

The Operation In the Triangle ♈ D F.
As ſ. D ♈ F——23° 30', the greateſt Declination ——— 9.6007000
  To Radius—————————————————— 10.0000000
So is ſ. DF—14 10; the preſent Declination ——— 9.3887109
To ſ. ♈ F‑‑37 52, the Diſtance from *Aries* ——— 9.7880109
The Compl. of 37° 52' to 360° is 322° 08'.
Which reduced into Signs, 10 Signs, 22° 08' or 22° 08' of *Aquarius.*

PROB. IV. The Sun's Declination given, to find the Right Ascension.

Example 1. The Sun's Declin. is 19° 30' North encreasing. To find his Right Ascension. Plate 3. Fig. 1.
In the Right-angled Triangle ♈ BC.
There is given the Leg BC 19° 30', the Sun's present Declination.
And the opposite Angle B ♈ C 23° 30', the greateſt Declination.
(by the 1ſt Case) to find the Leg ♈ B, the Right Ascension.

As

As Radius ———— —— —— ——————— 10 0000000
    To tc. B♈C 23° 30′ the greateſt Declination———— 10 3616981
    So is t BC 19 30, the preſent Declination————— 9 5491487
    To ſ ♈B 54 32, the Right Aſcenſion, from ♈ —— 19 9108468

The ſame Caution which was given for the right accounting the Sun's Place in the third *Problem,* ſerves for the Right Aſcenſion, only as that was given in Signs, degrees and minutes, this muſt be given in degrees and minutes from *Aries*

  Example 2. The Sun's Declin. is 14° 10′ South decreaſing.
  To find the Right Aſcenſion.   *Plate 3. Fig. 1.*

The Operation.
In the Right-angled Triangle ♈ D F.

As Radius ——— —— - - - —— Log. 10.0000000
    To tc D♈F —— 23° 30′, the Sun's greateſt Declin —10 3616981
    So is t. DF ——14 10, the preſent Declination ·· -9 4021237
    To ſ. ♈ D———— 35 29, the Right Aſcenſion ——— 19 7638218

The Complement of 35° 29′, to 360° is 324° 31′, the Right Aſcenſion from *Aries.*

PROB V. The Latitude of a Place, and the Sun's Declination being given, to find the Aſcenſional Difference.

Example. In the Latitude of 51° 32′, the Sun's Declination being 20° 12′, to find the Aſcenſional Difference.

In the Right-angled Triangle a b c   *Plate 3. Fig. 2.*

There is given the Leg bc 20° 12′, the Sun's Declination, and the oppoſite Angle b a c 38° 28′, the Compl. of the Latitude, or the Angle between the Equinoctial and Horizon (by the firſt Caſe) to find the other Leg a b, the Aſcenſional Difference.

The Operation.

As Radius ———— —— — — ——————Log. 10.0000000
    To tc. b a c 38° 28′ the Compl. of the Lat. ——— 10.0999135
    So is t. bc 20 12, the Declination ———— 9 5657633
    To ſ. ab—27 35, the Aſcenſional Difference ——— 19.6656768

PROB. VI. To find the Oblique Aſcenſion or Deſcenſion.

Firſt, Find the Aſcenſional Difference by the fifth Problem, and the Right Aſcenſion by the fourth Problem.

Secondly, If the Sun's Declination be Northerly, the Aſcenſional Difference ſubtracted from the Right Aſcenſion leaves the Oblique Aſcenſion; and added to the Right Aſcenſion, gives the Oblique Deſcenſion.

                           Thirdly

Thirdly, If the Sun's Declination be Southerly, the Aſcenſional Difference added to the Right Aſcenſion, gives the Oblique Aſcenſion; and ſubtracted theretrom, leaves the Oblique Deſcenſion.

Note; if the Right Aſcenſion be leſs than the Aſcenſional Difference, add 360° to the Right Aſcenſion, and then ſubtract it therefrom; or if the Sum of the Right Aſcenſion and Aſcenſional Difference, exceeds 360°, reject 360°, the Remainder is the Oblique Aſcenſion or Deſcenſion required.

PROB. VII. To find the Time of the Sun's Riſing or Setting; and conſequently the Length of the Day or Night.

Firſt, Find the Aſcenſional Difference by the fifth Problem, which reduced into Hours and Minutes of Time, by allowing for every 15° one Hour, and for every degree leſs than 15, 4 Min. of Time, and for every 15' one Minute of Time

Secondly, If the Sun's Declination be Northerly, the Aſcenſional Difference added to 6 Hours, gives the Time of Sun ſetting. ·

And ſubtracted therefrom, leaves the Time of Sun riſing.

On the contrary, if the Sun's Declination be Southerly, the Aſcenſional Difference added to ſix Hours, gives the Time of Sun riſing, and ſubtracted therefrom, the Time of Sun ſetting.

Thirdly, If you double the Time of Sun ſetting, it gives you the Length of the Day: And the Time of Sun-riſe doubled, the Length of the Night.

Example 1. In the Latitude 51° 32' North, the Sun's Declination 20° 12' North.

And the Aſcenſional Difference by the 5th Problem is 27° 35', which reduced into Time, makes 1 Hour 50 Minutes.

	Ho. Min.
Therefore the Time of Sun-ſetting is	7 50
The Time of Sun-riſing	4 10
The Length of the Day	15 40
The Length of the Night.	8 20

Example 2. In the Latitude 51° 32', the Declin. 20° 12' South.

And the Aſcenſional Difference is 27° 35', which makes (as before) 1 Hour 50 Minutes of Time.

	Ho. Min.
The Time of Sun-riſing	7 50
The Time of Sun-ſetting	4 10
The Length of the Day	8 20
The Length of the Night.	15 40

N

PROB

PROB. VIII.   The Latitude of a Place, and the Sun's Declination being given, to find the Sun's Amplitude.

Example In the Latitude 51° 32', the Sun's Declination being 20ᵒ
12', to find the Amplitude.

In the Right-angled Triangle abc, there is given the Leg b c, 20°
12', and the oppofite Angle b a c, 38° 28' (by the tenth Cafe) to find
the *Hypotheaufe* a c the Amplitude.   *Plate* 3. *Fig.* 2.

The Operation.

As f. b a c 38° 28' the Complement of the Latitude ———— 9.7938317

  To Radius —— —— —— —— — —— —— 10.0000000

  So is f. b c 20 12, the Declination ——————————— 9.5381943

  To f ac 33 43, the Amplitude ——— ———— —— 9.7443626

If the Sun's Declination be Northerly, the Amplitude is to the Northward of the Eaft or Weft; if the Declination be Southerly, to the
Southward.

PROB IX The Latitude of a Place and the Sun's Declination being given, to find what Time the Sun fhall be due Eaft or Weft.

Example In the Latitude 51° 32' North, the Sun's Declination, 20°,
12' North.

To find what time the Sun fhall be due Eaft or Weft.

In the Right-angled Triangle a d e, there is given the Leg d e, 20°
12', and the oppofite Angle d a e, 51° 32', (by the firft Cafe) to find
the Leg a e, the time from fix.   *Plate* 3 *Fig.* 2.

The Operation.

As Radius———— ————— ———————— Log. 10.0000000

  To tc. d a e 51° 32', the Latitude——————————— 9.9000865

  So is t. d e 20 12, the Declination ——————————— 9.5657633

  To f. a e—16 59, the Diftance from fix ——— —— 19.4658598

· Which being reduced into Time, makes one Hour eight Minutes *fere*,
which added to fix Hours, gives 7 Hours and 8 Minutes, at which time
the Sun comes to the Eaft; and fubtraƈted from fix Hours, leaves four
Hours 52 Minutes, the time of his being in the *Weft Azimuth*, or
Prime Vertical.

PROB X. The Latitude of the Place, and the Sun's Declination being given, to find the Sun's Altitude, being in the Eaft or Weft *Azimuth*, or *Prime Vertical.*

Example. In the Latitude 51 deg. 32 min. North, the Declination
20 degrees 12 minutes North, to find the Sun's Altitude, being due
Eaft or Weft.

In

In the right-angled Triangle a d e, there is given the Leg d e 20° 12' and the oppoſite Angle d a e 51 deg. 32 min. (by the tenth Caſe) to find the *Hypothenuſe* a d.   Plate 3. Fig 2.

The Operation.

As ſ. d a e 51° 32' the Latitude ———————————— 9.8937452

To Radius ———————————————————— 10.0000000

So ſ. d e 20 12, the Declination —————————— 9.5381943

To ſ. a d 26 10, the Alt in the *Prime Vertical* —— —— 9 6444491

PROB. XI. The Latitude of a Place, and the Sun's Declination being given, to find the Sun's Altitude at ſix of the Clock.

Example. In the Latitude 51 deg. 32 min. North, the Declination 23 deg. 30 min. North, to find the Sun's Altitude at ſix.

In the right-angled Triangle a b c, there is given the *Hypothenuſe,* a c 23 deg 30 min. and the Angle b a c, 51 deg. 32 min. (by the ninth Caſe) to find the oppoſite Leg b c.   Plate 3. Fig. 3.

The Operation.

As Radius —————————————— Log. 10 0000000

To ſ. a c, 23° 30' the Declination ——————— 9.6007000

So is ſ. b a c 51 32', the Latitude———————— 9.8937452

To ſ bc 18 11, the Altitude at ſix. ————— 19.4944452

PROB. XII. The Latitude of a Place, and the Sun's Declination, being given, to find the *Azimuth* at ſix.

Example In the Latitude 51 deg. 32 min. North, the Declination 23 deg. 30 min. North, to find the Sun's *Azimuth* at ſix of the Clock.

In the right-angled Triangle a b c, there is given the *Hypothenuſe,* a e, 23 deg. 30 min. and the Angle b a c, 51 deg. 32 min. (by the ſixth Caſe) to find the adjacent Leg a b.   Plate 3. Fig. 3.

The Operation.

As Radius ——————————————— Log. 10.0000000

To t. a c —23° 30' the Declination ———— 9.6383019

So is ſc. b a c 51 32, the Latitude ————— 9.7938317

To t. a b —15 08, the *Azimuth* from the Eaſt—— 19.4321336

PROB. XIII. The Latitude of the Place, the Sun's Altitude and Declination being given, to find his *Azimuth.*

Example 1 In the Latitude 51 deg. 32 min. North, the Declination 23 deg 30 min. North, the Altitude 49 deg. 40 min to find the Sun's *Azimuth*

In the oblique angled Triangle DPZ, there is given the three Sides, ZP 38° 28' the Compl. of the Latit. PD 66° 30' the Compl. of the

            De-

Declination, or the Sun's diftance from the elevated Pole, and DZ 40°
20' the Compl· of the Altitude (by the 11th Cafe) to fin·the Angle
DZP, the *Sun's Azimuth* from the North.   *Plate* 3 *Fig* 3·

The Operation.

The ⎰ ZD	40° 20' Sine	——	—Co Ar 0.1889391
Legs ⎱ ZP	38 28 Sine	——	—Co. Ar 0.206·683
The Bafe DP	66 30½ Sum 72° 39' Sine Log	——	—9.9797764
Sum—145 18	Rem 06 09 Sine	——	9 0299182

Ac 40°010 ½ Sum 72 39 ————————— Sum 19 0409880

    Rem. 06 09 fc——59 44 ——————— ½ Sum 9.7024005

    Which doubled,——59 44 produces

    The *Sun's Azimuth*—119 28 from the North.

Example 2. In the Lat. 51° 32' North, the *Sun's Declin.* is 15° 16'
South, and his *Altit.* 19° 37' , to find his *Azimuth* from the North.

    The Operation   *Plate* 3. *Fig.* 4·

In the Triangle *DPZ*,

    There is given *PZ* 38° 28'.

DZ 70° 23', DP 105° 16', and *DZP* required.

The ⎰ ZD	70° 23' Sine	——	—Co. Ar. 0.0259676
Legs ⎱ ZP	38 28 Sine	——	—Co. Ar. 0.2061685
The Bafe DP	105 16 ½ Sum 107° 03' Sine Log.	——	9.9804803
Sum——214 07	Rem. 01 47 Sine	——	8.4930398

    ½ Sum — 107 03 ——————————— Sum 18 7056562

    Rem. —— 01 47 fc.——76 59 ————— ½ Sum, 9.3528281

    Which doubled, ———76 59 produces

    The *Sun's Azimuth* 153 58 from the North.

Example 3. In the Lat· 51° 32' *South*, the *Sun's Declin.* 23° 30' *South*,
and his *Altitude* 49° 40' : to find his *Azimuth* from the *South*.

    In the Triangle *DPZ*, P muft reprefent the *South* Pole; then there is
given *PZ* 38 deg 28 min. the Compl. of the Latit· *DZ* 40·deg. 20 min.
the Compl. of the *Altitude*; *PD* 66 deg. 30 min. the Compl. of the
Declination, or the *Sun's* diftance from the elevated (or *South*) Pole, to
find *PZD*, the *Sun's Azimuth* from the *South*.   *Plate* 3. *Fig.* 3·

    The Operation is the fame with the firft Example; only as the *Azi-
muth* there was accounted from the *North*, this finds it from the South
part of the Horizon, which is 119 deg. 28 min.

    Example 4. In the Lat. 51 deg. 32 min. South, the *Sun's* Declina-
tion is 15 deg. 16 min. North, and the Altitude 19 deg. 37 min. to find
his *Azimuth* from the South.   *Plate* 3. *Fig.* 4·

In

In the Triangle DPZ, P reprefents the South Pole, as in the former Example.

Then there is given PZ 38 deg. 28 min. DZ 70 deg. 23 min. PD 105 deg. 16 min. and DZP required.

The Operation is the fame with the fecond *Example*, only the *Azimuth* found is to be accounted from the South, which will be found 153 deg. 58 min.

PROB. XIV. The Latitude of the Place, the Sun's Declination and Altitude being given, to find the Hour of the Day.

Example 1 In the Latit 51° 32' North, the Sun's Declin. is 23° 30' North, and his Altitude 49 deg. 40 min. to find the Hour from Noon.

In the Triangle DPZ, there is given PZ 38 deg. 28 min. DZ 40 deg. 20 min DP 66 deg 30 min and DPZ the Hour from Noon required. *Plate* 3. *Fig.* 3.

The Operation.

The ⎰ DP	66°	30' Sine			*Co. Ar.* 0.0376022	
Legs ⎱ PZ	38	28 Sine			*Co. Ar.* 0.2061683	
The Bafe DZ 40	20	½ Sum 72° 39'			Sine Log. 9.9797764	
Sum —— 145	18 Rem.	32	19		Sine	9.7280275
½ Sum —— 72	39				Sum	19.9515744
Rem. —— 32	19	fc. 18	57		½ Sum	9.9757872

The Double of 18 deg. 57 min. is 37 deg. 54 min. which being reduced into time, gives two Hours 31 min. from Noon ; fo that the Hour of the Day is either 2 hours 32 min. Afternoon, or 9 hours 28 min. before Noon.

Example 2. In the Latit. 51° 32' North, the Sun's Declin. 15° 16' South, and his Altit. 19° 37', to find the Hour P. M. Afternoon

In the Triangle DPZ, there is given the three fides, PZ 38° 28', DZ 70° 23', PD 105° 16', and DPZ required. *Plate* 3. *Fig.* 4.

The Operation.

The ⎰ DP	105°	16' Sine			*Co. Ar.* 0.0156029	
Legs ⎱ PZ	38	28 Sine			*Co. Ar.* 0.2061683	
The Bafe DZ 70	23	½ Sum 107° 03'			Log 9.9804803	
Sum —— 214	07 Rem.	36	40			9.7760897
½ Sum —— 107	03					19.9783412
Rem. —— 36	40 Sc.	12	44			9.9891706

Which doubled, produces 25 deg. 28 min. and that reduced into Time, makes 1 hour 42 min. *fere.*

PROB XV. The Latitude of a Place, the Sun's Declination, and the Hour of the day given, to find the Sun's Altitude.

Example

Example. In the Lat. 51 deg. 32 min. North, the Sun's Declination is 23 deg. 30 min. North; the Hour, 1 hour 53 min. Afternoon.

To find the Sun's Altitude.

1 hour 53 min. reduced, makes 28 deg. 15 min.

In the Triangle DPZ, there is given the two Sides, PZ 38 deg. 28 min. DP 66 deg. 30 min. and the contained Angle DPZ 28 deg. 15 min. and the third Side DZ required. (by Cafe the *9th*)

The Operation   *Plate* 3 *Fig* 3.

As Radius ——————————————————————— Log 10 0000000

   To fc DPZ   28° 15′ the contained Angle——— —— 9.9449220

   So is t PZ   38 28 the leffer Side———————— 9 9000865

   To t. ————34 59 a fourth Arch————————19 8450085

      From the other fide PD ——— ———— 66° 30′

      Subtract the fourth Arch ——— ——— — 34 59

      The Remainder is the refidual Arch————31 31

                                              Co. Ar.

As fc.——— — 34° 59′ the fourth Arch ——— ——— 0.0865471

   To fc. ————31 31 the refidual Arch ——— ——— 9 9306883

   So is fc PZ-——38 28 the leffer fide————— 9 8937452

   To fc. DZ- —— 35 27 the fide fought ——————19 9109806

Whofe Compl. 54 deg. 33 min. is the Altitude required.

PROB. XVI. The Latitude of a Place, the Sun's Declination, and the Hour given, to find the Sun's Azimuth.

Example. In the Latitude 51 deg. 32 min. North, the Sun's Delination is 15 deg. 16 min. South, and the Hour, 10 hours 18 min. in the Morning; to find the Sun's, Azimuth.

        The Time from Noon is 1 hour, 42 min.

        Which reduced, is 25 deg. 30 min.

In the Triangle DPZ, there is given the two Sides PZ 38° 28′, PD 105° 16′, and the contained Angle DPZ 25° 30′, to find one of the oppofite Angles, *viz.* PZD, (by Cafe the third.)

                                          Plate 3. *Fig.* 4.

              The Operation.

        PD   105° 16′

        PZ   38 28

        Sum 143 44½ Sum 71° 52′ DPZ   25° 30′

        Diff. 66 48½ Diff. 33 24 the half 12 45

                                           Ce.

Co. Ar.

As f. ½ Z cr³. DP and PZ — 71 52 ——————— 0 0221234
To f. ½ X cr ———————33 24 ————————— 9.7407421
So is tc. ½ DPZ————————1? 45 ——————— 10.6453598
To t. ½ X∠s PDZ and PZD 68 39————————— 10 4082263

Co Ar.

As fc. ½ Z cr¹ DP and PZ——71 52———————— 0.5069194
To fc. ½ X cr¹. —,———— 33 24 ——————— 9.9216073
So is tc. ½ DZP ——————— 12 45 ————— 10 6453598
To t. ½ Z∠s PDZ and PZD 85 10————————— 41.0738865

½ Z∠s   85° 10'
½ X ∠s   68 39
Sum   153 49 DZP required.

Which is the Sun's *Azimuth* from the North.

PROB ×VII. The Latitude of a Place, the Sun's *Altitude* and *Azimuth* given, to find the Hour.

Example. In the Latitude 51 deg. 32 min. the Sun's *Altitude* 49 deg. 40 min. his *Azimuth* 119 deg. 44 min. from the North; to find the Hour Afternoon.

In the Triangle DPZ, there is given the two Sides DZ 40 deg. 20 min. PZ 38 deg. 28 min. and the contained Angle DZP, 119 deg. 44 min. and the oppofite Angle DPZ required. (by Cafe the third)

The Operation.   Plate 3. Fig. 3.

DZ 40 20
PZ 38 28

Sum 78 48 ½ Sum 39° 24' ⌐DZP   119° 44'
Diff. 01 52 ½ Diff. 00 56 ⌐the half 59 52   Co. Ar.

As f. ½ Zcr³. DZ and PZ — ———39° 24' ——— 0.1974106
To f. ½ Xcr³. ————————00 56 ——— 8.2118949
So is tc. ½ DZP ———— — 59 52 ——— 9 7637702
To t. ½ X ∠s PDZ and DPZ ——— 00 51 ——— 18.1730757

Co. Ar.

As fc. ½ Zcr¹. DZ and PZ ——— — 39 24 ——— 0.1119702
To fc. ½ X cr¹ —————————00 56 ———— 9.9999424
So is tc. ½ DZP ── ————— 59 52 ——— 9.7637702
To t. ½ Z ∠s PDZ and DPZ——— 36 54——— 19.8756828

½ Z∠s 36° 54'
½ X∠s 00 51
Sum— 37 45 DPZ required.

Note

Note; DPZ is the greater Angle, becauſe oppoſite to the greater Side DZ; 37° 45′ reduced, makes the Time 2 hours 31 min. Afternoon.

PROB. XVIII. The Latitude and Longitude of a fixed Star being given, to find the *Right Aſcenſion* and *Declination*.

Example The Longitude of *Caſtor* is 15° 33′ of *Cancer*, and his Latitude 10° 02′ North; to find his *Right Aſcenſion* and *Declination*

In the Oblique Triangle DIP, there is given two Sides, IP 23 deg. 30 min. the Diſtance between the Pole of the *Equinoctial* and the Pole of the *Ecliptick*, ID 79 deg 58 min. the Complement of the Latitude; and the contained Angle DIP 15 deg. 33 min the Longitude from *Cancer*: To find one of the oppoſite Angles DPI, the Complement to 180° of the *Right Aſcenſion* from *Cancer*, and the third Side DP, the Complement of Declination.   *Plate* 3. *Fig* 5.

The Operation. For the *Right Aſcenſion.*

ID	79° 58′				
IP	23 30				
Sum	103 28 ½	Sum 51° 44′ ½	DIP	15° 33′	
Diff.	56 28 ½	Diff. 28 14 5 ½	DIP	07 46	

                                                Co. Ar.

As ſ. ½ Zcr². ID and IP ———— 51 44 ———— 0.1050547
To ſ. ½ X cr². ——— 28 14 ——— .9.6749194
So is tc. ½ DIP ——— 07 46 ——— 10.8652165
To t. ½ X ∠s DPI and IDP ——— 77 15 ——— 10.6451906

                                                Co. Ar.

As ſc. ½ Zcr². ID and IP ——— 51 44 ——— 0.2080832
To ſc ½ X cr². ——— 28 14 ——— 9.9449899
So is tc. ½ DIP ——— 07 46 ——— 10.8652165
To t. ½ Z ∠s DPI and IDP 84 31 ——— 11.0182896

½ Z ∠s 84° 31′
½ X ∠s 77 15
Sum 161 46 DPI

Whoſe Complement to 180 deg. is 18 deg. 14 min the *Right Aſcenſion from Cancer*; the *Right Aſcenſion* of *Cancer* is 90 deg. and therefore the *Right Aſcenſion* from *Aries* is 108 deg. 14 min.

For the *Declination.*   Co. Ar.

As ſ. DPI —— 161° 46′ the Compl. of the Right Aſcen. —— 0.5046117
To ſ DI — 79 58 the Complement of the Latitude — 9.9933068
So is ſ. DIP — 15 33 the Longitude from *Cancer* ——— 9.4282631
To ſ. DP — 57 32 the Complement of the Declin. —— 19.9261816
                                             Whoſe

Whofe Compl. 32 deg 28 min. is the *Declination* Northerly.

PROB. XIX. The Right Afcenfion and Declination of a fixed Star
being given, to find the Longitude and Latitude thereof.

· *Example.* The Right Afcenfion of *Caftor* is 18° 15′, and his Declination 32° 32′ North; to find his Longitude and Latitude.

In the Triangle IDP, there is given the two Sides, IP 23° 30′; PD
57° 28′, and the contained Angle DPI 161° 45′, to find the oppofite
Angle DIP, and the third Side DI. (by Cafe the third)

Plate 3. *Fig* 5.

The Operation. To find the Longitude.

PD   57° 28′
IP   23 30
Sum   80 58½ Sum 40° 29′ ⎰ DPI   161° 45′
Diff 33 58½ Diff. 16 59 ⎱½ DPI   80 52

	°	′	Co. Ar.
As f. ½ Zcr². PD and IP	40	29	0.1876035
To f. ½ X cr²	16	59	9.4655219
So is tc. ½ DPI	80	52	9.2062072
To t. ½ X∠s DIP and IPD	04	08	18.8593326

	°	′	Co. Ar.
As fc. ½ Zcr². PD and IP	40	29	0.1188466
To fc. ½ X cr²	16	59	9.9806349
So is tc. ½ DPI	80	52	9.2062072
To t. ½ Z∠s DIP and IDP	11	25	19.3056887

½ Z∠s 11° 25′
½ X∠s 04 08
Sum—15 33 DIP the Longitude from *Cancer.*

To find the Latitude.   Co. Ar.

As f. DIP — 15° 33′ the Longitude from *Cancer*	0.5717369
To f. DP—57 28 the Complement of Declination	9.925868⅟
So is f. DPI 161 45 the Compl. of the Right Afcenfion	9.4957716
To f. DI—80 01 the Complement of Latitude	19.9933766

PROB. XX. The *Diftance* of a *Planet, Comet,* or *New-Star,* from two
known fixed Stars being given, to find the unknown *Star's* Longitude
and Latitude

Example. The unknown *Star's* Diftance from the *Swan's Beak* is 49°
05′ and from *Perfeus's Side* 88 deg. 57 min. to find the Longitude and
Latitude thereof.

Long. ⎰ Of the *Swan's Beak,* ♑ 26° 39′ ⎱ Lat. ⎰49° 02′ N.
      ⎱ Of *Perfeus's Side,* ♉ 27 12 ⎰   ⎱30 05 N.

O   Here

Here IK Reprefents the Poles of the *Ecliptick,* A the *Swan's Beak,* D *Perfeus's Side,* B the unknown *Star;* then,

1. In the Triangle ADI there is given two Sides, AI 40 deg. 58 min. the Complement Latitude of the *Swan's Beak,* DI 59 deg 55 min. the Complement Latitude of *Perfeus's Side,* the contained Angle AID 120 deg 33 min the Difference of Longitude between the two Stars; and the Angle DAI, and the Side AD required   *Plate 3 . Fig 6. .*

The Operation.

		o '		Co Ar.
As f ½ Zcr. AI and DI	—	50 26	—	0 1130110
To f ½ X cr.	—	09 28	—	9 2160967
So is tc. ½ ∠ AID	—	60 16	—	9 7567587
To t. ½ X∠s DAI and ADI	c6 56	—		19 0858664

		o '		Co Ar.
As fc. ½ Zcr AI and DI	—	50 26	—	0.1958772
To fc. ½ X cr	—	09 28	—	9 9940449
So is tc ½ AID	—	60 16	—	9 7567587
To t. ½ Z ∠s DAI and ADI	—	41 29	—	19 9466808

The Angle DAI is 48 25

			Co. Ar.
As f. DAI	—	48 25	0 1261035
To f. DI	—	59 55	9.9371653
So is f AID	—	120 33	9 9350969
To f. AD	—	85 02	19.9983657

2. In the Triangle ADB there is given three Sides, AD 85 deg 02 min. the Diftance between two known Stars, AB 49 deg. 05 min the unknown Stars Diftance from the *Swan's Beak,* BD 88 deg. 57 min the Diftance from *Perfeus's Side;* and the Angle DAB required

The Operation.   *Plate 3 Fig. 6.*

AD	85°	02' Sine	Co Ar. 0 0016337
AB	49	05 Sine	Co. Ar. 0 1216719
BD	88	57 ½ Sum 111° 32' Sine	9 9685783
Sum	223	04 Rem. 22 35 Sine	9 5843615
½ Sum	111	32	Sum 19 6762454
Rem.	22	35 Sc. 46 28 ½ Sum	9 8381227

Which being doubled, makes 92° 56', the Angle DAB required.

Which being added to the Angle DAI, the Sum is the Angle BAI 141 deg. 21 min

3. In the Triangle ABI there is given, the two Sides, AI 40 deg. 58 min. AB 49 deg. 05 min. the contained Angle BAI, 141 deg. 21 min. and

and the Angle AIB, the difference of Longitude between the unknown Star, and the *Swan's Beak*, and the Side BI, the Compl. of the unknown Star's Latitude required.　　　　　　　　　　*Plate 3. Fig. 6.*

The Operation.

		°	′	Co. Ar.
As f. ½ Zcrᵃ. AI and AB	——	45	01	—— 0.1503887
To f. ½ Xcrᵃ.	——	04	03	—— 8.8489707
So is tc. ½ BAI	——	70	40	—— 9.5451193
To t. ½ X∠s ABI and AIB	——	02	00	—— 18.5441787

　　　　　　　　　　　　　　　　　　　　　　Co. Ar.

		°	′	Co. Ar.
As fc. ½Zcrᵃ. AI and AB	——	45	01	—— 0.1506414
To fc. ½ X crᵃ.	——	04	03	—— 9.9989141
So is tc. ½ BAI	——	70	40	—— 9.5451193
To t ½ Z ∠s ABI and AIB	——	26	20	—— 19.6946748

The Angle AIB is 28 deg 20 min. which added to the Longitude of the *Swan's Beak*, ♑ 26 deg. 39 min makes the unknown Star's Longitude to be ♒ 24 deg 59 min.　　　　　　　　　　*Co. Ar.*

		°	′	Co. Ar.
As f. AIB	——	28°	20′	—— 0.3236719
To f AB	——	49	05	—— 9.8783281
So is t. BAI	——	141	21	—— 9.7955752
To f BI	——	83	57	—— 19.9975751

Whose Complement to 90° that is 6° 3′ is the unknown Star's Latitude Northerly.

PROB XXI. The *Meridian Altitude* of an unknown Star or Planet, and the Diftance from a known fixed Star being given; to find the unknown Star's Latitude and Longitude.

Example In the Latitude 51 deg. 32 min. North, the Meridian Altitude of an unknown Star is 30 deg. 36 min. and his Diftance from the Star in *Cepheus's Girdle* is 84 degeees 32 minutes, to find his Longitude and Latitude:

The Meridian Altitude of the Star being given, his Declination is also given.

For the Meridian Altitude fubtracted from the Complement of the Latitude 38° 28′, there remains 7° 52′, the Declination South.

First, Therefore in the Triangle AOP, there is given the three Sides OP, 20 deg. 52 min the known Star's Diftance from the *North Pole,* AP 97 deg. 52 min. the unknown Star's Diftance therefrom, AO 84 deg. 32 min. the Diftance between the two Stars, and the Angle APO required, being the Difference of Right-Afcenfion between the two Star's. (by Cafe the 11*th.*)　　　　　　*Plate 4. Fig. 7.*

　　　　　　　　　　　　　　　　　　　　　　　　　The

The Operation.

OP	20° 52' Sine		Co Ar.	0.4483129
AP	97 52 Sine		Co. Ar.	0.0041164
½ Sum	101 38 Sine			9.9909859
Rem.	17 06			9.4684069

            Sum, 19.9118221

Sc   25 23   ½ Sum—9.9559110

Which doubled is 50 deg 46 min the Angle APO

The *Right Aſcenſion* of *Cepheus*'s Girdle is 321° 02', to which adding 50° 46' (the unknown Star being to the Eaſtward of the known Star) produceth the *Right Aſcenſion* of the unknown Star 11° 48'

Secondly, Then having the unknown Star's *Right Aſcenſion* and *Declination*, you may find his Longitude and Latitude by *Prob* 19

PROB. XXII Having the Latit. of the Place, the Sun's *Right Aſcenſion,* and the Altitude of a known fixed Star, to find the Hour of the Night.

Example In the Latitude 51° 32', the Sun's *Right Aſcenſion* being 228° 45', and the *Altitude* of *Aldebaran* 38° 58', to the Eaſtward of the Meridian; to find the Hour of the Night.

The *Right Aſcenſion* of *Aldebaran* is 64 deg. 10 min and his *Declination* 15 deg. 46 min.

In the Triangle APZ, there is given the three ſides PZ 38° 28', the Compl of the Latitude; AZ 51° 02', the Compl. of the Star's *Altitude*; AP 74° 14', the Compl. of his Declination, to find the *Angle* APZ, the Difference of *Right Aſcenſion* between the *Medium Cœli* and *Aldebaran.*   Plate 4. Fig 8.

The Operation.

AP	Sine 74° 14'		Co. Ar	0.0166551
PZ	Sine 38 28		Co. Ar.	0.2061683
½ Sum,	Sine 81 52			9.9956095
Rem.	Sine 30 50			9.7097299

            Sum, 19.9281628

Sc. 22 59   9.9640814

Which doubled, produces 45° 58',

This ſubtracted from the Right Aſcenſion of *Aldebaran*, leaves 18° 12'. the Right Aſcenſion of the *Mid-Heaven* Add 360 deg. to 18 deg. 12 min. and from the Sum Subtract the Sun's Right Aſcenſion 228 deg. 45 min. the Remainder 149 deg. 27 min. reduced into Time, makes 9 Hours, 57 Minutes, 48 Seconds, the Hour of the Night ſought.

PROB. XXIII. Two unequal Altitudes of the Sun taken in one Day, with the Time between the Obſervations, and the Sun's Declination

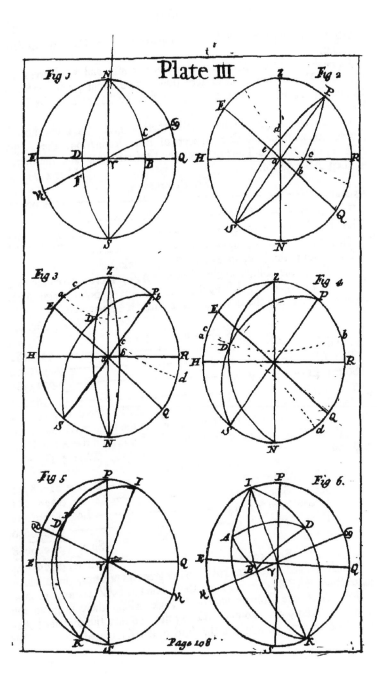

Plate III

Fig 1   Fig 2

Fig 3   Fig 4

Fig 5   Fig 6.

nation, being given; to find the Latitude of the Place of Obfervation.

Example The two Altitudes are 43 deg 6 min. and 56 degrees 34
min. the Time between the Obfervations is two Hours, and the Sun's
Declination 20 deg. 14 min. North; to find the Latitude of the Place
Northerly

In the Right angled Triangle ABP, there is given the Hypothenuse
AP 69 deg 46 min. the Complement of the Declination, the Angle
APB 15 deg. half the Time between the Obfervations, and the oppo-
fite Leg AB required.   *Plate 4 Fig 9.*

The Operation.

As Radius		10 0000000
To f. APB —— 15° 00'		10 0000000
So is f. AP —— 69 46		9 4129962
To f AB —— 14 03		9 9723380
		19 3853342

Which being doubled, gives AE 28 deg. 6 min.
Secondly, In the oblique angled Triangle APE, there is given the two
Sides AE 28 deg. 6 min EP 69 deg. 46 min. the oppofite Angle APE
30 deg 00 min. and the other oppofite Angle EAP required.

Plate 4. Fig. 9.
The Operation.

As f. AE —— 28° 06'		Co. Ar.
To f APE —— 30 00		0.326968 L
So is f. EP —— 69 46		9.6989700
To f EAP —— 84 54		9 9723380
		19.9982761

Thirdly, In the Oblique-angled Triangle AZE, there is given the
three Sides AZ 33° 26', the Complement of the greater Altitude, EZ
46° 54', the Complement of the lefler AE 28° 06', and the Angle EAZ
required.

Plate 4. Fig. 9.
The Operation.

AZ Sine 33° 26'		Co. Ar. 02588750
AE Sine 28 06		Co. Ar. 0.3269681
½ Sine Sum 54 13		Log. 9.9091461
Rem. Sine 07 19		9.1050096
	Sum,	19.5999988
	half Sum;	9.7999994

Sc. 50 52
Which doubled, produces EAZ 101 degrees 44 minutes, from which
fubtracting EAP 84 deg 54 min. there remains PAZ 16 deg. 50 min.
Fourthly, In the Oblique-angled Triangle APZ, there is given the
two Sides AP 69 deg 46 min. AZ 33 deg. 26 min. the contained Angle PAZ 16 deg. 50 min. and the third Side PZ required.   *The.*

As Radius ——————————————————————— 10.0000000

　To fc. PAZ ——————— 16° 15' —————————— 9.9822938

　So is t. AZ——————— 33　26 ——————————— 9.8196844

　To t. of a fourth Arch—— 32　22 ——————————— 19.8019782

　　　　　　　　　　°　　　'　　　　　　　　　Co. Ar.

As fc. of the fourth Arch——32　22 ——————————— 0.0733286

　To fc. of the Refidual——37　24 ——————————— 9.9000472

　So is fc. AZ —— — —— 33　26——————————— 9.9214406

　To fc PZ———————38　17 ——————————— 19.8948164

Whofe Complement ———51　43 is the Latitude Northerly.

PROB. XXIV. Two unequal Altitudes of the Sun, and the Difference of their correfpondent *Azimuths* taken in one Day, and the Sun's Declination being given, to find the Lat. of the Place of Obfervation.

Example. The firft *Altitude* is 43 deg. 6 min. and the fecond *Altitude* 56 deg. 34 min the Difference of *Azimuths* 39 Degrees 16 Minutes, and the Sun's Declination is 20 Degrees 14 Minutes North; to find the Latitude of the Place Northerly

Firft, In the Oblique-angled Triangle AEZ, there is given the two Sides AZ 33 Degrees 26 Minutes, EZ 46 Degrees 54 Minutes, the contained *Angle* AZE 39 degrees 16 minutes, the Difference of the *Azimuths*; and the *Angle* EAZ, and the third Side AE required

　　　　　　　　　　°　　　'　　　　　　　　　Co. Ar.

As f. ½ Z cra. AZ and EZ —— 40　10 ——————— 0.1904314

　To f. ½ X cra. ————06　44 ——————— 9.0691074

　So is tc. ½ AZE———————19　38 ——————— 10.4476486

　To t. ½ X∠s EAZ and AEZ 27　00————————— 19.7071874

　　　　　　　　　　°　　　'　　　　　　　　　Co. Ar.

As fc. ½ X cra. AZ and EZ——40　10 ——————— 0.1168092

　To fc. ½ X cra. ————— 06　44 ——————— 9.9969941

　So is tc. ½ AZE ——————19　38 ——————— 10.4476486

　To t. ½ Z∠s EAZ and AEZ 74　39 ————————— 10.5614519

　　　　　　The *Angle* EAZ 101° 39'.　　　　Co. Ar.

As f. EAZ——— ——————101　39 ——————— -0.0090412

　To f. EZ ——————— 46　54 ——————— 9.8634194

　So is f. AZE ——— ——39　16——————— 9.8013561

　To f. AE—— ———— 28　09 ——————— 19.6738167

Secondly, In the Right-angled Triangle ABP, there is given the *Hypothenufe* AP 69 deg. 46 min. the Leg AB 14 deg. 04 min. the half of AE, and the adjacent *Angle* BAP required.　　　　　*The*

The Operation.

As Radius ———————————————— 10.0000000
To tc. AP 69° 46' ——————————— 9.5665424
So is t. BA 14 04——————————— 9.3989191
To ſc BAP 84 42 —————————— 18.9654615

From the *Angle* EAZ 101 deg. 39 min ſubtract the *Angle* EAP 84 deg. 42 min. there remains the *Angle* PAZ, 16 deg. 57 min.

Thirdly, In the Oblique-angled Triangle PAZ, there is given the two Sides AP 69° 46'. AZ 33° 26', the contained *Angle* PAZ 16° 57', and the third Side PZ required. *Plate 4. Fig 9.*

The Operation.

As Radius ———————————————— 10.0000000
To ſc. PAZ ———16° 57' —————————— 9.9807120
So is t. AZ ——————— 33 26 ——————— 9.8196844
To t. of a fourth Arch—32 16 —————— 19.8003964

Co. Ar.

As ſc of the fourth Arch——— 32° 16'———— 0.0728491
To ſc. of the Reſidual ——— 37 30 ——— 9.8994667
So is ſc AZ- ———————— 33 26——— 9.9214406
To ſc. PZ- ——————— 38 28½——— 19.8937564
Whoſe Compl. ——————— 51 32 is the Latitude North.

S E C T. III. *Containing the general Aſtronomical Theories.*

The Ptolomaick Syſtem.

THE *Ptolomaick Syſtem* is that which was by *Ptolomy* invented, and ſuppoſeth the Earth to be fixed as the Center of the World, and that all the Celeſtial Bodies move round the ſame in their Diurnal and Annual Revolutions.

The World is ſuppoſed to be divided principally into two parts, Elementary and Celeſtial.

The Elementary admits of four Diviſions.

The firſt is the *Earth.*

The ſecond is the *Water* ; both which make one entire Body or Globe whereon we dwell.

The third is the *Air*, encompaſſing the *Earth*

And the fourth is *Fire*, which according to the Opinion of ancient Philoſophers, is contained in that ſpace between the *Air* and the Sphere of the Moon ; as you may ſee in the following Figure.

The

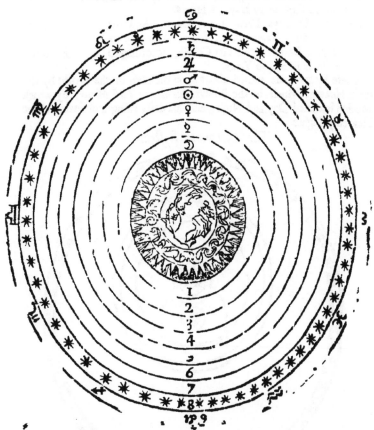

These Four Elements are subject to a continual Change and Alteration one into another, according to the Proverb, *Omnia Sublunaria mutabilia.*

The Cœlestial Part is that which is without these Elementary Parts, void of all Changes, and is by the ancient *Astronomers* divided into ten Parts or Heavens.

The first of which, next to the Region of Fire, is the Heaven, or Orb of the *Moon.*

The second of *Mercury.* The third of *Venus.* The fourth of the *Sun.* The fifth of *Mars.* The sixth of *Jupiter.* The seventh of *Saturn.* The eighth of the *Fixed Stars.* The ninth is called the *Chriftalline Heaven.* The tenth the *Primum Mobile.*   The

The Magnitude of thefe Heavens is known by the Courfes which thofe great Bodies within them make round the Poles of the *Zodiack.*

The *Moon* runneth through the Heavens by her own natural Courfe from *Weft* to *Eaft*, in 27 Days, 8 Hours.

Mercury in 88 Days. *Venus* in 225 Days. And the *Sun* in a Year. *Mars* in 2 Years. *Jupiter* in 12 Years. *Saturn* in 30 Years.

The *Eighth Heaven* perfects its Courfe, according to the Affirmation of *Tycho Brahe* in 25400 Years.

Thefe Heavens are turned about upon the *Axis* of the World by the tenth Heaven, which is the *Primum Mobile*, or *Firft Mover*, by which Motion is caufed Day and Night, and the daily rifing and fetting of the Heavenly Lights

The Tychonean Syftem.

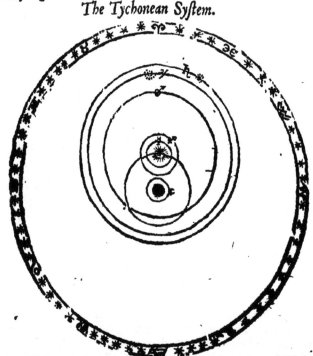

This *Hypothefis* derives its Name from the Author thereof, *Tycho Brahe*, a Nobleman of *Denmark*, the moft famous *Aftronomical* Obfervator in the World in his Days ; who by his own Obfervations did rectify

tify

tify the Places of moſt of the *Fixed Stars*, which appeared in that *Hor.zou* wherein he lived. This famous Man, according to his preſent Apprehenſion, framed this *Hypotheſis* of the Heavenly Motions, wherein he ſuppoſeth, that *Venus, Mercury, Mars, Jupiter, Saturn,* in their Motion reſpect the *Sun* as their Center ; and the *Sun* and *Moon* the *Earth* : and that *Saturn* in *Oppoſition* to the *Sun,* is nearer to the *Earth* than *Venus* in *Apogeon* ; and that *Mars* in *Oppoſition* is nearer the *Earth* than the *Sun* it ſelf ; as may appear in the ſaid *Hypotheſis.*

The Copernican Syſtem.

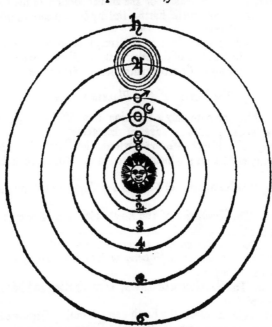

This *Hypotheſis* was firſt invented by *Pythagoras,* and revived by *Copernicus* a famous *Aſtronomer* of *Germany,* who lived in the Year 1500, who ſuppoſes,

1. That the Sun is placed in the midſt of the World, in or about the Centre of the Sphere of the Fixed Stars, and hath no Circular Motion but Central only.

2. The

2: The primary Planets are each of them in their proper Syftems moved about the Sun, and accomplifh their Periodical Revolutions moft exactly in their determinate and appointed Times.

3. That the *Earth* is one of the Planets, and with her annual Motion about the *Sun* defcribeth her Orb in the middle between the Orbs of *Mars* and *Venus*.

4. That the fecundary Planets are ordinarily moved about the primary Planets refpecting their Bodies for their common Nodes and Centers.

5. That the fecundary Planet, the *Moon* is moved about the Earth as her Center, where, by reafon of the annual Motion of the Earth, fhe hath not only relation to the Earth, but by confequence to the Sun, as have the other Planets.

6. That as this primary Planet, the Earth, is invironed with the Sphere of the *Moon*; fo are fome of the other primary Planets, who have in like manner their Moons or Concomitants encompaffing them.

The Motion of the Planetary Syftem.

Firft, The *Sun* hath only a Rotation from *Weft* to *Eaft*, upon his own *Axis*, in the fpace of 26 days, or thereabouts.

Secondly, The Planet *Mercury* performs his Revolution about the Sun in eighty eight days; which is noted in the Scheme with the Figure 1 ☿.

Thirdly, The Revolution of *Venus* in 225 days, noted by the Figure 2 ♀.

Fourthly, The Revolution of the *Earth* with the *Moon* in one Year; noted by the Circle 3 ⊕.

Fifthly, The Revolution of *Mars* in two Years; noted by 4 ♂.

Sixthly, The Revolution of *Jupiter*, with his four Companions, in 12 Years; noted with 5 ♃.

Seventhly, The Revolution of *Saturn*, with his Ring and Moon, in 30 Years; noted 6 ♄.

The *Moon* circumvolveth the Earth every Month; *Jupiter's* four Attendants him, in time correfponding their Diftance from him.

The firft, and next him, in one day 18 hours.

The fecond next without that, in 3 days 13 hours.

The third in 7 days 4 hours.

And the fourth and outmoft, in 16 days 8 hours.

Saturn's Moon moves about him in 16 days; and all from *Weft* to *Eaft*, according to their Revolutions about the Sun.

Saturn, Jupiter, Mars, the *Earth, Venus,* and *Mercury* (whofe Revolutions refpect the *Sun* only) are call'd *Primary Planets*

The reft (that move again about *Saturn, Jupiter,* and the *Earth,*) are *Secondary Planets*

The *Earth* hath a Revolution upon her *Equinoctial* Poles in 24 hours, from *Weft* to *Eaft.*

The *Secondary Planets* are all of them much lefs in Magnitude than their *Primary,* and all the *Planets* together much lefs than the *Sun,* from whom they all receive their Light, Virtue, and principal Power of Motion.

Far without the *Planetary Syftem* are placed all the *Fixed Stars,* in feveral Diftances, but all unto us incommenfurable. The *Parallax* of the *Earth's* Orb being infenfible in any of their Places.

A Defcription of the Golden Number, Cycle *of the* Sun, Roman Indiction, Epact, *and* Leap-Year.

THE *Golden Number,* or *Prime,* is a Circular Revolution of 19 Years, in which Term of Years it hath been Anciently fuppofed, that the *Sun* and *Moon* do make all the variety of Afpects one to another.

The *Cycle* of the *Sun* maketh its Revolution in 28 Years, becaufe in that time all the variety of the *Dominical Letters* and *Leap-Years* are expired, and the 29th Year the Cycle doth begin again, which Number is to find out the *Dominical Letter* for any Year paft, prefent or to come.

The *Roman Indiction* confifteth of 15 Years, and is fet down in the Charters and Writings of the *Protonotaries* of the Pope of *Rome*; for once in 15 Years the Nations were to pay Tribute to the *Romans.*

The *Epact* is a Number never exceeding 30 days, it is the 11 days and fix hours, which added to the *Lunar Year,* being 354 days, do make it equal to the *Solar Year,* which is 365 days.

The *Leap-Year* is every 4th Year, which hath one day more in it than a common Year, this day is made up in 4 Years, by the odd 6 hours that are over and above 365 days, which day is added after the 24th of *February.* So that in the Leap-Year *February* hath 29 days. And here note, that the *Prime* and *Dominical-Letters,* and the *Cycle of the Sun,* change the firft of *January*; and the *Epact* the firft of *March*; and the *Roman Indiction* the firft of *September.*

Memorial Verfes on the Ecclefiaftical and Civil Kalendar, &c.

To know if it be Leap-year.

Divide the Year by 4, What's left fhall be,
For Leap-Year 0, for paft, 1, 2, or 3.

Here

H E R E you may omit the Hundreds of the Year of our Lord, and divide the Refidue by 4.

For Example.

Anno 1725, omitting the Hundreds, I divide the Refidue, which is 25, by 4, and there remains 1, which fhews it is the firft after *Leap-Year.*

To find the Dominical-Letter.

Divide the Year its 4th, *and* 4 *by* 7 ;
What's left fubtract from 7, the Letter's given.
A 1. B 2. C 3. D 4. E 5. F 6. G 7.

Example.

Of the Year of Chrift—————————	1725
The 4th part (omitting Fraction) is—————	431
To both which I add the Number——————	4
The Sum is ———————————————	2160

Which divided by 7, there is left 4, which fubtracted from 7, there refts 3 ; which fhews the Dominical Letter, for the Year 1725 is the 3d in order of the Alphabet, that is C.

But the Leap-Year hath two Dominical Letters ; the latter found by this Rule ferveth from St. *Matthias's* day to the Years end, and for finding *Eafter* , the former (next following in order from A to G, and beginning again at A) ferveth from *New-Year's Day* unto St. *Matthias.*

For the Golden Number, Cycle of the Sun, and Indiction.

When 1, 9, 3, *to 'th Year hath added been,*
Divide by 19, 28, 15.

Example.

To 1725 I add 1, the Sum 1726 I divide by 19, and there remains 16, which is the Golden Number for the Year 1725.

Again, to 1725 I add 9, and the Sum 1734 I divide by 28, the Refidue 26 is the Cycle of the Sun *Anno* 1725.

Laftly, To 1725, I add 3 the Sum 1728 divided by 15, the Remainder 3, which fhews it is the third Year of the Indiction for the Year 1725.

The Prime, or Golden Number being given, to find the Epact.

Divide by 3, for each one left add 10 ;
30 reject. the Prime makes Epact then.

Example.

Anno 1725, the Golden Number 16, I divide by 3, and there is left 1 : therefore ten times 1, which is 10, added to 16, the Sum is 26, the

the Epact for the Year 1725, which Sum had it exceeded 30, 30 must have been taken from it.

By the nineteen Epacts, to find the Day of Easter-Limit from the beginning of March *inclusively.*
>	The Epacts take from 47 ; but two,
>	The greatest take from 77 ; 'twill do.
>			*Example*

Anno 1725. The Epact being 26, I subtract it from 47, and the Residue 21 is *Easter-Limit, Anno* 1725, that is *March* 21st, reckoned from the beginning of *March* inclusively.

But when the Epact is 28 or 29, it must be subtracted from 77, that so the Limit may remain. And the next following Sunday after the Limit is always Easter-Day.

Easter Limit, and the Dominical Letter being given, to find Easter-Day.

>	*The Letter more by 4 from Limit take ;*
>	*What's left from nearest Sevens, shall Easter make.*

Or thus ; Take the Number of the given Letter more by 4 from the given Limit, and the Residue from the nearest greater Sum of Sevens ; the last Remainder added to the Limit ; the Sum, or its Excess above 31, is Easter-Day in *March* or *April*.

Example. Anno 1725, the Dominical Letter is C, which is the third Letter in order, which more by 4 is 7 ; which take from the Limit 21, the Residue is 14 ; this take from the nearest greater Sum of Sevens, which is 21, and there remains 7, which being added to the Limit 21, the Sum 28, therefore the 28th of *March* is Easter-Day, 1725.

For the Days of the Month on which the Sun entreth the twelve Signs.
>	*Twice 9, twice 10, four 12's 11 ;*
>	*Then 10, then 9, then 8, or 7:*
>			Anno 1725 ☉ in

♈	♉	♊	♋	♌	♍	♎	♏	♐	♑	♒	♓
Mar.	Apr.	May	June	July	Aug.	Sep.	Oct.	Nov.	Dec.	Jan.	Feb.
9.	9.	10.	10.	12.	12.	12.	12.	11.	10.	9.	8.

For the Degree of the Sun's Place on any Day.

From the Day of the Month on which the Sun's Place is required, if you may, or else from the Sum of that and 30, subtract the Day of his Entrance into the Sign of that Month, the Remainder will be the Degree of his Place in that or the next preceeding Sign.

For the Age of the Moon, or Day of her Change.

> *Janus* 0, 2, 1, 2, 3, 4, 5, 6;
> 8, 8, 10, 10, *these to the Epact fix* :
> *The Sum* ('bate 30) *to the Month Day add,*
> *Or take from* 30, *Age or Change is had.*

Or thus, add to the Epact in

Jan.	Feb.	Mar.	Apr.	May,	Jun.	Jul.	Aug.	Sept.	Oct.	Nov.	Dec.
0.	2.	1.	2.	3.	4.	5.	6.	8	8.	10.	10.

The Sum, if it be less than 30, or else the Excess above 30, added to the Day of the given Month (rejecting 30 if need be) gives the Age of the Moon that Day; but subtracted from 30, leaves the Day of the Change in or from the beginning of that Month.

For the Day of the Full-Moon, add or subtract 15, to or from the Day of the Change.   *Example.*

1. For the Age of the Moon, *Anno* 1725, *May* 29; the Number for the Month 3, added to the Epact 26, makes 29; which added to 29 (rejecting 30 from the Sum) gives 28 the Age of the Moon required.

2. For the Day of the Change, (or *New-Moon*) in *May* 1725, the Epact 26, with the Month 3, makes 29, as before; which subtracted from 30, the Residue 1, is the Day of the New-Moon, in *May* 1725.

3. To which 15 being added, gives 18, the Day of Full-moon in *May* 1725.

To find the Day of the New Moon, and the Entrance of the Sun into the Signs, for Time past, or to come.

> 312, 131————————————————
> *Past, add; to come, subtract for Moon and Sun.*

Or thus, for every 312 Years past, add 1 Day to the time of the New-moon found above; for 312 Years to come, subtract 1 Day.

Likewise for 131 Years past, a Day is to be added to the former account of the Sun's Entrance; and for 131 Years to come, subtracted.

To find the Distance of the Sun from the Nodes of the Moon perpe-
tually in all Lunations; Remember,
Year 17 hundred, Node, Sign 4, Degree
27, 3, 800, 43.

1 Take the Interval between the given Time, and 1700 compleat in Years and Days, allowing 12 Months to the Year, and 30 Days to a Month, and the Account will suffice for this Work.

2 Multiply the Years of the Interval by 43, and divide the Product by 800, the Residue multiply by 9, then take the half of this Product, and distinguish the last Figure from the rest by a Point. So have you the Degrees, and 10th Part of a Degree, answerable to the Years of Interval Also multiply the Days of the Interval by 43, and divide by 800; this Quotient shews the Degrees, and the Remainder divided by 80, the 10th part of a Degree of the Motion for the Day of Interval Then collect the former and latter Degrees and Tenths into one Sum, and reduce it into Signs, Degrees, and Tenths.

3. For times afore 1700 compleat, add the Signs, Degrees and Tenths thus found, to 4^s, 27°, 3 Tenths; but for Time after 1700 compleat, subtract them from 4^s 27°, 3 Tenths, and the Sum or Remainder shall be for the place of ☊, adding 1 Degree for the Tenths, if they exceed 5, else rejecting them

Always in Additions omit Cycles (to wit, 12^s or 360°) but in Subtractions add one Cycle, if need be, to the Number from which you are to subtract.

Next by the common Rule for 1700, without any Correction for time past or to come, find the Sign and Degree of the Sun's Place and subtract the last found Place of ☊ from it; the Residue is the Distance of ☉ from ☊ required.

The Limits of Eclipses of the Sun and Moon, in Degrees from
☊ *or* ☋.

Within 16 *the Sun, and* 10 *the Moon,*
Suffers Eclipse, above 18, 12, *none.*

To find the Length of Days and Nights in the Latitude
52 deg. *for ever.*
To 15, 1; 1, 16; 2, 6, 3;
1, 2, 3, 4 *hours;* 4 *and half agree*

*

T☉

To the given Diſtances of the Sun from the next Equinoctial Point, the anſwerable Hours are theſe ; to 15°, 1 Hour : to 1 Sign 2 Hours ; to 1 Sign 16°, 3 Hours ; to 2 Signs 6°, 4 Hours ; and to 3 Signs, 4 Hours and a half ; which Hours added to 12, the Sum is from the Vernal Equinox to the Autumnal, the juſt length of the Day ; but from the Autumnal to the Vernal, the Length of the Night in thoſe Diſtances.

And for all other intermediate Diſtances of ☉ from the Equinoctial Points, the Proportion is, As 15, 16, or 20° to 60′, or as 20° to 30′; So are the degrees of the Exceſs of the intermediate Diſtances above 0ˢ, 15′ 1ˢ. 1ˢ, 16°, or 2ˢ, 6°, and not exceeding 2ˢ 26°, to the Minutes of the length of the Day or Night, above 12, 13, 14, 15 or 16 Hours : Always allowing 4 degrees or Days afore and after the Ingreſs into ♋ and ♑, for Solſtice.

The length of the Day and Night taken together is 24 Hours, from which if the one be ſubtracted, there will remain the other ; And,

Half the Length of the $\left\{ \begin{matrix} \text{Night,} \\ \text{Day,} \end{matrix} \right\}$ is the time of $\left\{ \begin{matrix} \text{Sun-riſing.} \\ \text{Sun-ſetting.} \end{matrix} \right.$

To find the Hour of the Moon's coming to the South, and High-water at London.
The Moon's Age multiply by 4 ; Divide
By 5 for Southing, Add 3 for the Tide.

But when the Age of the Moon exceeds 15 days, you may reject 15; As in this Example.

Anno 1725, the Moon being 27 days old, out of which reject 15, the Remainder is 12, which being multiplied by 4 makes 48, which divided by 5, the Quotient is 9, and 3 the Remainder : which ſhews that the Moon cometh to South at 9 of the Clock, and 3 times 12′ paſt, which is 36 minutes. (And here note, that for every Unit in the Remainder, you muſt reckon ſo many times 12′; which muſt be added to the hour found in the Quotient, as in the Example aforegoing) to which I add 3 hours, and the Sum is 12 hours 36′ the time of full Sea at *London*.

But it is here to be noted, that by manifeſt Experience it is found, that when the Moon is in either of the Quarters, then the Tides do not hold out their full time, but it is High-water ſooner than is found by the Rule which may partly be occaſioned by the weakneſs of the Tide at ſuch a time, and the Length of the River. For by the foregoing Rule you may find, that when the Moon is 7 days old, the time of High-water will be at 9 of the Clock, when upon true Obſervation it will be found to be an hour ſooner ; and therefore to know the true time of High-water, you muſt ſubtract ſome Minutes from the time found by the precedent Rule, according to the Age of the Moon, as you may plainly ſee in the annexed Table.　　　Q　　　　*　*Example*

The M-n's Age			H. M.
1	14 16 29		0　0
2	13 17 28		0　5
3	12 18 27	Subtract	0　10
4	11 19 26		0　20
5	10 20 25		0　30
6	09 21 24		0　45
7	08 22 23		1　00

Example. The Moon being 7 days old, it is high Tide (by the Rule) at *London*, at 9 of the Clock; then in this Table look for the Figure 7, which is in the firſt Column, and right againſt it in the two laſt Columns, under the Title of Hour and Minute, you will find one Hour, which muſt be ſubtracted from the Hour found by the Rule, and the Remainder is 8, the true Time of High-water.

A Table ſhewing the time of the Moon's coming to the South, any day of her Age.

M-n's Age.		Moon's Southing
Days.		H.　M.
1	16	0　48
2	17	1　36
3	18	2　24
4	19	3　12
5	20	4　00
6	21	4　48
7	22	5　36
8	23	6　24
9	24	7　12
10	25	8　00
11	26	8　48
12	27	9　36
13	28	10　24
14	29	11　12
15	30	12　00

The Uſe of the Table, to find the Time of the Moon's coming to South. The firſt and ſecond Columns ſhew the Days of the Moon's Age; in the 3d and 4th the hour and minute of the Moon's coming to South.

Example. The Moon being 10 days old, I would know at what time the Moon will be South. I find 10 under the Title of the Moon's Age, in the firſt Column, and right againſt it in the third and fourth Columns, you have 8 hours 00 min. which ſheweth that the Moon being 10 days old, cometh to South at 8 of the Clock, and 00 Minutes; unto which if you add the time of flowing at Full and Change, the Sum will be the time of Full Sea at the ſame Place. As here at *London*, the time of Flowing at Full and Change is at 3 of the Clock, which you are to add to the Moon's Southing, and the Sum is 11, which is the time of High-water when the Moon is 10 days old.

To find the Hour of the Night by the ſhadow of the Moon upon a Sun-Dial.

Firſt, find her coming to South as before; then ſee how many hours and minutes the ſhadow wants of the hour of 12; which hours and minutes take from the hour and minute of the Moon's coming to South; and the Remainder is the hour of the Night; but if the ſhadow be paſt the hour of 12, then you muſt add ſo many hours and minutes as the ſhadow is paſt 12, to the hour and minutes of the Moon's coming to South, and that will be the hour of the Night.

Ex-

Example. On the 4th of *December* 1725, I find the Moon to be 11 days old, and therefore she comes to the South 48′ after 8 of the Clock ; and suppose the same Night you look upon a Sun-Dial, and should find the shadow to fall upon half an hour past 1, which is an hour and a half past the Line of 12 ; which 1*h* 30*m*. must be added to 8*h*. 48*m*. the Moon's Southing, shews it is 18′ past 10 of the Clock.

Again, Suppose the same Night the shadow had fallen upon half an hour past 11, which wants half an hour of 12 which is to be subtracted from 8*h*. 48*m*. the Moon's Southing, and the Remainder will be 18*m*. after 8 of the Clock.

CHAP. IX.

Of the MARINER's COMPASS.

Of the *Variation* of the *Compass*, and the probable Causes thereof. Some Observations to find the *Variation*. The Description and Use of the *Azimuth Compass*; And the *Universal Ring-Dial*.

SECT. I. *Of the Original Discovery, and Invention of the* Mariner's Compass, *and the Excellency thereof.*

THE original Invention of this most useful Instrument, (by the help whereof the glorious Gospel hath been transmitted into the most dark Corners of the Earth.) Some attribute to one *John Goia* (or *FlaviaGoia,* as others stile him) of *Amalphi* in *Campania,* in the Kingdom of *Naples,* who only accommodated the *Superfices* thereof with 8 Points, that is four Cardinal and four Collateral ; and so left the Improvement of this Invention to be attempted by Posterity. Others do entitle the Invention thereof to the People of *China*. Dr. *Gilbert,* in his Book *de Magnete,* asserts, that *Paulus Venetus* transported it first into *Italy,* in the Year 1260, having learnt it from the *Chineses*. And *Ludi Vertomannus* affirms that when he was in the *East Indies,* about the Year 1500, he saw a Pilot of a Ship direct his Course by a Compass fashioned and framed as those which now are commonly used.

And Mr. *Barlow,* in his Book intitled, *The Navigator's Supply, Anno* 1597, relateth a Story of two *East Indians,* that he had personal Conference with, (one of them was of *Mamilia* in the Isle of *Laxon,* the other of *Miaco* of *Japan*) who declared that instead of our Compass,

they

they ufe a Magnetical Needle of fix inches, and longer, upon a Pin, in a Difh of white *China* Earth filled with Water, in the bottom whereof they have two crofs Lines for the principal Winds, the reft of the Divifions being left to the Skill of their Pilots. Alfo he there relates, that the *Portuguefe*, in their firft Difcoveries of the *Eaft Indies*, got a Pilot of *Malindo*, that brought them from thence in 33 days within the fight of *Calecut*, by which it appears that then they had the Ufe of the Compafs.

But let the Invention be attributed to whom it will, 'tis manifeftly known to have received its abfolute Perfection in thefe Parts of the World: But more particularly, the compleating of this Invention is due to the People of *Antwerp* and *Bruges*, and alfo to our own Nation, by annexing to the Compafs twenty four fubordinate Winds or Points; and alfo on the Limb thereof 360 degrees, which are numbred from North and South, towards the Eaft and Weft, with 10, 20, 30, &c. So that it appeareth, that every point containeth 11° 15'. Upon the North Point there is a *Flower-de-luce*, to diftinguifh it from the reft of the Points.

Before the Invention of this rare Inftrument, Men were directed in their Voyages by certain Stars they took notice of, efpecially the *Pleiades* or *Seven Stars*, by *Charles's Wain*, and the Pole Star and Guards in the *Little Bear*, which were therefore called *Load-Stars*. Alfo Travellers in the Defarts of *Arabia*, and thofe of *Tartaria*, were guided by fome fixed Stars in the Night-time, to fteer their Courfes in thofe pathlefs ways. So Seamen were directed by the like Heavenly Guides, in the unbeaten Paths of the Ocean, before this excellent Artifice was difcovered. But if the Sky happened to be overcaft, then the moft experienced Mariner was at a lofs, and was conftrained to come to an Anchor, or to lie by, to wait the appearance of his Cœleftial Directors. Alfo *Plinly* tells you of the Inhabitants of *Sumatra*, who becaufe they could not behold the *Pole Star* to fail by, carried certain Birds to Sea, which they often did let fly; and as thofe Birds by natural Inftinct applied their Flight always to Land, fo the Mariners directed their Courfe after them.

To thefe and the like Difficulties were Men expofed before the Invention of this marvellous Inftrument; and by it Pofterity is furnifhed with a noble Remedy againft this grand Inconvenience, and a Method difcovered, as by an immediate Meffenger from Heaven, to fteer an infallible Courfe in the moft gloomy Nights, and tumultuous Seas, and by the Providence of the Almighty be fafely conducted to the defired Port.

Yet the Mariners Compafs is not fo abfolutely perfect (by that acquired Virtue it receives from the Loadftone) but that it requires fome Improvements, becaufe it doth not conform it felf to the true Meridian in

all

all Places, but varies in some places more, in some less, from the direct Position of the true North, and South. This Variation of the Compass augments the Mariner's Care, and ought to be constantly observed in all Voyages, the neglect of which may expose them to many Dangers

A Discourse of the Variation, and of the probable Conjectures of the natural Cause thereof, is handled in that which follows. I thought it necessary (for Method-sake) to subjoin the Figure of the *Mariner's Compass*

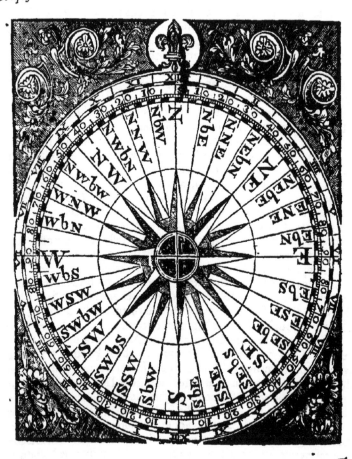

SECT. II. *A Discourse of the* Variation *of the* Compass, *and of the Natural Cause thereof* With Observations *on the* Variation.

THE *Variation* of the *Compass* is an Angle intercepted between the Magnetical and true Meridian, the Horizon determining its Quantity and Quality. These Meridians sometimes are coincident in such Places where there is no Variation: Sometimes again they are different, and then that part of the Horizon wherein the northern Extremity of the Needle lies, denominates its Quality: for if it be to the Eastward, then it is Easterly Variation; if to the Westward then Westerly.

This *Variation* of the *Compass* was formerly supposed to remain the same, which I suppose hath given rise to the Opinion of the first Author hereof, Mr. *Seller*, who (as it appears by former Impressions of this Book) supposed the Variation of the Compass to be occasioned by the *Excavation of some Parts of this Terrestial Globe*; and *by Megnetical Veins, Collaterally respecting the Needle,* &c. but now the Variation is known to vary in all Places, as appears by the following Observations of the *Variation* of the *Compass* near the City of *London*, for above an hundred Years last past.

Mr. *Burroughs*, comparing several Observations, made at *Lime-house*, *October* 16. 1580. found the *Mean Variation,*   11° 17'

By Mr. *Gunter's* Observations at *Lime-house*, *June* 13. 1622. the *Mean Variation* was then,   5 55

Mr. *Gillibrand* by his Observation made at *Deptford*, *June* 12. 1634. found the *Mean Variation* to be,   4 6

——And *July* the 4th, 1634. he found by his Observations at *Pauls Cray* in *Kent*, the *Mean Variation*,   4 1

Mr. *John Seller*, by Observations made at the *Hermitage*, near *London*, *June* the 4th, 13th, and 14th, 1666. found the *Mean Variation* to be,   0 34

The Worshipful Sir *Nicholas Millet*, at his House in *Battersey*, comparing several Observations made *May* 28. 1670. found the *Mean Variation*,   2 6

(marginal: Easterly; Westerly)

If we compare the first of these Observations, *viz.* that of Mr. *Burroughs*, in the Year 1580. with those of the famous Capt. *Halley*, who in the Year 1701. found the Variation in all Parts of the Channel to be 7° 30' Westerly (it being observed nearly the same at *London*) the Mean Motion of the Variat. between those two Observations, will be found to be about 11$\frac{44}{35}$ Minutes in a Year; but comparing the two first Observations, *viz.* Mr. *Burroughs*, and Mr. *Gunters*, the *Mean Variation* is 8° 36' East,

Eaft, and its *Mean Motion* is but $7\frac{5}{7}$ Minutes in a Year ; and by the Obfervations of the aforefaid Captain *Halley*, when the Variation was about $7\frac{1}{4}$ deg. Wefterly it increafed about 10 minutes in a Year; all which feems to Import, that the Motion of the Variation is floweft when it is neareft its Period, or greateft Deviation, according to the following Theory of Mr. *Bond*; *And how far this may tend to the confirming of the Opinion of thofe who think that the Pofition of the Wires of the Compafs (nearly) parallel to the Axis of the World, is occafioned by the Attraction of Magnetical Poles, which have a Regular Motion about (and at fome diftance from) the Poles of the World, we muft leave to Time, and future Obfervations to determine : But in the mean time, it feems inconfiftent with Reafon (if not impoffible in Nature) that the Variation of the Needle fhould be occafioned by the Excavation of fome part of the Globe of the Earth, fince fuch Excavations muft be allow'd to be always the fame, contrary to our Hypothefis of the Variation ; which by above 120 Years Obfervation compared, is found to have a General (and perhaps Regular) Motion.*

Mr. *Bond's* Theory of the Motion of the Variation.							
Years.	Variation Weft	Years.	Variation Weft.	Years.	Variation Weft.	Years.	Variation Weft.
	D. M.		D. M.		D. M.		D. M.
1689	5 29	1696	6 34	1703	7 36	1710	8 33
1690	5 39	1697	6 43	1704	7 45	1711	8 41
1691	5 48	1698	6 52	1705	7 53	1712	8 49
1692	5 57	1699	7 01	1706	8 01	1713	8 56
1693	6 06	1700	7 10	1707	8 09	1714	9 04
1694	6 16	1701	7 19	1708	8 17	1715	9 11
1695	6 25	1702	7 28	1709	8 25	1716	9 $17\frac{1}{2}$

SECT. III. *The Defcription and Ufe of the Azimuth Compafs.*

THIS Compafs doth derive its Name from its Ufe, being principally to find the *Magnetical-Azimuth* of the Sun, and is in feveral refpects like unto another Compafs, only with fuch neceffary things added, as are moft convenient for that purpofe.

Upon the round Box, wherein, are the Fly and Needle, is faftned a broad Circle of Brafs, the one half of the Limb thereof is divided into 90 degrees numbred from the middle of the faid Divifions both ways, with 10, 20, 30, &c. unto 45 degrees; which degrees are alfo fubdivided into minutes by *Diagonal* Lines, and by certain *Excentrical Circles* interfecting one another, for thefe degrees are drawn from the oppofite part of the Limb whereon the Indix moveth, cutting thofe degrees. On this Indix is erected a Sight, which for conveniency is to fall down with a
Hinge,

Hinge, and to set up upon occasion, and from the top of this Sight, down to the middle of the Index is fastned a Thread or Lute-string, to shew the shadow of the Sun upon a Line that is on the middle of the said Index.

And by this means of placing the Index upon the Circumference, the degrees come to be as large again as they would be, if it be moved upon the Center, the Truth hereof is evidently demonstrated in the Third Book of *Euclid*, Prop. 20.

This broad Circle is crossed at Right Angles, with two strings, and commonly from the Terminations of these strings are drawn four small black Lines on the Inside of the Box, for rectifying the Instrument in time of Observation, by the four Lines that are also drawn at Right Angles, on the Superfices of the Fly.

This Compass being thus fitted, is hung in strong Brass Rings, and those also fastned into a square Wainscot Box, fit for that purpose; which you may more plainly perceive in this following Figure.

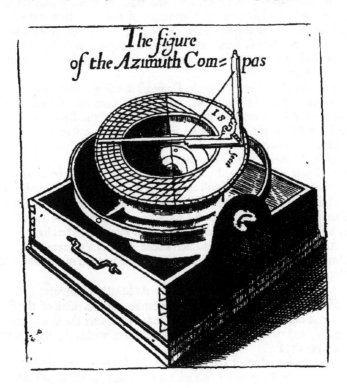

The figure
of the Azimuth Com=pas

The Use of the Azimuth-Compass.

First, you must rectify the Brass Limb on the Edge of the Box (by the Needle and Fly within the Box) according as the nature of the Observation doth require. For if the Observation be in the Forenoon, then you must put the Center of the Index upon the West Point of the Chard or Fly within the Box; and so, that the Four Lines on the Edge of the Chard, and the Four Lines by the inside of the Box, do always concur.

The Instrument being thus rectifyed, turn the Index towards the Sun, until the shadow of the *Hypothenusal Thread* fall directly into the very slit of the Sight, that is on the Index, and also upon a Line that is in the middle of the Index; then at the same time will the inner Edge of the Index cut the degree and minute of the Sun's Magnetical Azimuth from the East, to the Northward or Southward.

As for Instance Suppose the Instrument be rectifyed, as before is shewn, for an Observation in the Forenoon, and that the Index should cut ten degrees upon the Limb to the Northward of the East, then is the Azimuth of the Sun 80 degrees from the North, or else 100 degrees from the South. So likewise if the Index had cut ten degrees to the Southwards of the East, then would the Azimuth be 80 degrees from the South, and 100 from the North.

And here also observe, that the Compass standing in this Position, and if the Azimuth of the Sun be less than 45 deg. from the Meridian, and you turn the Index towards the Sun, it will go off the Divisions on the Limb, and there can be no use made thereof as it now stands.

Therefore you must turn the Instrument just one Quadrant, or quarter of the Compass, *viz.* Place the Center of the Index on the North or South Point of the Chard, according to the Sun's Position from you, and then the Edge thereof will cut the degree of the Sun's Azimuth from the North or South. That which is said as to the Use of the Azimuth Compass, when the Sun is on the East-side; the like is to be understood with the same reason when he is on the West-side of the Meridian.

And also Note, That the Observations of the Sun's Azimuth are best when the Sun is near the Horizon, because the Motion of the Sun in his Altitude is more easily observed.

To take an Amplitude by the Azimuth-Compass.

If the Amplitude be taken in the Morning, at the rising of the Sun, then you must turn the Center of the Index right over the West point of the Fly, and rectify the Instrument by the Lines within the Box, to the Lines on the Fly.

Then looking through the Sight, turn the Index towards the Sun, until you cut the Body of the Sun with the Thread; at the same time will

R

the

the Edge of the Index shew the degree of the Sun's Magnetical Amplitude, upon the Limb of the Instrument, from the East, either Northerly or Southerly.

But if you take the Amplitude in the Afternoon, at the setting of the Sun, then you must turn the Index over the East Point of the Fly, and proceed as before

But because the Refraction, (besides allowing for the Parallax) causeth the Sun to appear in the Horizon, when indeed he is about 30 minutes below it; and consequently makes him seem to rise further to the Northward in North Latitude (and the contrary) than really it doth; therefore to prevent any mistake thereby, let the Center of the Sun be about 30 minutes above the Horizon, when you observe for the Amplitude, which will be when the lower Edge of the Sun is almost half his Diameter above the Horizon, for the Sun's apparent Diameter is about 32 minutes, therefore when his lower Limb is just in the Horizon, his Center is 16 minutes above it, and when the lower Limb appears 14 minutes (which is almost half his Diameter) above the Horizon, his Center appears about 30 minutes above it, which (for the reason before given) is the time to observe for the Amplitude.

Having found the Magnetical Azimuth or Amplitude, by the Compass, find the Sun's Azimuth by *Problem* 13. *Chap.* 8 and the Sun's Amplitude by *Problem* 8 *Chap* 8.

Then find the Difference between the Sun's Azimuth or Amplitude, and the Magnetical Azimuth or Amplitude, by subtracting the one from the other, this Difference is the Variation of the Compass And to know whether the Variation be Easterly or Westerly, observe these following Rules.

Rules for casting the Variation.

I. By the Observation of the *Azimuth*

In the Forenoon. 1. If the Angle of the Sun's Azimuth (by Calculation) from the North, be greater than the Magnetical Azimuth (by Observation) then is the Variation Easterly.

2. If the Angle of the Sun's Azimuth from the North, be less than the Magnetical, then is the Variation Westerly.

In the Afternoon. 3. If the Sun's Azimuth from the North be greater than the Magnetical, then is the Variation Westerly.

4. If the Sun's Azimuth from the North be less than the Magnetical, then is the Variation Easterly.

Example 1. Suppose on the 4th of *June* 1716, in the Forenoon, I set the Sun with my Azimuth Compass, and find his Magnetical Azimuth to be 90° 48' from the North, at the same time the Sun's Azimuth, by Calculation is 84° 20' from the North part of the Meridian.

The

The Difference of these Azimuths (which is the Variation) is 06° 18'; I demand which way the Compass varies?

Answ. Westerly; because that Observation being made in the Forenoon, and I find the Sun's true Azimuth from the North to be less than the Magnetical, according to the second Rule aforegoing.

Example 2. Admit that in the Afternoon, at the same time that I find the Sun's Azimuth to be 102° 00', I find his Magnetical to be 96° 00' from the North

The Difference is 06° 00'; I demand which way the Compass varies?

Answ Westerly, because the Observation being made in the Afternoon, I find the Sun's Azimuth from the North to be greater than the Magnetical, according to the third Rule

Note, These four Rules for casting the Variation, by Observation of the Sun's Azimuth, are the same in South as in North Latitude, the Sun's Declination being either Northerly or Southerly

II. By the Observation of the Amplitude.

At Sun-rising 1. If the Sun's Amplitude be nearer to the North than the Magnetical, then is the Variation Westerly.

2. If the Sun's Amplitude be farther from the North than the Magnetical, then is the Variation Easterly.

At Sun-setting. 3. If the Sun's Amplitude be nearer to the North than the Magnetical, then is the Variation Easterly.

4. If the Sun's Amplitude be farther from the North than the Magnetical, then is the Variation Westerly.

Example. Admit that by the Azimuth Compass, at Sun setting, I find the Magnetical Amplitude to be 19 deg. 00 min. and the Sun's Amplitude to be 24 deg. 00 min. from the West Northerly; I demand which way the Compass varies?

Answ. Easterly; because by an Observation at Sun-setting, the Sun's Amplitude is nearer to the North than the Magnetical, according to the third Rule.

Having by the former Rules found the Quantity and Quality of the Variation it yet remains there be some Directions for rectifying the Course.

The manner that I shall here set down is performed by a Compass-Chard (having Degrees on the Limb,) and a pair of Compasses; which tho' it be mechanical, yet it's facile and demonstrative, and in my Opinion exact enough for Nautical Uses; however, any One may use the Pen if he please

But before we deliver the Rule for Operation, it will not be amiss for plainness sake, to give these Cautions.

R 2   1. **That**

1. That when a Man directly beholds the North part of the Horizon, the East is on the Right Hand, and the West on the Left ; and therefore when the North-point of the Compass (and consequently all the other Points) vary from the true North or Meridian to the Eastward, then the Variation is reckon'd to the Right Hand ; and for the same Reason, if the Variation be Westerly, it's accounted to the Left.

2. That in the Use of the Compass Chard, you must always observe, that you place the Course, or Point on which you steer, right from you.

The Rule.   Take the Quantity of the Variation in Degrees, from the Limb of the Chard, between the Compasses (the Chard lying before you as is directed) placing one Foot of the Rhomb or Course ; if the Variation be Easterly, turn the other Foot towards the Right Hand ; but if Westerly, to the Left   The Number of Degrees in which the Point of the Compass stays, shews the true Course from the North or South, either Easterly or Westerly, the Quantity and Quality of the Variation being allow'd.

As for Example.   1. Let the Magnetical Rhomb, or Point of the Compass, be North-East, and the Variation 10 Degrees Easterly ; I demand the true Rhomb?

The Chard lying as is directed, take the Extent of 10 Degrees between the Compasses, and place it from the N. E. toward the Right-Hand, because the Variation is Easterly, that shews the true Course to be N. E. 55 degrees, or N. E. by E. a little Easterly.

2. Let the Course by the Compass be West and by South, (*i. e*) S.W. 78 deg. 45 min. and the Variation 10 deg Easterly, as before, I demand the true Rhomb?

Take the extent of 10 degrees between your Compasses, and place it from W. by S. towards the Right Hand ; it shews the true Rhomb to be S. W. 88 deg. 45 min. or almost West.

3 Let the Magnetical Rhomb be West, and the Variation 10 deg. Easterly; I demand the true Course ?

Take the Extent of 10 degrees, as before, set it off from the West towards the Right Hand, it gives the true Rhomb N. W. 80 deg. 00 min. or almost West by North.

4. Let the Magnetical Rhomb be N. N. W. the Variation 10 deg. Westerly ; I demand the true Rhomb?

Take the Extent of 10 degrees, place it from the N. N W. towards the Left-hand, because the Variation is Westerly, it gives the true Rhomb N. W. 32 deg. 30 min. or almost N. W. by N

5. Let the Course by the Compass be West, the Variation 10 deg. Westerly, I demand the true Course?

Take

Take the Quantity of the Variation 10 deg. place it from the Weſt
towards the Left-hand, which ſhews the true Rhomb to be S. W. 80 deg.
or almoſt W. by S.

The Deſcription of the Univerſal Ring-Dyal.

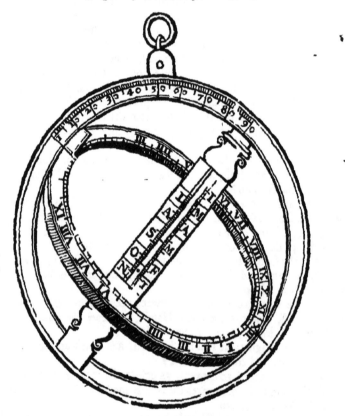

THIS Inſtrument conſiſts chiefly of two Rings, cloſely fitting within
each other, and a Bridge, and is made either of Braſs or Silver.
The outermoſt Ring repreſents the Meridian of the Place, and on
the fore-ſide has one of its upper Quadrants divided into 90 Degrees :
likewiſe on the back-ſide a Semi-circle is divided into the like Number of
Degrees from the Hole or Center in the Circumference. On the Convexity of this Ring is fitted a Nut with a Wire-ring to it, having a ſmall
Line

Line drawn in the middle of it, to move to any of the Degrees on the forefide.

The inner Ring (when they are open at Right-angles) reprefents the Equinoctial Circle, on the infide of which is drawn a Line in the very midft, and thereon are divided the Hours into Halves and Quarters, and are number'd with their proper Figures on the upper fide of this Ring.

The Bridge reprefents the Axis of the World, in the middle whereof there is cut a long flit, upon one fide are plac'd the Days of the Month, on the other the Degrees of the Sun's Declination · Upon the Bridge is contriv'd a fliding Nut, which directs a fmall Plate moving within the flit; this Plate is crofs'd with a fine Divifion, and in the midft thereof is drill'd a fmall Hole.

To find the Hour of the Day by the Ring-Dial

Place the Hole that is on the fmall Plate on the Bridge, to the Day of the Month, or the Sun's Declination, and fet the Nut upon the Convexity of the outer Ring, to the Degrees of the Place's Latitude (whether Northerly or Southerly) 'on the forefide of the Ring · Open the Rings to Right Angles, and then having your Inftrument on your Finger, turn the upper end of the Bridge towards the elevated Pole, and place the flat fide of the Bridge againft the Sun, that his Rays may the better tranfpierce the little Hole ; then turn the Inftrument to the Sun, until the Sun-beams (by the little Hole) fall exactly upon the Line drawn on the infide of the Equinoctial, or inner Ring, then is fhewn the Hour of the Day according to the Capacity of the Inftrument.

The dividing the Degrees of the Sun's Declination on the Bridge of this Inftrument (which I purpofely omitted) is Geometrically defcrib'd by the Worthy Mr. *Edward Wright*, in his *Correction of Errors*, who, I think, was the firft Contriver of this Univerfal Dial, altho' differing from this here difcourfed of.

To find the Sun's Altitude.

To perform this, you muft firft fet the Line in the midft of the Nut, upon the outer Ring, to the beginning of the Degrees on the forefide of the fame; then put a Pin in the Center-hole, and hanging your Dial upon your Finger, turn the Edge of the outer Ring towards the Sun, fo as the Shadow of the Pin may fall upon the Divifions on the back-fide; the Degrees cut by the Shadow is the Sun's Altitude.

Note, If you ufe the Ring-Dial in South Latitude, you muft place the Hole in the fliding Plate on the Bridge, to the Sun's Declination, ufing the South Declination inftead of the North, and the contrary.

CHAP.

CͪAᴴᴾ. X.

Containing the Uſe of the Croſs-ſtaff, *and* Quadrant: *Likewiſe how to find
the Latitude of a Place by the Meridian Altitude and Declination of the Sun.
And the Uſe of the* Nocturnal.

The Figure of the Croſs-ſtaff, *and the manner of the Obſervation.*

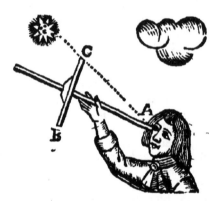

THIS Inſtrument is of ſome Antiquity in Navigation, and is commonly uſed at Sea to take the Altitude of the Sun or Stars, which
it performs with ſufficient exactneſs, eſpecially if it be leſs than 60 deg.
but if it exceed 60, it is not ſo certain, by reaſon of the length of the
Croſs, and the ſmalneſs of the Graduations on the Staff.

The Staff is made ſtraight, four-ſquare, and commonly of Box or Pear-
tree, and graduated on the Sides with Degrees and Minutes.

The Croſſes, uſually four, are commonly made of the ſame Wood
with the Staff, of a convenient breadth, and of length Proportional to
the Graduations, fitted to ſlide evenly upon the Staff, without jogging.

On one ſide of the Staff, the Graduations beginning about Three Degrees, and proceeding towards the Center or Eye-end, increaſe by every
10 Minutes to 10 Degrees; and this ſide is called the Ten-ſide; ſome-
times the breadth of the Thirty-Croſs ſupplies the place of the Ten-
Croſs.

On another ſide of the Staff, the Diviſions begin at about 10°, and
increaſe upwards to 30°; this is called the Thirty-ſide.

On another ſide of the Graduations begin about 20; and increaſe towards the Eye-end of the Staff to 60°; this is named the Sixty-ſide.

The

The remaining and fourth Side hath the Divisions beginning at 30° and increasing upwards to 90°, from thence it is named the Ninety-side and his Cross (the longest) the Ninety-Cross.

Sometimes the several sides of the Staff are numbred likewise with their Complements to 90° in small Figures, viz. at 90° stands 00, against 80° 10°. at 70° stands 20°. and so of the rest.

The Use of this is to take the Complement of the Altitude, or Zenith distance from the Staff, without Subtraction.

A Table of the Lengths and Half Lengths of the Crosses, shewing the Measure of each Cross by the Graduation on the Staff, proving whether they be rightly made or not.

Crosses 10 30 60 90	From	10 30 60 90	to	Whole Length of the Crosses.		Half Length of the Crosses.	
				Degrees	Minutes	Degrees	Minutes
		10		08	31	09	02
		30		19	47	23	52
		60		30	00	40	13
		90		36	52	53	07

An Example of the Sixty-Cross.

The length of the Sixty-Cross, if rightly made, must reach from 60° to 30° 00'; and his half Length to 40° 13'.

There are two ways principally for the graduating the Cross-Staff, one by Geometrical Projection, the other by Arithmetical Calculation.

I will give you an Example of the latter, by which you may divide any Staff, or at least be able to examine one that is already graduated.

Example.

Suppose the Length of the Sixty-Cross to be 10 $\frac{2}{10}$ Inches, and the half Length 5 $\frac{1}{10}$ Inches, I desire to know the distance of 45° 33' from the Center of the Staff proportional to this Length of the Cross. Take half of 45° 30', that is 22° 45'.

The Proportion is,

As the Tangent of 22° 45' ————————————9.622561
Is to half the length of the Cross 5 $\frac{1}{10}$ Inches, ————0 707570
So is the Radius ————————————————10 000000

To the distance required. 12. 16 Inches,————————1.085009

This gives the distance from the Center of the Staff, to the Division, representing 45° 30' to be 12. 16 (or $\frac{16}{100}$) Inches.

But if you propose to graduate a Staff, the more ready and expedite way is divide the half length of the Cross into 100 or 1000 equal

parts

parts, and taking only the Tangent Complement of half the Angle required, out of a Cannon of Natural Tangents, gives the Diſtance required.

Example. Suppoſe as before, the half length of the Sixty-Crofs to be 5 7/10 Inches, and it is required to know the Diſtance from the Center to 45° 30'?

The half-length of the Crofs being divided into 100 equal parts, or into as many as conveniency admits of, (the reſt ſupputated by Eſtimation) look in the Tables of Natural Tangents, for the Tangent Complement 22° 45', (the half of 45° 30') and you will find 23 8472; then cutting off two Figures toward the Right-hand, the Remainder 2384 ſhews the Number of equal Parts (whereof the half Crofs contains 1000) which muſt be taken, to ſet off the Diſtance from the Center to 45° 30', that is twice the half length of the Crofs, and 384 Parts more.

The like you may perform for any other Degree, to every tenth or fifth Minute, or lefs, according as the Staff will admit of the Diviſions; and as you ſee in the Example of this Crofs, ſo the like may be perform'd for any Crofs of what length ſoever.

The Ufe of the Crofs-ftaff.

To make a forward Obfervation of the Sun's Meridian Altitude at Sea.

When you intend to take the Meridian Altitude at Sea (in order to the obtaining of the Place's Latitude) it is convenient that you be preparing your ſelf for your Obſervation ſome competent time before Noon; and conſider what the Sun's greateſt Altitude may be that Day, accordingly to uſe thoſe Croſſes that may be moſt fit for your purpoſe.

As ſuppoſe the Meridian-Altitude for that Day be judged to be 20° then uſe the Thirty-ſide of the Staff, and the Thirty-Crofs; if you think it will be 30°, or more, then take the Sixty-Crofs.

There is another requiſite fit to be underſtood before you proceed to Obſervation, and that is, how to place your Fore-ſtaff to your Eye, to prevent an Error mentioned by Mr. *Wright* in his *Correction of Errors*; to avoid which, take theſe few Hints.

Firſt, Place the Center of the Staff at A, to the out ſide of the Corner of your Eye, as near your Eye as conveniently you can, without hindring your Sight, letting the end reſt upon your Eye-bone, reſpecting as it were the Eye's Center, and cauſe the viſual Rays to concur with the middle Parallels drawn on each ſide of the Crofs-Staff, and then is your Staff rightly placed for Obſervation But becauſe this is ſomewhat difficult plainly to be deſcribed, and perhaps that which is already ſaid may not be ſo obvious to the Reader as I could wiſh it. I will therefore give an eaſy Illuſtration, which may be verifyed by Experience.

S

H

Having firſt of all ſatisfyed your ſelf in the truth of the Diviſions on the Staff, and likewiſe of the exact Length, and Half-length of your Croſſes, then put on the Sixty-Croſs, and place it to 30° on his proper Side, and alſo ſlip on your Ninety-Croſs parallel with the former, and put that to 30° likewiſe, on his peculiar Graduations, then bring the End of the ſtaff to the Corner of your Eye (as is directed) and remove it ſo that you ſee each End of the two Croſſes at once, exactly to concur and agree with the viſual Lines proceeding from your Eye; that is the place of your Staff in time of Obſervation, and may eaſily be found by frequent Trial.

Having thus prepared for your Obſervation, and acquainted your ſelf with the holding of your Inſtrument, being upon the Deck, turn your Face towards the Sun, and place your Staff to your Eye, holding the Croſs up-right, look at the upper end of your Croſs at C for the Sun, and at the lower at B for the Horizon · But if the Sea obſcure the Horizon from your Sight, then remove the Croſs a little further from your Eye: if on the contrary, your Sight do not extend ſo low as the Horizon, but the Sky only appears inſtead thereof, then move the Croſs a little nearer your Eye, until by the upper part thereof you ſee the Center of the Sun, and by the lower the Horizon, exactly at the ſame time; then look upon the proper Side of the Staff (for the Croſs you uſe) the Sun's preſent Altitude will be cut by the ſame; and this if it were for one ſingle Obſervation either of the Sun or any Star, were ſufficient.

But the Sun's greateſt Altitude being that you are to take, you muſt therefore wait (making Obſervation as your Judgment ſhall direct you) until the Sun be upon the Meridian, ſtill ſliding the Croſs nearer your Eye as the Sun riſes, until you perceive it to be at the higheſt; for ſo ſoon as the Sun is to the Weſtward of the Meridian, and falling, if you make your Obſervation again, you will find the Sea to obſcure the Horizon from your Sight, and then in no Caſe remove your Croſs, but let it remain fix'd, and finiſh your Obſervation for that Day.

Then caſt your Eye upon that Side of the Staff belonging to the Croſs you uſe, the Degrees and Minutes cut thereby, and numbred with larger Figures, (decreaſing always from the Center of the Staff) gives the Sun's Meridional Altitude, and the ſmall Figures underneath, the Complement of the Altitude, or the Zenith Diſtance.

In obſerving forward by the Croſs-Staff, 'tis uſual to take a piece of Red Glaſs to defend the Sight from the Luſtre of the Sun in time of Obſervation, and it would, in my opinion, be better to have the Glaſs fitted in a piece of Braſs, and ſo to be put upon the End of any of the Croſſes, as occaſion requires. Thus much for a forward Obſervation.

After the ſame manner you muſt obſerve the Altitudes of the Stars.

To

To make a backward Observation of the Sun's Altitude by the Cross-Staff.

These Observations are frequent at Sea, especially with the *Hollanders*; and to perform this, you must have a Horizon-Vane, the inner-side of which fits upon the Center of your Staff, or else a sliding one, according to the *Dutch* fashion.

Likewise there is a Shoe of Brass to fit on the End of any of the Crosses, whose Use is the same with the Horizon-Vane in the Quadrant.

Having a Staff thus fitted, place the Horizon-Vane upon the Center or Eye-end of your Staff, and put on a Cross fittest for your purpose: fix the Brass Shoe at the lower End thereof, then turn your Back to the Sun, and looking thro' the Sight (made by the Brass Shoe) on the end of your Vane, elevate or depress the end of your Staff, until the Shadow made by the upper-end of the Cross, fall upon the upper-part of the Sight in the Horizon-Vane, then look through that Sight for the Horizon: But if the Sea obscure the Horizon from your sight, then remove your Cross a little nearer to the Horizon-Vane; but if on the contrary your Sight doth not extend so low as the Horizon, but the Sky only appears instead thereof, then remove the Cross further from the Horizon-Vane, till you see the Shadow fall upon its due place, and perceive the Horizon exactly at the same time, then have you the Sun's present Altitude.

If you observe for the Latitude, you must reiterate your Observation as before; and when you perceive the Sun to be past the Meridian, desist, and concluding your Observation, account your Degrees and Minutes, either of the Altitude, or its Complement as is before shewn.

To use the Staff in a backward Observation, after the *Dutch* Fashion, there must be a Horizon-Vane fitted to slide evenly upon the Staff, and then all the variety from the former manner of Observation will be this·

Place any of your Crosses that you intend to use upon the Center of the Staff turning the Nut inward, then slide on your Horizon-Vane with the Nut inwards, and fix on the Brass-Shoe to the lower-end of your Cross, then proceed with your Observation, removing the Horizon-Vane, as before you did the Cross, and the Degrees and Minutes cut by the Edge of the Horizon-Vane, upon the side peculiar to the Cross you use, is the Sun's Altitude, or Complement thereof, as you reckon it in the greater or lesser Figures.

SECT. II. *The Description and Use of the* QUADRANT.

THIS *Quadrant* is of a very commodious Form and Contrivance, being at present the best approv'd, and most general Instrument that is in use, for observing the Sun's Meridian Altitude at Sea.

S 2

The

The Parts of this Inftrument are principally Three Vanes, and Two Arches, which Arches together contain 90 Degrees, and give it therefore the Denomination of a *Quadrant*.

This Inftrument is faid to be firft contriv'd by Captain *Davis*, (that was employ'd in Queen *Elizabeth's* time to difcover the North Weft Paffage) and therefore call'd *Davis's Quadrant*, and by the *French*, the *Englifh Quadrant*.

The Figure of the Quadrant, *and Manner of Obfervation.*

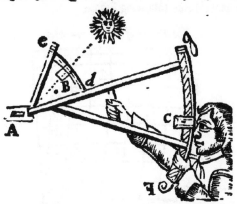

Of the Three Vanes : That which in time of Obfervation refpects the Horizon, in this annex'd Figure reprefented by A, is call'd the Horizon-Vane ; that which gives the Shadow, noted by B, is nam'd the Shadow-Vane, and that through which you are to look for both Shadow and Horizon, diftinguifh'd with C, is call'd the Sight-Vane.

Of the Arches : The leffer noted with *d e*, is nam'd the Sixty-Arch, becaufe it ufually contain'd but 60°, but of late it commonly contains 65 (and the greater Arch 25) it is of a fmall Radius (advifedly fo contriv'd) for the more apt placing of the Vane B thereon, that the Shadow thereof falling upon the Horizon-Vane A, at this fhort Diftance, might become the ftronger, and the more perfpicuous to the Eye of the Obferver.

This Arch is commonly divided but to every Degree, and numbred from the upper-end of the Arch downwards to the Line of Partition, (which is a Line drawn on the middle of the upper Leg of the Quadrant, between the Two Arches) with 5, 10, 15, &c. And this is the Complement of the Altitude. Sometimes this Arch is figur'd with the Altitude from the Line of Partition upwards towards the higher end of the Arch; with 5, 10, 15, &c. to 60 ; but this is not frequently ufed.

The

The greater Arch, here denoted by the Letters *fg*, is call'd the Thirty-Arch; this Arch is of a large Radius, the better to be divided and subdivided into Degrees and Minutes, the Limb whereof is of a competent breadth; and thereon are ufually defcrib'd feveral Concentrick Circles, interfected with Diagonal Lines, for the more facile and exact dividing the Degrees into every 5th or every 2d Minute; and hereby the Subdivifions are confpicuous, and may readily be computed by the Obferver.

But becaufe poffibly this manner of Divifion may not be underftood by every One that has occafion for this Inftrument, for their fakes therefore I have annex'd this following Figure.

The Figure of part of the Arch.

The foregoing Figure is part of the Limb of this Arch, as 'tis ufually drawn upon the Limb of the Quadrant, each Degree being fubdivided into 5 Minutes: Upon the Plane of this Arch are defcribed 6 concentrick Circles, and are noted with the Figures, 1, 2, 3, 4, 5, 6. And in the Limits of each Degree are drawn 2 Diagonals, interfecting thefe Circles; and thofe Diagonals divide each Degree into 2 Parts, *viz.* into 30 Min. and the concentrick Circles fubdivide each of thefe Diagonals, reprefenting 30 Minutes into 6 other Parts, being 5 Minutes a-piece: Therefore the 1ft Interfection at 5, is 5 Minutes; the 2d at 10, is 10 Minutes; the 3d at 15, is 15 Minutes; the 4th at 20, is 20 Minutes; the 5th at 25, is 25 Minutes; the 6th at 30, is 30 Minutes: The 1ft again at 35, is 35 Minutes; the 2d at 40, is 40 Minutes; at 45 is 45 Minutes; at 50, is 50 Minutes; at 55, is 55 Minutes, and at 60, 60 Minutes, or 1 Degree. And the like is to be underftood of the reft, always as they afcend, increafing 5 Minutes.

And take for a General Rule: Firft count how many concentrick Circles there are, which are 6 or 10, and are to be computed as is here fhewn, and noted by the Figures at the end of this Scheme; then fee how

how many Diagonal Lines are drawn within the Extent of each Degree, which are 2 or 3, then multiply the Number of concentrick Circles by the Number of Diagonals in 1 Deg and by the Product divide 60, (the Min in a Degree) the Quotient will give you the Number of Min. that each Interfection increafes by, and is more than the precedent. As fuppofe the concentrick Circles to be 10, the Diagonals in each Degree 3; then multiply 10 by 3, the Product is 30, by which if you divide 60, the Quotient is 2, which fhews that the Interfections increafe by 2 Min. the first reprefenting 2 Min and fo 4, 6, 8 Min. &c. to 58 and 60 Min. or 1°, and the 1° 2', 1° 4', 1° 6', &c. And the like is to be understood of the reft.

The Use of the Quadrant.

This Inftrument is commonly ufed to obferve the Sun's Meridian Altitude, which to perform we will briefly defcribe.

First, Put the Horizon-Vane on the end of the Quadrant on A, and then the Sight-Vane upon the Thirty-Arch in the precedent Figure, and laftly, the upper-edge of the Shadow-Vane upon the Sixty-Arch, to a certain number of Degrees moft proper for your prefent Obfervation; which readily to perform, take this Caution.

Confider what will be the Complement of the Meridian Altitude that Day, then place the Shadow-Vane fo, that the Degrees cut by the upper-edge of the Vane, be always lefs by 10 or 15° then you judge the Complement of the Sun's Meridian Altitude will be that Day in the place of Obfervation.

For Inftance: Suppofe that the greateft Altitude of the Sun for the time in the place of Obfervation, be eftimated to be 45°, the Complement is 45°; then place the Shadow-Vane at 30 or 35 deg. which are proper for our prefent Obfervation.

Having thus prepared your Inftrument, and being ready upon the Deck, turn your Back towards the Sun, and holding the Quadrant as upright as you can, place the Sight-Vane to your Eye, and looking thro' the Sight, bring the Shadow of the upper edge of the Shade-Vane, to fall upon the upper part of the flit, or open Sight in the Horizon-Vane, and at the fame time look thro' the faid flit for the Horizon; and if the Sea obfcure the Horizon from your Sight, then flide the Sight-Vane a little lower down towards *f*, but if on the contrary, your Sight doth not extend fo low as the Horizon, but if the Sky only prefents it felf to your Eye, then remove your Sight-Vane a little higher towards *g*; then make Obfervation again, continuing to move your Sight-Vane higher or lower according to thefe Directions, until looking thro' the Sight-Vane, the Shadow fall upon his due place, and that at the fame time you exactly fee the Horizon through the Sight in the Horizon-Vane, then have

you

you the Sun's prefent Altitude. But it being the Meridian or greateft Altitude that you are to obferve, you muft therefore continue to make Obfervation as often as you fhall think fit (but efpecially you are to tend your Obfervation, when you perceive the Sun almoft upon the Meridian) until the Sun be to the Weftward of the Meridian, and is leffening his Altitude, for then, if you make Obfervation, the Sky will be feen, and not the Horizon, and in this Cafe you muft not alter your Sight-Vane, but letting it ftand, conclude your Obfervation for that Day: Then caft your Eye upon the Thirty-Arch, and fee how many Degrees and Minutes are cut by the infide of the Sight-Vane, and thereto add the Degrees at the upper edge of your Shadow-Vane, the Sum is the Complement of the Altitude, or the Sun's Diftance from the Zenith.

Note, The fmall Arch in fome Quadrants contains 70°, and the greater 20°, whofe Sum is 90. Thefe Arches are numbred and divided like the former, and if that be well underftood, this will not feem to obfcure, and therefore it is needlefs to fay any more of this Alteration.

And here note: That there is a late Contrivance with a fmall Convex-Glafs to be let into the Shadow-Vane, which may be ufed when the Sun is hafey, and will not ftrike a clear fhadow upon the Horizon-Vane; then this Glafs will contract the Beams of the Sun, and reflect a fmall Speck of Light upon a fmall black Line drawn on the Horizon-Vane, which refpects the Center of the Sun. And further *Note,* That in thofe Obfervations made by the upper-edge of the Shadow-Vane, it is proper to fubtract 16 min. or fomewhat lefs, from the Sun's Altitude, or add it to the Zenith Diftance (for the Semi-diameter of the Sun;) but in ufing the Glafs you are not to make any fuch Allowance, becaufe the Speck reprefents the Center of the Sun.

Sect. III. *Rules for finding the Latitude of the Place by Obfervation of the Sun's Meridian Altitude, or Zenith Diftance, by help, of the Table of the Sun's Declination.*

BEcaufe it is common to work the Obfervation of the Sun, taken by the Quadrant, and other Inftruments now in ufe, by the Complement of the Meridian Altitude, or the Sun's Diftance from the Zenith, I fhall therefore give Rules, illuftrated with Examples, for that purpofe.

Rule 1. If the Sun comes to the Meridian in the South, and have South-Declination, fubtract the Declination from the Complement of the Meridian Altitude, the Remainder is the Latitude of the Place of Obfervation Northerly: But if the Declination exceed the Zenith Diftance, then fubtract the Zenith Diftance from the Declination, the Remainder is the Latitude Southerly.

Ex-

Example 1. Admit you are at Sea, and the Sun being upon the Meridian in the South, is 37 d. 30 m. diftant from the Zenith, and at the fame time hath 12 deg. 00 min. South Declination ; I demand the Latitude of the Place,

The Operation.

Complement of the Meridian Altitude————————37° 30'
The Sun's Declination South, fubtract————————12 00
The Latitude of the Place ————————————25 30 North.

Exampl 2 Admit (being at Sea) the Sun being on the South part of the Meridian is 10 deg. diftant from the Zenith, and the Declination 20 deg. 30 min. South : I demand the Latitude of the Place.

The Operation.

The Sun's Declination ——————————————20° 30'
The Diftance from the Zenith, fubtract————————10 00
The Latitude ————————————————10 30 South.

Rule 2 If the Sun be upon the Meridian in the South, and hath North Declination, then add the Declination to the Zenith Diftance the Sum is the Latitude Northerly.

Example Admit a Ship at Sea, and the Sun on the South part of the Meridian is 30 deg. 30 min. from the Zenith, and the Declination is 15 deg. 30 min. North, I demand the Latitude?

The Operation.

The Complement of the Altitude or Zenith Diftance is — 30° 30'
The Declination added————————————————15 30
The Latitude————————————————— 46 00 North

Rule 3. If the Sun be on the Meridian in the North, and have North Declination, then fubtract the Zenith Diftance from the Declination, the Remainder is the Latitude Northerly: But if the Zenith Diftance exceeds the Declination, then fubtract the Declination therefrom, the Remainder is the Latitude Southerly.

Example 1. Suppofe the Declination were 20 deg. North, and the Zenith Diftance 12 deg. 30 min. the Sun being upon the Meridian in the North, I demand the Latitude ?

The Operation.

The Sun's Declination North————————————20° 00'
The Zenith Diftance fubtracted————————————12 30
The Latitude of the Place————————————07 30 North.

Example 2. Suppofe the Sun's Declination to be as before, 20 deg. North, and that being upon the Meridian to the Northwards, his Zenith Diftance is 40 deg. 15 min. I demand the Latitude ?

The

The Operation.

The Zenith Diftance of the Sun is——————————40° 15'
The Declination North fubtract ——————————20 00
The Latitude ————————————————————— 20 15 South.

Rule 4. If the Sun be upon the Meridian in the North, and hath South Declination, then add the Declination to the Zenith Diftance, the Sum is the Latitude Southerly.

Example. Admit the Sun's Declination were 16° 45' South, and the Zenith Diftance 29° 45', I demand the Latitude.

The Operation

The Declination of the Sun South——————————16° 45'
The Zenith Diftance add——————————————29 45
The Latitude——————————————————————46 30 South.

Rule 5. If the Sun have no Declination then the Complement of the Altitude is the Latitude of the Place ; and if the Sun be on the Meridian in the South, your Latitude is Northerly, if in the North, Southerly. This needs no Example.

Rule 6. If the Sun be in the Zenith, *i e.* 90° above the Horizon, then the Declination either Northerly or Southerly, is the Latitude of the Place . This likewife needs no Illuftration.

Rule 7. If you be within the Artick or Antartick Circles, and obferve the Sun upon the Meridian under the Pole, then add the Sun's Declination to the Complement of the Altitude, and fubtract the Sum from 180°, the Remainder is the Elevation of the Pole.

Note, If your Inftrument wherewith you obferve give only the Meridian Altitude, then fubtract that Altitude from 90° the Refidue is the Zenith Diftance or Co-Altitude of the Sun ; and the Operation is the fame as the precedent Examples.

For the Stars

What hath been here delivered in thefe Rules, concerning the Sun's being upon the Meridian, the fame is to be underftood of any Star whofe Declination is known.

Admit you fhould obferve the bright Star *Arcturus,* whofe Declination is 20 deg. 58 min. North, when he is upon the Meridian in the South, and find his Altitude to be 65 deg. 25 min. the Compl. thereof 24 deg. 35 min. is the Zenith Diftance ; then adding 20 deg. 58 min. to 24 deg. 35 min. the fum 45 deg. 33 min. is the Latitude Northerly, according to the fecond Rule foregoing.

But if you obferve by any of the Stars near the North Pole, whofe Polar-diftance is fet down in the Tables of Declination ; and if they be on the Meridian under the Pole, add the Complement of the Declination, or Polar-Diftance, to the Meridian Altitude found, the fum is the Latitude Northerly.   . T   but

But, *Secondly*, If you obferve any Star that is upon the Meridian in the North above the Pole, then from the Meridian-Altitude of that Star, fubtract the Complement of the Declination, or Polar-diftance, the Remainder is the Latitude Northerly ; But if the Complement of the Star's Declination cannot be fubtracted from his Meridian-Altitude fubtract the Meridian Altitude therefrom, the Remainder is the Latitude Southerly.   The fame may be underftood of Stars near the South Pole.

Here I thought it neceffary to mention fomething of the *Crofiers*, which are certain Stars that are of good ufe in the Southern Navigation ; they are fo called, becaufe they do fomewhat refemble the Form of a Crofs, according to the annexed Figure.

The Figure of the Conftellation called the Crofiers.

The Head   A   Declination from the South-
                     *   Pole 34° 45'.

                *   *

                     * C

The *Cock's Foot*, Declination from South-Pole 28° 45'.

The Star at C, call'd the *Cock's-Foot*, or rather the *Crofs-Foot*, whofe Declination, according to the Obfervation of Mr *Edmund Halley*, at St. *Hellena*, is 61° 15' Southerly , and fo the Complement of the Declination or Polar-diftance, is 28 deg. 45 min. By this Polar-diftance, and the Meridian-Altitude of this Star, when he is either above or below the Pole, you may find the Latitude of the Place, by the Rules of the Stars laft mention'd, The Polar-diftance of the Head of the Crofs, is 34 deg. 45 min.

To know when thefe Stars are fit for Obfervation, hold up a Thread and Plummet ; and when the Thread cuts the Star at A, and that at C both at the fame time, then they are upon the Meridian, and fit to be obferved.

Sect. V. *The Defcription and Ufe of the* Nocturnal.

THIS Inftrument confifts of Three Parts :

Firft, The broadeft and greateft, which we may call the unmoveable Part, which hath a handle to hold it by, in time of Obfervation.

Secondly, The firft Moveable, or middle Part.

Thirdly, The long Index, that is to turn to the Pofition of thofe Stars for which they are made, *viz.* the Guards of the *Little* or *Great Bear*.

The forefide of the firft, or unmoveable Part, hath the Limb or outward Circle divided into 12 Months, and each Month fubdivided into its refpective Days, and are counted towards the Left-hand, and mark'd with their Names, or the firft Letter thereof, as *J* for *January*, F for *February*,

February, M for *March, &c* And upon fome of them there are two
other Circles, the outermoft of which is divided into 24 equal Parts or
Hours; and the other into 29 Parts and a half, or Days of the Moon's
Age, by which the Moon's Southing may be known by Infpeⅽtion, and
thereby a Computation of the Tides.

Of thefe *Noⅽturnals* there are two forts, one for the Guard of the
Little, the other for the Guards of the *Great-Bear,* or *Charle⸲'s Wain,*
commonly call'd the *Two Pointers* Now to know for which of thefe
Conftellations any Noⅽturnal is made, you may obferve, that the Noⅽturnals that are for the Guards of the *Great-Bear,* have the 17th of *February* on the Top, and if it be for the Guard of the *Little-Bear,* then
you will find the 21ft of *April* there. The back-fide of this Part is divided into the 32 Points of the Compafs, which are to fhew the bearing
of the Guards, thereby to know what Declination the North-Star hath
upon any Point of the Compafs.

The fecond and moveable Part hath a Tooth proceeding from it,
with the edge continued in a Right Line from the Center; which is to
be turn'd to the Day of the Month at Pleafure; and on the Superficies
thereof is a Circle divided into 24 equal Parts or Hours; which when
the faid Tooth is fet to the Day of the Month, and the Index turn'd to
the Pofition of the Guards, the ftraight fide of the Index will fhew the
Hour of the Night upon the faid Circle.

The third and upper moveable Part, is call'd the Index, having one
fide thereof proceeding from the Center, which is to be turn'd to the
Guards in time of Obfervation; and through which you are to fee the
North-Star, and at the fame Time the Index is to be turn'd to the
Guards.

*The Figure of the Stars, as they fhew themfelves in the Heavens, for which
the Noⅽturnals are made.*

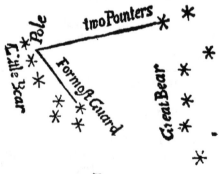

But if you will be better fatisfyed in the Forms of the Stars in each Conftellation, I refer you to the new Hemifpheres and Planifpheres of the Heaven, that are very ufeful for knowing of the Stars; fold by Mr. *Mount* on *Great Tower-hill.*

The Figure of the Nocturnal.

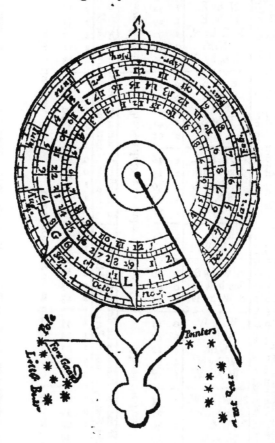

A Table of the Declination of the North-Star, *upon every Point of the Compass the Guards are upon, fitted for both sorts of Nocturnals.*

	Points of the Compass	For the Guard of the Little Bear.			For the Guards of the Great Bear, called the two Pointers.			
		D	M			D	M	
If the former of the Guards be Ascending from the North or lower Part of the Meridian	North.	2	09	Above the Pole.	If the after Wheels, or two Pointers be Ascending from the North, or lower Part of the Merid	2	20	Above the Pole.
	N. by E.	1	52			2	30	
	N. N. E.	1	29			2	35	
	N. E by N.	1	02			2	33	
	N. E.	0	35			2	26	
	N. E. by E.	0	06			2	13	
	E. N. E.	0	22	The North Star is under the Pole.		1	55	The North Star under the Pole.
	E. by N.	0	52			1	33	
	East	1	18			1	07	
	E. by S.	1	41			0	38	
	E. S. E.	2	01			0	08	
	S. E. by E.	2	16			0	22	
	South East.	2	25			0	52	
	S. E. by S.	2	30			1	20	
	S. S. E.	2	29			1	44	
	S by E.	2	22			2	04	
If the former of the Guards be descending, from the South, or upper Part of the Merid	South.	2	11		If the two Pointers be descending from the South, or upper Part of the Merid	2	20	
	S. by W.	1	55			2	30	
	S. S. W	1	34			2	29	
	S. W. by S.	1	10			2	27	
	South West.	0	43			2	23	
	S. W. by W.	0	14			2	13	
	W. S. W.	0	15	Above the Pole.		1	55	Ab. the Pole.
	W. by S.	0	44			1	33	
	West.	1	11			1	07	
	W. by N.	1	36			0	38	
	W. N. W.	1	58			0	08	
	N. W. by W.	2	14			0	22	
	North West.	2	25			0	52	
	N. W. by N.	2	30			1	20	
	N. N. W.	2	29			1	44	
	N. by W.	2	22			2	04	

The manner of holding the Nocturnal *in Time of Observation.*

Take the handle in your Hand, with the foreside towards you, holding of it upright in your Hand, (which you may discern by the Tip that is on the very top of the Nocturnal) then looking through the Hole in the Center to the North Star, you must turn the upper Edge of the Index (which cometh from the Center) to the Guards; this being understood, you may now proceed to the several Uses thereof.

To find the Hour of the Night by the North Star, *and the Guards either of the* Little *or* Great-Bear, *and upon what Point of the Compass they are.*

To perform this, you must first set the Index of the second moveable Part to the Day of the Month, (then if it will not stay of it self, you must stay it with your Thumb) holding it as you are before directed ; find the North Star through the Hole, and turn the Index to the Guards, and then upon the second moveable Part, the Edge of the Index shall cut the Hour of the Night. at the same time you will find on the back-side what Point of the Compass the Guards are upon, so that you may know also what Distance the North Star hath at that time, either above or under the Pole.

In Nocturnals made for both Bears, the use is the same, only these have on the second moveable Part two Indexes, one marked G for Great Bear, the other marked L for Little Bear; and likewise on the back-side there is two Circles distinguished by the same Marks, but their Use is the same as before taught; only if you observe for the hour of the Night by the Guards of the Little Bear, use the Index marked L, or if you seek the height of the Pole Star, look in the Circle (on the back-side) marked L: But if you observe by the Pointers of the Great Bear use the Index and Circle marked G, &c.

To find the Time of the Moons coming to the South any Day of her Age, and also the Time of High-water that Day.

First, find the Moon's Age on the moveable Part, and right against it in the Circle of Hours, you will find the Time of the Moon's Southing.

Suppose the Moon were eight days old, I demand the Time of her coming to South.

Therefore look for 8 on the Circle of her Age, and right against it you will find in the Hour-circle, almost half an Hour past 6 of the Clock in the Evening (because that always between the Change and the Full she cometh to South in the Evening, but after the Full she cometh to the South in the Morning): So having found the Moons Southing, if you add thereto the hour of the flowing at any place, it will shew you the Time of High-water that Day.

Ex-

Example. Suppose here at *London*, the Moon being 8 Days old, I find by the Nocturnal that the Moon cometh to the South at almost half an Hour past 6 of the Clock; to which I add three Hours, the Time of High-water at the Full and Change, which makes Nine of the Clock, and almost half an Hour past, the Time of High-water at *London*-Bridge, that Day of the Moon's Age.

And if those Numbers being added together should exceed 12, that 12 must be subtracted from it, and that will be the Time of Full-Sea.

As suppose the Moon should be 13 Days old at which time I find by the Nocturnal that the Moon cometh to the South at 10 of the Clock, and almost half an Hour, unto which if you add 3 it makes 13 Hours and a half, from which if you take 12, there remains 1 of the Clock, and almost half an Hour, the Time of High-water, at *London*-Bridge, according to the common way of Computation.

And to know the Time of Full-Sea at any other Place I refer you to the Tide-Tables.

CHAP. XI. *Containing the Use of the* Plain-Scale; Gunter's Scale, Plain Chart, Mercator's Chart, *and of both Globes.*

The Description and Use of the Plain-Scale.

THE Use of this Instrument is facile and delightful, and serves the Construction of Problems in *Navigation* and *Astronomy*.

The Lines on a *Plain-Scale*, are usually a Line of equal Parts, Chords, Rhombs, and Longitude; but on this here described, are likewise a Line of Sines, Tangents, and Seeants.

We shall here insert the Projection of these Lines on the Scale.

The Line of Rhombs.

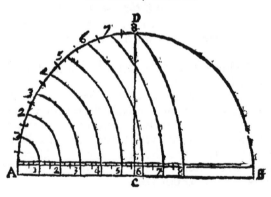

The

The Projection of the Line of Rhombs.

For the dividing of the Line of Rhombs, first draw the Line A C B and upon the Point C describe the Semi-Circle A D B, and divide the Quadrant A D into 8 equal Parts. which being done set one Foot of your Compasses in the Point A, and with the other Foot extend to each of those Divisions, and transfer those extents unto the Line A C B, which will divide the said Line into 8 unequal Parts, which will be a Line of Rhombs, and to number with 1, 2, 3, 4, &c. unto 8: And so the Halves and Quarter-Points of the Compass are to be inserted.

The Line of Longitude.

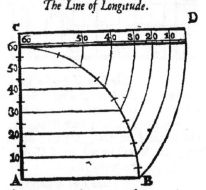

The Projection of the Line of Longitude

First, draw the Quardrant C A B, and divide the Side C A, into 60 equal Parts, then through each of those equal parts draw Lines parallel to the Side A B, until they touch the Quadrant C B, which being done, set one foot of your Compasses in the Point C, and extend the other foot unto each respective Point of Interse&ion in the Quadrant B C, and then transfer them to the Line C D (wich is to be the Distance between C and B, or the Chord of 90 Degrees ;) so shall those Interse&ions divide the Line C D into 60 unequal Parts, which is called the *Line* of *Longitude.*

The Proje&ion of the Line of Sines.

The Proje&ion of the Line of Sines is thus to be performed; First draw the Line A C B, and upon C draw the Semi-circle, and one of the Quadrants divide into 90 Degrees, as the Quadrant A D C, then draw a Line through each tenth Degree of the Quadrant parallel to the Line A C B it will divide the Line D C into 90 unequal Parts, which will be a Line of Sines, to be numbred from C towards D, with 10, 20, 30 &c. unto 90

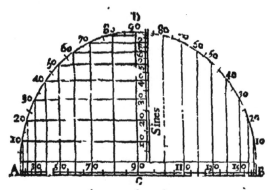

The Line of Verſed Sines.

The Projection of the *Line of Verſed Sines*, is thus to be effected: Firſt, draw the Line ACB, and upon C deſcribe the Semi-circle ADB, which divide into 180 Degrees; then through each Deg. drawing Right Lines parallel to the Line DC, they will divide the Line AB into 180 unequal Parts, which will be a Line of Verſed Sines, to be numbred with 10, 20, 30, 40, *&c.* unto 180.

The Line of Chords.

For the Projection and Diviſion of the Line of Chords, you muſt firſt draw the Diameter ACB in the following Scheme, and upon the Center C deſcribe the Semi-circle ADB; which Semi-circle divide into two Quadrants by the Point D, then divide the Quadrant DA into 90 equal Parts or Degrees, this being done, ſet one Foot of your Compaſſes in the Point A, let the other be extended to each Degree of the Quadrant AD, which Extents transfer unto the Line ACB, as you may ſee the Arches lead in the following Figure. This Line, ſo divided into 90 unequal Diviſions, is called a *Line of Chords*. After this manner you make it of what Radius you pleaſe, and number it with 10, 20, 30, *&c.*

The Line of Tangents.

Firſt draw the Quadrant, as in the following Scheme, and divide it into 90 Degrees, and from the Point B erect a perpendicular Line, as the innermoſt Line T B; then from the Center C draw Lines through each Degree of the Quadrant CDB, until they touch the line T B, and thoſe Interſections will divide the Line TB, into a Tangent, to be numbred with 10, 20, 30, *&c.*

The Line of Secants.

Having drawn thoſe Lines in the following Scheme, through each reſpective degree of the Quadrant, from the Center C, until they touch

†   U   the

the line **TB**, extend your Compasses from the Center **C** to the extremity of each respective Line, and the foot of the Compasses still remaining in the point **C**, transfer the said Lines unto the line **CDS**, so shall they divide the said line into unequal Parts, which is a *Line of Secants,* and number them with 10, 20, 30, *&c.*

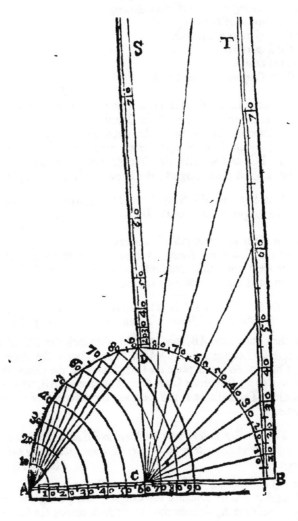

Problems of Plain Sailing by the Plain-Scale.

PROB. I. *A Ship sails N. E. by E.* 108 *Leagues; I demand the Difference of Latitude and Departure.*

In the following *Problems of Plain Sailing,*
AC reprefents the *Diftance failed.*
AB the *Difference of Latitude.*
BC the *Departure.*
BAC the *Courfe.*
ACB the *Complement of the Courfe.*

Plate 5 *Fig.* 13

Draw the occult Line AB, take off 60 from the Line of Chords, and fweep the prick'd Arch d e. Set off the Courfe five Points, taken from the Line of Rhombs, from d to e, then draw the Line A e C, and fet off 108 Leag. by the Line of equal Parts, from A to C; let fall the Perpendicular BC, and fo finifh the Triangle ABC, in which you will find the dift. Lat. A B 60 Leagues; the Departure B C 90 Leagues.

PROB. II. *A Ship fails N. E. by E until her difference of Latitude be* 60 *Leagues ; I demand the Diftance and Departure?*

Plate 5. *Fig.* 13.

Draw AB of the given Length 60, and raife the occult Perpendicular BC, fet off the Courfe five Points, as in the former Problem. Draw AC until it meet with BC, and finifh the Triangle; the Diftance is 108 Leagues, and the Departure 90 Leagues.

PROB. III. *A Ship fails S W. by W. until her, departure be* 90 *Leagues ; I demand the diftance and difference of Latitude ?* *Plate* 5 *Fig.* 14.

Draw the occult Line AB, and raife the Perpendicular BC of the given Length 90 Leagues; then upon the Point C fweep the Arch d e with the Chord of 60°, and place the Complement of the Courfe three Points from d to e; then draw C e A until it meet with AB, and finifh the Triangle. The Diftance is 108 Leagues, the difference of Latitude 60 Leagues.

PROB. IV *A Ship fails between the North and Eaft* 108 *Leagues until t'e difference of Latitude be* 60 *Leagues ; I demand the Courfe and Departure?* *Plate* 5. *Fig.* 15.

Draw AB 60 Leagues, and raife the occult Perpendicular BC, take off the Length of AC the Diftance 108 Leagues, and placing one point of your Compafles at A, defcribe the Occult Arch cutting the Line BC at the point C, by which draw AC, and finish the Triangle; the Departure BC is 90 Leagues; with a Chord of 60° sweep the Arch d e, which measured upon the Line of Rhombs, will be found five Points the Course Sought.

PROB. V *A Ship sails between the North and the East 108 Leagues, until her Departure be 90 Leagues; I demand the Course and Difference of Latitude?*   *Plate 5. Fig 15.*

Draw the occult Line AB, and raise the Perpendicular BC of the given Length 90 Leagues; take AC 108 Leagues, and setting one Point of the Compasses at C, describe the occult Arch, cutting the Line AB at A, by which draw AC, and finish the Triangle. The Course is found five Points, measured as in the former Problem, the difference of Latitude 60 Leagues.

PROB VI *A Ship sails between the North and East, until the difference of Latitude be 60 Leagues, and the Departure 90 Leagues, I demand the Course and Distance?*   *Plate & Fig 18.*

Draw AB 60 Leagues, raise the Perpendicular BC 90 Leagues, and by the Points A and C draw AC, and finish the Triangle. The Course is found 5 Points, as in the 4th Problem, the Distance 108 Leagues.

Traverse by the Plain-Scale

PROB VII *A Ship sails S S W 40 Miles, then S W 60 Miles, then S by E 63 miles, then W S W 49 Miles, then S E· by S 56 Miles; I demand the Course, Distance, Difference of Latitude, and Departure made good?*   *Plate 1 Fig 7.*

First, draw the Line AB at pleasure, and (as you are taught in Prob 1 of this *Chapter*) set off S S W. 40 Miles from A to D, and for the rest of the Courses observe this general Rule,

Find how many Points it is between the Course you are next to lay down, and the Point opposite to the Course last laid down, for that is the Points for laying down; thus the Course last sailed when the Ship is at D, is S S W. its opposite Point is N. N. E The next Course is S. W. the Points between N. N. E. and S. W is 14 Points, or 157° 30', therefore with the Chord of 60° and one foot in D describe the Arch AK, upon which set off 14 Points from A to K, and draw the Line D K E, which will be a South West Line, and upon that set off the second Distance 60 Miles from D to E, the Point the Ship is in at the end of the second Course

But when the Course last laid down and the Course next to be laid down, makes so great an Angle with each other, as here A D and D E

makes

makes an Angle of 14 Points at D; you may continue the Line AD obscurely to R, and with the Chord of 60° draw the Arch RK; and because ADR is a S.S.W. Line, and your next Course is to be S W. set off two Points from R to K, and through K draw the Line DE, and set the second Distance 60 Miles from D to E, and so by one or other of these Methods, always chusing to set it off that way that requires the least extent of the Compasses, (for then you are less subject to Errours) which being done you will find that from A the first Course S. S. W. 40 Miles, brings her to D, and from thence S. W 60 Miles to E; and after sailing S by E 63 Miles she arrives at F, and then W S. W. 49 Miles, brings her to G, and S E by S 56 Miles to C, where the Course, Distance, Difference of Latitude, and Departure made good is required. For the finding of which let fall the Perpendicular CB upon the Line AB, and draw AC, and with the Chord of 60° and one foot in A describe the Arch P O from the Line AC to the Line AB, then PO measured on the Chords, shews the Course South 16° 12′ Westerly; or S. by W almost half W The Distance A C 211 Miles, the Difference of Latitude AB 203, and the Departure BC 59 Miles, and this is sufficient for all varieties of Traverses in plain Sailing, which serves only in short Distances, or near the Equinoctial, and therefore shall forbear to enlarge here, and the rather because in a few Pages further we shall shew the Use of the Plain Scale in *Mercator's* Sailing, and how to lay down a Traverse both in the Latitude and Longitude, to which I refer you for more entire satisfaction

Oblique Sailing by the Plain Scale.

PROB VIII *There are two Ports that bear S W. by S. and N. E. by N. distance 40 Leagues, A Ship sails from the Northermost of them, first South, and then West by South, sometimes upon one of those Courses, sometimes upon the other, until she arrive at the Southermost Port; I demand how many Leagues she hath sail'd upon one Course, and how many upon the other.* Plate 5 Fig. 16.

Let A represent the Northermost Port, and E the Southermost, AE their distance, AD the distance sailed upon the South Course, DE the distance upon the W. by S Course.

Draw the Line AE 40 Leagues, being a N. E. by N. and S W. by S. Line, describe the Arch f g, setting off three Points, and draw the occult Line AD, being a South Line; then sweep the Arch h l, and set off four Points, drawing the occult Line DE, until it meet with AD, and so finish the Triangle ADE. The Distance sailed South is 29 Leagues, and W. by S is 22½ Leagues. **PROB**

PROB. IX. *There are two Islands that bear East and West, and are di-stant 40 Leagues, A Ship sails from the Westermost N. E by E and then sailing 22 Leagues and a half farther, arrives at the Eastermost Port, I demand the Distance sailed upon the first Course, and what was the second Course?*   *Plate 5. Fig. 16.*

Let A reprefent the Weftermoft Port, E the Eaftermoft, D the Place where the Ship altered her Courfe, making the beft of her way, AD the N. E by E. Courfe; DE the other Courfe unknown · Draw AE 40 Leagues, fet off an Argle of three Points, and draw AD, the N E. by E. Line occultly, take the diftance 22 Leagues and a half, and placing one Point of your Compaffes in the Point E, crofs the Line AD in the Point D, draw DE, and finifh the Triangle The Diftance upon the firft Courfe is 29 Leagues, the Angle at E is fourPoints, therefore the fecond Courfe is S E.

PROB X. *Two Ships fail from the fame Ifland, the firft fails N W by N. 22 Leagues and a half, the fecond W by N. 40 Leagues, and arrive at their feveral Ports, I Demand the Bearing and Diftance of thofe Ports*   *Plate 5 Fi. 16.*

E reprefents the Ifland, D the Northermoft Port, A the Weftermoft. Draw AE 40 leagues, and fet off the Angle at E four Points, and draw DE 22 leagues and a half, then by the Points D and A draw AD, and finifh the Triangle. The Angle at A is three Points, which fhews the bearing of the Ports to be E. N. E. and W. S W. and the Diftance AD almoft 29 leagues.

PROB. XI. *A Ship fails from a certain Port W N.W. 22 Leagues, and a half, and then more Southerly 29 Leagues, and then fhe is forced back a-gain to the Port from whence fhe came 40 Leagues; I demand her Courfe from the fecond Place to the third, and how fhe fteer'd back again.*

        Plate 5 Fig 16.

E reprefents the firft Port, D the Place where the Ship altered her Courfe, A the Place where fhe was driven back.

Draw the Line DE 22 Leagues and a half, take the Diftance AD 29 Leagues, placing your Compaffes in D, defcribe the occult Arch at A, and take the diftance AE 40 Leagues, defcribe another occult Arch from E croffing the former in the Point A; draw AE and AD, and finifh the Triangle. The Arch m n is 9 Points, therefore the Courfe from the fecond Place to the third, is S W. by S. and fhe fteer'd back again to the firft Port E N. E

Here follow fome *Problems* of *Mercator's Sailing*, wrought two ways. Firft, By the *Plain-Scale* only, by taking the middle Latitude; which

        is

is not exactly true, but may serve as an Approximation in a single Course, provided the Distance be but small, otherwise it is too grofs.

The *second* Way is by the *Meridional Parts*, which will be exact according to the Capacity of the Instrument.

The Use of the Plain-Scale in Mercator's *Sailing by middle Latitude.*

PROB. I *A Ship being in the Latitude of 40°, fails a N. Wefterly Courfe, until she come into the Latitude 45° 30', the difference of Longitude 90 Leagues; I demand the Courfe, Distance, and Departure?*

Plate 4. Fig. 10.

For the Solution thereof by the *Plain-Scale*, first draw the Line ACB, and upon the Center C defcribe the Semi-circle A D B, and crofs the Line ACB at Right-angles with the Line ECD, then find the middle Latitude, by taking the Half Sum of both Latitudes added together, which you will find to be 42° 45', which middle Latitude fet off from D to M and L both ways, and draw the Line M L; then fet the Diftance DF from B to G, then fet off the Difference of Latitude 110 Leagues from B to H, and from G to A, and upon the Point A erect a Perpendicular as A K, and from A fet off the Difference of Longitude in Leagues which is 90, to K, and from the Point K draw the Line KG, then from the Point H erect an occult Perpendicular, as the Line HI, then laying a Ruler from the Point B to the Point E (where the Line BK doth cut the Line EC) and draw the Line B I, then upon the Point B defcribe the occult Arch Cn, which being meafured on the Line of Chords will be found to be 31° or two Points three Quarters, which is the Courfe required, N. N W. three Quarters Wefterly; and the Line BI is the Diftance required, which being meafured upon the Line of Leagues, will be found to be 129 Leagues, and the Departure H I 66 Leagues.

PROB. II. *A Ship being in the Latitude 40° North, fails N N W three quarters (or 7°) Wefterly until she come into the Latitude of 45° 30'; I demand the Diftance run, the Difference of Longitude and the Departure?*

Plate 4 Fig 10.

In the Solution of this *Problem* by the *Plain Scale*, draw the Line AB, at any convenient Length, and upon C defcribe the Semi-circle A D B, and find the middle Latitude as before, and fet it off from D to M and L, and draw the Line ML, and upon the Point B defcribe the obfcure Arch Cn, and fet off the Courfe given, (which is two Points three quarters, or 31° and a quarter) from C to n, and fet the Diftance CE from C to G, and from B fet off the Difference of Latitude 110 Leagues, and the fame Diftance from G to A, and from the Points H and A erect

erect the two Perpendiculars HI an AK, then through the Point n, draw the Line BI, which being measured in the Scale of Leagues, will be found to be 129, then laying a Ruler from G to the Intersection of the Lines at E, draw the Line GK, and note where it intersecteth the Line AK, which is at K · So the Distance AK being measured upon the Scale of Leagues, will be found to be 90 Leagues, the Difference of Longitude sought, and HI the Departure 68 Leagues

PROB. III. *A Ship being in the Latitude* 40° *North, sails between the North and the West, until she arrive to the Latitude of* 45° 30', *and that her Distance run be* 129 *Leagues; I demand the Course, Difference of Longitude and Departure?*   *Plate* 4. *Fig.* 10.

First, draw the Line A C B at any convenient length: and upon C describe the Semi-circle A D B, and set off the middle Latitude as before, and likewise the Distance CF from C to G, also the Difference of the Latitude in Leagues from B to H, and from G to A ; then erect the two Perpendiculars at H and A, then take the Distance between the Compasses, and set one foot of the Compasses in B, and extend the other foot towards I, until it doth intersect the Perpendicular rais'd from H, in the Point I, and draw BI , then laying a Ruler upon the Point G, unto the intersection of the Lines at E, draw the Line GK and note where it doth intersect the Perpendicular rais'd from A, which will be at K , then the Distance KA being measured on the Scale of Leagues, will be found to be 90, the Difference of Longitude sought · Then for finding of the Course, with the Radius of your Scale and one foot in B, draw the obscure Arch Cn, and that being measured on the Line of Chords, will be found to be 31°, or two Points three Quarters, the Course required, which is N. N W three Quarters Westerly, and the Departure H I 66 leagues.

PROB IV *A Ship being in the Latitude* 40° *North, sails N N.W. three quarters (or* 7°) *W.* 129 *Leagues; I demand the Latitude of the second Place, the Difference of Longitude and Departure?*

                                                Plate 4. *Fig* 10

First, draw the Line BA of any convenient length, then from one end thereof, as B, describe the occult Arch Cn, and set off 31°, or two Points three Quarters from C to n, then by the Point n draw the Line BI, the Distance 129 leagues, and from the end thereof as at I, let fall the Perpendicular IH, then measure the Difference of Latitude HB, which you will find to be 110 leagues, or 5° 30'; the Latitude of the second Place is 45° 30'. Then having the two Latitudes find the middle

middle Latitude, as is before directed; then upon the Line BA, and upon the Center C, describe the Semi-circle BDA, and drawing the Line DE from the Point D set off the middle Latitude 42° 45′ both ways to M and I, and draw the Line ML; then take the distance DF in your Compasses and set it off from B to G, and from H to A; then upon the Point A erect an occult Perpendicular as M K; then by the Point E, draw the Line G K, till it intersect the Perpendicular at K, then draw the Line A K, which being measured in the Line of Leagues, will be found to be 90 Leag. or 4° 30′, the Diff. of Long. and H I the Dep 67 Leagues.

See other Ways of Projecting Middle Latitude Sailing. *Chap. 6.*

PROB V. *A Ship being in the Latitude 40°; sails in that Parallel, until her Difference of Longitude be 6°: I demand the Distance run?*

To resolve this Problem by the Line of Longitude on the *Plain-Scale*, you must understand, that according to the Globe, the Meridians do incline nearer together, until they concur and intersect each other in the Poles, so that hereby the degrees of Longitude are not 60 of the Equinoctial Minutes in any Parallel on the North or South side of the Equinoctial, but the nearer to either of the Poles you approach, the more they decrease; so that in the Latitude of 60 deg. there are but 30 min of the Equinoctial to one Degree of Longitude; and in the Latitude of 84 Degrees, there are but 6 Minutes, which doth shew the Errors of the *Plain Chart*, And therefore in sailing, it ought to be rectified according to the Globe, and to that end was this Line of Longitude contrived, which is thus to be used.

If you desire to know how many Miles there are in a Degree of Longitude in any Latitude, you must extend the Compasses from the Center in the Line of Chords, to the Degree of the Latitude of the Place, and the same extent will reach from the Center at 60 on the Line of Longitude, to the number of Miles answering to a Degree of Longitude in that Latitude.

Therefore for the Solution of the fifth Problem here proposed, extend your Compasses upon the Line of Chords, from the Center to the Latitude of the Place, which is 40°, and the same extent will reach from the Center at 60, in the Line of Longitude, to 46, which shews that 46′ make a degree of Longitude in that Latitude, which 46 being multiplied by 6, the Degrees of Longitude, gives 276′, the Distance run which was required.

PROB. VI *A Ship being in the Latitude of 40°, sails in that Parallel 276′; I demand her difference of Longitude?*

For the Solution of this Problem, find how many Miles make a degree of Longitude in the Latitude of 40°, (as in the last Problem)

X   which

which is 46, therefore if you divide 272 (the Diftance run) by 46 (the Miles in a Degree of Longitude in that Latitude) the Quotient will be 6°. the Difference of Longitude required.

Parallel *Sailing by the Plain-Scale.*

But if you would find the things required by Projection, or would have your Queftion fo laid down, that what is given or fought may be meafured by Scale and Compaffes, a very proper method (which is alfo a Demonftration of the Proportions we have made ufe of in working *Parallel-Sailing* by a Canon) is as follows.   *Plate* 2. *Fig.* 7

Upon the *Plain-Scale*, take in your Compaffes the S of 90° (which is equal to the Chord of 60) and fet from A to B, and at B raife the Perpendicular B C; and fet the Sine of the Complement of Latitude from A to b, and raife the Perpendicular b c, and if Difference of Longitude be given, fet it on the Line B C from B to C, but if the Diftance be given, fet it off upon the Line b c, from b to c, and through C or c draw the Hypothenufe A C, fo is A b the Sine Complement of the Parallel of Latitude, b c the Diftance, B C the Difference of Longitude. So that in three things, *viz.* the Latitude of the Parallel, the Dift. and Diff. of Longitude ; if any two be given, the third may be found.

Example 1 A Ship in Latitude 60° 00' fails due W till her Difference of Longitude be 7° 17', or 437. I demand how far fhe hath failed in that Parallel

Draw A B equal to the Sine of 90, and take in your Compaffes the Sine of the Complement of Latitude, which here is 30 (the Latitude being 60) and fet from A to b, and raife the Perpendicular B C; upon which fet off the Difference of Longitude 437, from B to C, and draw A C ; and at b erect the Perpendicular b c, to cut A C in c ; and b c meafured, will be found to be 218 ½, the Diftance required.

Example 2. A Ship in Latitude 42° 10', fails W. 397 Miles I demand her Difference of Longitude?   *Plate* 2. *Fig.* 8.

With the Sine of 90° draw the Line A B as before, fet the Sine of the Complement of Latitude from A to b, and raife the Perpendicular b c, upon which fet off the Diftance 397 Miles. Erect alfo the Perpendicular B C, and from A through the Point c draw A C, till it cut B C in C, fo is B C, the Difference of Longitude 536' or 8° 56'.

Example 3 A Ship fails Weft 597 Miles, her Difference of Longitude 769 Minutes, or 12° 49'. I demand what Latitude fhe failed in.   *Plate* 2. *Fig.* 9.

Having drawn A B (the Sine of 90°) raife the Perpendicular B C, upon which fet off the Difference of Longitude 769, from B to C, and draw A C, then take in your Compaffes the Diftance 597 Miles and with
one

one foot at (or near) the end of the Line A B, as at A, fweep the pricked Arch d, and with one foot in (or near) B, and the fame extent
fweep the fmall Arch e, lay a Ruler from the Extremity of both thefe
Arches, it will cut A C in c; from c let fall the Perpendicular c b to cut
A B in b, the extent A b taken in the Compaffes and applied to the
Line of Sines, reacheth to 50° 56' the Complement of Latitude. So
that the Latitude is 39° 4', which was required.

And becaufe the Triangles B A C and b A c are fimilar (having one
Right *Angle*, and the *Angle* at A being common to both) therefore their
Sides are proportional, by *Eucl. Lib. 6. Prop.* 4. that is, As Bafe A b
to Bafe A B; So Perpendicular b c, To Perpendicular B C. Or by
altering the Terms it is, As A b, to b c, So A B, to B C. And becaufe in this way of Projecting *Parallel-Sailing* A b is Sine Complement
of Latitude, b c the Diftance, A B Radius, and B C the Difference
of Longitude, it will follow that, As Sine Complement of Latitude
A b, to the Diftance b c; So is Radius A B, To the Difference of Longitude B C   Which is the Proportion we made ufe of in our Trigonometrical Operations in *Parallel-Sailing*; which is hereby clearly de-
monftrated, and this Proportion altered or inverted as occafion requires,
ferves in all Cafes, for reducing Miles Eafting or Wefting, to Minutes
or Degrees of Longitude, and the contrary.

Queftions in failing in a *Parallel*, may alfo be laid down by a Right
angled Plain-Triangle, with only one Perpendicular, making the Perpendicular equal to the Diftance failed in the *Parallel*, and the *Angle* at
the Bafe equal to the Complement of Latitude; fo fhall the Hypothenufe be equal to the Difference of Longitude.   *Plate* 1. *Fig.* 3.

Example. Suppofe a Ship fails Weft 206 Miles, in Latitude 56° 15',
make B C 206, the *Angle* B A C 33° 45', equal to the Complement of
Latitude, and having finifhed the Triangle it is, As Sine of B A C
Complement of the Latitude, To Side oppofite B C the Diftance failed;
So is Radius, To the Hypothenufe A C. The Difference of Longitude,
372' or 6° 12', and this way alfo you may by any two things given, lay
it down and find the third

Another way to work Mercator's *Sailing by the Plain-Scale, and the*
Meridional Parts.

PROB. I. *A Ship fails* S. S. E. *from the Latitude* 40° *North, to the*
Latitude 37° 35' *North; I demand the Diftance failed, the Departure and*
difference of Longitude.   *Plate* 5. *Fig.* 17.

Having the two Latitudes 40° North, and 37° 35' North, find the
Meridional Difference of Latitude by the Table of *Meridional Parts,* which
is 186' and fubtracting the one Latitude from the other, the difference
is 2° 25', or 145'.   X 2   To

To work this Problem, draw the Line AbB, then place 145 from A to b, and 186 from A to B; raise the two occult Perpendiculars, b c and B C, set off the Course two Points and draw the Line AcC, producing it until it cut both the Perpendiculars in the Points c and C, and so finish the two Triangles A b c, and ABC The distance Ac is 152, the Departure b c 58, and the difference of Longitude BC 77'.

PROB II. *A Ship sails from the Latitude* 40° *N to the Latitude* 42° 20' *N. until her Difference of Longitude be* 77' *Westerly ; I demand the Course, Distance and Departure?*   *Plate* 5. *Fig.* 17.

The Meridional Difference of Latitude is, as in the first Problem, 186', the proper Difference of Latitude 140'.

Draw AB 186', place 140' from A to b, raise the Perpendicular BC of his given length 77', and also the occult Perpendicular b c, by the Points A and C draw AC, and finish the two Triangles. The Course the Angle at A is two Points, or N N.W. the Distance Ac 152', the Departure 58'.

PROB. III. *A Ship sails N. Westerly* 152' *from the Latitude of* 40° *North, to the Latitude of* 42° 20' *North; I demand the Course, Departure, and Difference of Longitude?*   *Plate* 5 *Fig.* 17.

The *Meridional Difference of Latitude* is 186 Minutes, the proper *Diff. Lat* 140 Minutes.

Draw AB 186', and Ab 140', as before, and raise the two occult Perpendiculars b c and BC , take the Distance 152' ; and placing one Point of your Compasses in the Point A, cross the occult Line b c in the Point c, and draw Ac, producing it until it concur with BC, and finish the Triangles. The Course is two Points, or N.N.W. the Departure 58', the Difference of Longitude 77'.

PROB IV. *A Ship sails N N W.* 152', *from the Latitude* 40° *North ; I demand the Latitude, Departure, and Difference of Longitude ?*
                    Plate 5. *Fig.* 17.

Draw the occult Line AB, and set off the Course two Points, and the Distance Ac 152', let fall the Perpendicular b c, and so finish the Triangle A b c. Then Ab will be found 140', or 2° 20', which makes the other Latitude 42° 20', by which you will find the *Merid. Difference of Latitude* to be 186' Place 186' from A to B, and raise the occult Perpendicular BC, until it meet with A c C continued, and so finish the Triangle ABC: The Departure b c is 58 min. The difference of Longitude BC 77 min.

The

The Uſe of the Plain Scale, *in laying down and working a* Traverſe, *according to* Mercator'*s Projection.*

A Ship in Latitude 43° 25′ North, bound for a Port in Latitude 40° 00′ N. Difference of Longitude Weſterly ; from the Northermoſt Port to the Southermoſt is 4° 52′, or 292′, ſhe ſails S W. by S 47 Miles, then S S. W. half W 51 Miles, then S by E. half E. 62 Miles, then W N. W. three quarters W 61 Miles, and laſtly W. S. W. a quarter W. 51 Miles. I deſire to know the *Latitude* come to, with the true *Courſe* and *Diſtance* made good ; and alſo the *Courſe* and *Diſtance* from the Ship to the Port bound for. *Plate* 2 *Fig* 10.

Firſt, (As you are taught in Prob. 1. of the Uſe of the *Plain-Scale* in *Mercator'*s Sailing by Meridional Parts) having both Latitude sand Difference of Longitude between the Ports, find the Meridional Difference of Latitude, which is 274, which ſet upon the line A D, from A to D, and raiſe the perpendicular D E, upon which ſet the Difference of Longitude 292 from D to E, and draw A E : Set alſo the Difference of Latitude between the Ports 205 from A to d, and erect the perpendicular d e, to cut A E in e; which done, A repreſents the Port ſailed from, A e the true diſtance between the Ports meaſured upon a Scale of equal Parts, according to Plain Sailing ; E the Port bound for as it is repreſented in the *Mercator'*s *Chart* ; D E the Difference of Longitude 292′, and here only lies the Inconveniency that attends *Mercator'*s *Charts,* that altho' E repreſents the Port bound for in the *Mercator'*s *Chart,* yet A e meaſured upon a Scale of equal Parts ſhews the true Diſtance ; but when the two Ports A and E, are placed each in its proper Longitude and Latitude there is ſo much difficulty attends the common Way of finding the true Diſtance, that I ſuppoſe has chiefly if not only diſcouraged many Perſons from the frequent Uſe of the *Mercator'*s *Chart,* and made them to return to the old but erroneous Practice of Sailing by the *Plain Chart ;* but to remedy this Inconveniency, and to encourage our *Engliſh* Sailors to abandon it (as being owned by all that know it to have no better Foundation than Falſhood it ſelf) you ſhall have in the Uſe of the *Mercator'*s *Chart* a Method whereby without much Puzzle or Trouble to make a Scale for every *Mercator'*s *Chart,* whereby you may with one Extent of the Compaſſes, and one Application to the Scale, as in *Plain Sailing,* meaſure any Diſtance : And I hope they that can make their own Charts will not be unwilling to be at very little more Pains to make a Scale to render ſuch a true and uſeful Invention, as the *Mercator'*s *Chart,* both Eaſy and Practical.

Having

Having thus laid down the two Ports, and conflituted the Triangles A de and A DE, fet off your firft Diftance S W. by S 47 Miles from A to g, and S S W half W 51 Miles from g to h, &c. as you are taught in *Prob.* 7 of *Plain Sailing* by the *Plain Scale*, and having laid down your feveral Courfes from h to k, and thence to m, the next Courfe, which is the laft propofed in the Queftion brings her to c, and the Dift. made good is A c, 204.2 Miles, the difference of Latitude A b 146 Miles, and confequently the Latitude come to is 40° 59', by which you find Meridional Difference of Latitude A B 198, from B erect the perpendicular B C, to cut A c (produced) in C, then is B C 191' the difference of Longitude made good, and C reprefents the Place that the Ship is in, in a *Mercator's Chart*, therefore draw C M parallel to B D, and draw C E, then is,

C M the Meridional Difference of Latitude, ⎫
M E the Difference of Longitude,   ⎪ Between the
C L the Difference of Latitude,   ⎬ Ship and the
C R the Diftance,   ⎪ Port.
R C L the Courfe   ⎭

When we come to fhew the Ufe of *Mercator's-Chart*, we fhall do it by a Traverfe laid down by the Scale above propofed, whereby the Ship is brought to her proper Place in the *Mercator's Chart*, without regarding Departure, or proper Difference of Latitude.

PROBLEMS of Great Circle Sailing.

PROB I. *Two Places both in one Latitude, the Difference of Longitude being given, to find by what Latitudes and Longitudes the Arch paffes, and the Courfes and Diftances from Place to Place, in the Arch of a Great Circle.*

Example. Suppofe the *Lizard* and *Penguin* Ifland on *New-found-Land*, both in the Latitude 50° North, the Difference of Longitude between them 47°; I demand by what Latitudes and Longitudes the Arch paffes, and the Courfes and Diftances from Place to Place?

Plate 4 *Fig.* 11.

Draw the Line A E and place the Tangent of 40 deg. the Complement of the Latitude from A to B: with 60 deg. of the Chords fweep the Arch D E, and fet off 47 deg. the Difference of Longitude from E to D, and draw the Line *A D*, and place the Tangent 40 deg. the Complement of the Latitude from *A* to *C*; then draw the Line *B C*, and upon the Arch *D E*, fet off every 05 deg. from E to D, and draw the

prick'd

prick'd Lines *A b*, *A e*, *A d*, &*c*. and where thefe Lines interfect *B C*, place the Letters *b, e, d, f, g,* &*c* The diftances, *A b*, *A e*, *A d*, &*c*. being meafured on the Line of Tangents, are Tangents Complement of the Latitude as follow.

Compl	Lat.	The Latitudes.	
A b	39		51
A e	$38\frac{1}{2}$		$51\frac{1}{2}$
A d	38	Therefore the *Lat.* arc,	52
A f	$37\frac{1}{2}$		$52\frac{1}{3}$
A g	$37\frac{1}{2}$		$52\frac{1}{2}$
A n	$37\frac{1}{4}$		$52\frac{1}{4}$
A o	38		52
A u	$38\frac{1}{2}$		$51\frac{1}{4}$
A t	$39\frac{1}{2}$		$50\frac{1}{2}$

Thefe are the Latitudes by which the Arch paffes at every 5 deg. of Longitude, from B reprefenting the *Lizard*, to C which reprefents the *Ifland*

Having thefe Latitudes and Longitudes, you may find the Courfe and Diftance from place to place, according to *Mercator's Sailing* , as you are taught *Chap* 7. *Prob.* 1. of this Book, where you have the fame Queftion anfwered by *Arithmetical Calculation*, to which (to avoid needlefs Repetitions) we fhall refer the reader for a Proof of his Work in this and the following Problem

PROB. II. *Two Places differing both in Latitude and Longitude, to find the Latitude and Longitude by which the Arch paffes, and the Courfes and Diftances from Place to Place.*

Example. Suppofe the two Places be *Trinity-Harbour* in *Virginia,* in Latitude 36° North, and the *Lizard* in Latitude 50° North, the Difference of Longitude between them 68 degrees. I demand by what Latitudes and Longitudes the Arch pafles, and what is the Courfe and Diftance from place to place? *Plate* 4. *Fig.* 12.

Draw the Line A F, place the Tangent of 40°, the Complement of the *Lizards* Latitude from A to C; and with 60° of the Chords, and one foot in A, defcribe the Arch E F, fet off 68° from F to E, and draw the Line A E; then place the Tangent 54° the Complement of *Trinity-Harbour's* Latitude from A to B, and draw BC, letting fall the Perpendicular A d ; then fet off every 5 deg. from E towards F, (becaufe we fail from B) draw the prick'd Lines A 1, A 2, &*c.* the Diftance A 1, A 2, A 3, &*c.* meafured on the Line of Tangents, gives the Complements

ments of the Latitudes, by which the Arch paſſes at every 5° Difference of Longitude from B, repreſenting *Trinity-Harbour*, towards C, which is the *Lizard*

And thus having the Latitudes and Longitude by which the Arch paſſes, you may alſo find the Courſes and Diſtances, as in the ſecond *Prob Chap* 7. which for a help to Memory, you may Collect into a ſmall Table, as in the foregoing Example, *&c.*

Aſtronomical Problems wrought by the Plain-Scale

PROB. I *The Sun's Place or Diſtance from the next Equinoctial Points, and the greateſt Declination being given, to find the preſent Declination.*

Example, The Sun's Place is 26 deg ¾ of *Taurus*, that is 56 deg ¾ from the *Equinoctial* Point *Aries*, I demand his Declination?

Plate 5 *Fig* 18.

With the Chord of 60 deg deſcribe the Semi-circle B D C, and raiſe the Perpendicular A D, and from the Point C ſet off the greateſt Declination 23¼ deg from C to E, and draw the line AE, then for the Sun's Longitude ſet off the Sine 56 deg. ¾ upon the line AE, from A to F; then from the Point F, take the neareſt Diſtance F I to the line A C, which meaſured on the line of Sines, is 19 deg. ½ or elſe through the Point F draw G H parallel to B A C, then A C meaſured on the Sines, or C H on the Chords, gives 19½ deg. the Sun's preſent Declination Northerly.

PROB. II. *The Sun's greateſt and preſent Declination being given; to find his Place or Longitude*

Example, The Sun's Declination is 19°½ North, increaſing; the greateſt Declination (as before) 23'½ I demand the Sun's true Place.

Plate 5. *Fig* 18.

Draw B C and deſcribe the Semi-circle B D C, raiſe the Perpendicular A D, and draw the line A E, as in the former *Problem,* place the Sun's Declination 19 deg. ½ from B and C to H and K; draw the Line HK, which interſects A E in the Point F, the diſtance A F is the Sine of 56°¾ the Sun's diſtance from *Aries*; ſo that the Sun's Longitude is 26°¾ of *Taurus*

PROB III. *The Sun's Place and greateſt Declination being given, to find his Right Aſcenſion.*

Example. The Sun's place is 26¾ of *Taurus*, the greateſt Declination, as before, I demand his Right Aſcenſion?   *Plate* 5. *Fig.* 18.
Deſcribe

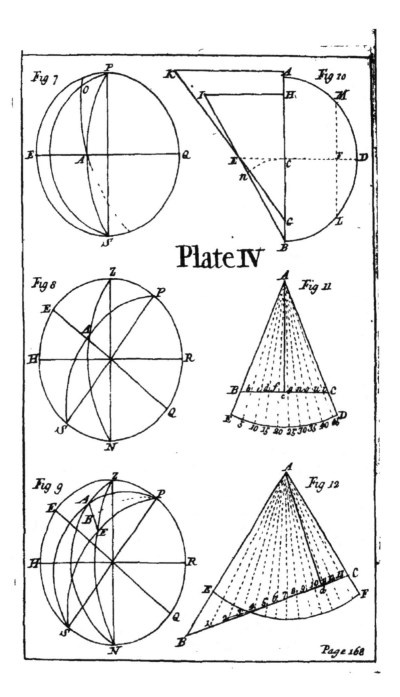

Plate IV

Describe the Semi-circle, draw A D and A E, as before, place the Sine of 56¾, the Sun's distance from *Aries* ; from A to F ; through the Point F draw the Parallel H K ; then is F G the Sine of the *Right Ascension*, GH being Radius, which you may Measure after this manner : Place the Distance H G from A to o ; upon o as a Center, with the distance F G, describe the occult Arch at m ; a Ruler laid from A until it touch the Arch, will cut the Semi-circle B D C in the Point N ; the Arch C N is the Measure of F G 54½°, the *Right Ascension*.

PROB. IV. *The Sun's Declination given, (the greatest Declination being known) to find the Right Ascension.*

Example. The Sun's Declination is 19° ½ North increasing ; I demand the *Right Ascension*, Plate 5. *Fig* 18.
Describe the Semi-circle B D C, and draw the Line A D and A E as before ; place the Declination 19° ½ from B and C to H and K, drawing H K ; F G being measur'd, as in the third Problem, gives the *Right Ascension* (as before) 54°½.

PROB. V. *The Latitude of the Place, and the Sun's Declination being given, to find his Amplitude.*

Example. In the Latitude 51° ½ North, the *Sun's Declination* being 17° ¾ N I demand the *Sun's Amplitude* ? Plate 5. *Fig.* 19.
Draw *BAC*, and the Semi-circle *BZC*, the Perpendicular *A Z* : place the Latitude or Height of the Pole 51° ½ from C to P, and draw *A P* ; set off the Complement of the Latitude 38° ½ from B to Q and draw *A Q* the Equinoctial ; place the Chord of the Declination 17°¾ from Q to D, and the Sine thereof from A to G, and draw the Parallel of declination *D F.* *A F* measured on the Line of Sines is 29°¼ the *Amplitude* required.

PROB. VI. *The Latitude of the Place, and the Sun's Declination being given, to find the Ascensional Difference ?*

Example. In the Latitude 51 deg. ½ North, the Sun's Declination 17°¾ North ; I demand the *Ascensional Difference* Plate 5. *Fig.* 19.
Describe the Semi-circle *BZC*, and draw the Line *A Z*, *A P*, *A Q*, and *D F*, as in the fifth Problem ; *FG* is the Sine of the *Ascensional Difference*, to the Radius *D G*, which is thus measured : Place *DG* from A to o ; upon o, as a Center, with the distance *F G* describe the Arch at E ; a Ruler laid from A until it touch the Arch, gives the Point I, and B I, 23deg. ¾ is the measure of the *Ascensional Difference*.
What the *Ascensional Difference* is, and the Use of it, may be seen *Prob.* 5, 6, and 7, *Chap.* 8.

I

PROB.

PROB VII. *The Latitude of the Place, and the Sun's Declination being given, to find when the Sun shall be due East or West*

Example. In the Latitude 51°½ North, the Sun's Declination 17°¾, North; I demand at what time he shall be due East or West?

Plate 5 Fig 20.

Describe the Semi-circle B Z C, and draw the Lines A Z, A P, A Q, and D O, as before; E O is the Sine of the time from 6, that the Sun is East or West (to the Radius D O) to measure which, place D O from A to a, and upon the Center a, with the Distance E O describe the Arch at g; a Ruler laid from A, until it touch the Arch, gives the Point L. and B L 14 deg ¾ is the measure of E O, which reduced to time (See. *Prob.* 7. *Chap* 8.) makes 59'; which shews that the Sun is due East at 59' past 6 in the Morning, and due West at one minute past 5, or 59 min. before 6 at Night.

PROB. VIII. *The Latitude of the Place, and the Sun's Declination being given to find the Altitude of the Sun, being due East or West*

Example. In the Latitude 51°½ North, the *Sun's Declination* being 17¾ N. I demand the Sun's Altitude, being due East or West?

Plate 5. Fig. 20.

Describe the Semi-circles *B Z C*, and draw the Lines *A Z, A P, Q A,* and *D O*, as before. A E being measured on the Line of Sines, is 23° *fere, Sun's Altitude* being due East or West.

PROB. IX. *The Latitude of a Place, and the Sun's Declination being given to find the Sun's Altitude at six.*

Example. In the Latitude 51°½ North, the *Sun's Declination* being 17°¾ N I demand his Altitude at six?   Plate 5. Fig. 20.

Describe the Semi-circle B Z C, draw the Lines A Z, A Q and D O, and through the Point O draw the Line l o b parallel to B C; B L or C b measur'd on the Chords, or A I on the Sines, gives 13°¾, the Altitude of the Sun at Six.

PROB. X. *The Latitude of the Place, and the Sun's Declination being given, to find the Sun's Azimuth at Six.*

Example. In the Latitude 51°½ North; the Sun's Declination 17°¾ North; I demand the *Sun's Azimuth* at Six.   Plate 5. Fig. 20.

Describe the Semi-circle BZC, and draw the Line A Z, A P, A Q and D O, as before; draw l o b as in the Ninth Problem: I o is the Sine of the Sun's Azimuth to the Radius I L which is thus measured; place I L from A to e, with the distance I o upon the Center e; describe the
occult

occult Arch at d; a Ruler, laid to touch the Arch, gives the Point b and C b meaſured is 11 deg. ¼ the Azimuth from the Eaſt or Weſt. So that the Sun is E. by N. at 6 in the Morning, and W. by N. at 6 at Night.

PROB. XI. *The Latitude of the Place, the Sun's Declination and Altitude given, to find the Sun's Azimuth.*

Example. In the Forenoon, in the Lat. 51 deg. ½ North, the Sun's Declination is 20 ¼ deg N. and his Altitude 43 deg I demand his Azimuth ?   *Plate 5. Fig. 21.*

Deſcribe the Semi-circle B Z C, and draw the Lines AZ, AP, AQ and D F, the Parallel of Declination, as in the former Problems; place the Altitude 43 deg. from B and C to d and e, and draw the Parallel d e, which interſects the Parallel DF in the Point G, I G is the Sine of the Sun's Azimuth from the Eaſt towards the South, I d being the Radius; which to meaſure, place I d from A to c, and thereon with the diſtance I G deſcribe the Arch at f; a Ruler laid from A to touch the Arch, gives the Point h, B h 24 deg. ½ is the Meaſure of I G, Eaſt Southerly. So that the Sun's Azimuth is S. E. 65 deg. ½.

PROB. XII. *The Latitude of a Place, the Sun's Declination and Altitude being given, to find the Hour from Noon.*

Example. In the Afternoon, in the Latitude 51 deg. ½ N. the Sun's Declination is 20 deg. ½, the Altitude 43 deg. I demand the Hour ?
Plate 5 Fig 21.

Deſcribe the Semi-circle BZC, and draw the Lines AZ, AP, A Q, DF, and d e, as in the 11*th Problem*; F G is the Sine of the Hour from Six, which to meaſure, place DF from A to u, and thereon with the diſtance FG ſweep the Arch at K, a Ruler laid to touch the Arch, gives the Point o, and C o is the meaſure of FG 45 deg. which reduc'd into Time, gives three Hours, the time Afternoon

---

SECT. II. *The Uſe of Gunter's Scale.*

I Shall not ſay much of the Deſcription of the Scale, nor of the Projection of the Lines thereon, being the Logarithms of Numbers, Sines, Tangents, &c. placed upon a Scale, only obſerve, that the common *Gunter's-Scales* have eight Lines, the uppermoſt is called Sine-Rhombs, marked at the end towards the Right-hand SR, and numbred towards the Right-hand, 1, 2, 3, 4, 5, 6, 7, 8; and is only the Sine of the Degree and Minute that anſwers to the Rhomb, as the Sine of 3 on the Rhombs, is equal to the Sine of 33° 45′ on the Sines; becauſe 33° 45′ is equal to 3 Points, &c.   Y 2   The

The next Line marked T R, is the Tangent of the Rhombs, and is numbred towards the Right-hand, 1, 2, 3, 4, and back again 5, 6, 7, the same Directions are to be observed in taking the Tangent of a Rhomb of this Line, as were given in taking the Sine of any Rhomb.

The third is the Line of *Numbers,* marked *Numb* the fourth is *Sines,* the fifth is *Versed-Sines,* marked *V Sine,* the sixth is *Tangents,* marked *Tang* the seventh the *Meridian-line,* marked *Merid* and the lowest is a *Line of Equal Parts,* of all which in order, and first of the Line of *Numbers*

To find a Whole Number on the Line of Numbers.

Among the Figur'd Divisions, look for the first Figure of your Number, then for the second Figure count so many tenths from the long Divisions on towards the end of the Rule, as the Units in the second Figure amount to   Then for the third Figure, count from the last Tenth so many Centesms as the Figure hath Units, and so likewise for the fourth Figure, count from the last Centesm so many Millions (or Thousands) as the same 4th Figure contains Units, this done, that shall be the Point where the Number propounded is represented on the Line of Numbers.

The Number given being 12, *to find the Point on the Line of Numbers that doth represent the same.*

Therefore according to the Rule, 1 being the first Figure of this Number, I take the Division at the Figure 1 (in the middle of the Line) for the first Figure, then the second Figure being 2, I count two tenths from that 1, and that is the Point representing 12, where commonly there is a small Brass Center because it is often in use

Suppose the Point representing 144 *were required to be found on the Line of Numbers.*

For the first Figure in the Number being 1, I take (as before) the middle 1 ; then for the second Figure which is 4, I count 4 tenths onwards, and from the tenth I count 4 Centesms, or hundred parts further, and that is the Point representing 144.

To find the Point representing 1728, first (as before) for 1000 I take 1 in the middle of the Line; secondly, for the second Figure being 7, I reckon 7 Tenths onwards, and that is 700 ; thirdly, for the third Figure being 2, I reckon 2 Centesms from the 7 Tenths, which represeseteth 20, and then lastly, for 8 you may reasonably estimate 8 Millions, or Thousand parts, from the last two Centesms, and that Point last found will be the Point representing the Number 1728.

To find a Fraction, or broken Number, on the Line of Numbers.

The Fractions that are to be found on the Line of Numbers, ought always to be Decimal Fractions, $\frac{1}{10}$, $\frac{1}{100}$, $\frac{1}{1000}$, (or 1, 01, 001) either

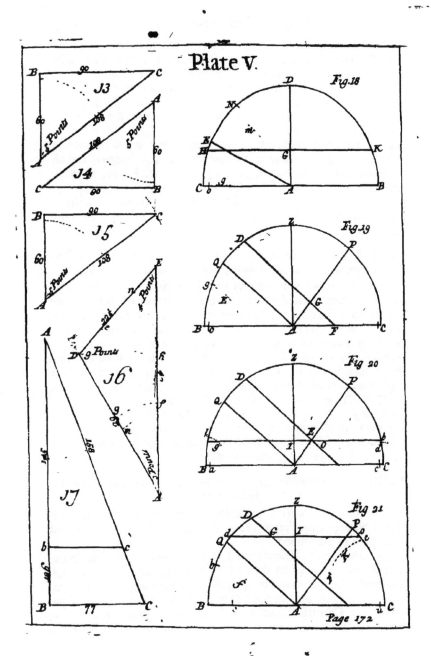

Plate V.

J3

J4

J5

J6

J7

77

Fig.18

Fig.19

Fig 20

Fig 21

ther Inches, Feet, Yards, Perches, or of any other Denomination; all other Fractions must be reduced into Decimals, and being thus considered, they are expressed as Whole Numbers upon the Line.

Note, If you call 1 at the beginning of the Line one tenth of any Integer, then 2 following must be two tenths, 3, 3 tenths, &c. and the 1 in the middle, one Integer, 2, two Integers, &c. and the 10 at the end must be 10 Integers.

But if one at the beginning be one Integer, then one in the middle must be 10 Integers, and 10 at the farther end 100 Integers, and all the intermediate Figures, 20, 30, 40, 50, 60, 70, 80, 90, so many Integers, and every longest Division between, as 21, 22, 23, 24, 25, 26, &c. single Integers, and the shortest of those Divisions, Tenths of those Integers; and so in Proportion, as $\frac{1}{10}$, 1, 10, 100, 10, 100, 1000, 100, 1000, 10000, &c

PROB. I. *Two Numbers being given, to find a third in a Geometrical Proportion, and to a third, a fourth, and to a fourth a fifth,* &c.

Example. Let the two Numbers given be 2 and 4, unto which it is required to find a third Proportional, &c. Therefore for the performance hereof by the Line of Numbers, extend the Compasses from one of the Numbers given to the other, this done, if you apply the same extent either upwards or downwards from either of the Numbers propounded, the moveable Point of the Compasses will fall upon the third Proportional required; and so the same extent being applyed the same way from the third, the moveable Point of the Compasses will fall upon the fourth Proportional, and from the fourth to a fifth, &c. and so to more, as you please; for if you extend the Compasses from 2 to 4, and turn the Compasses upwards, with one Point resting on 4, the moveable Point will fall on 8, the third Proportional, and from 8 to 16, from 16 to 32, from 32 to 64, and so forward.

PROB. II. *One Number being given to be multiplied by another Number, to find the Product.*

To resolve this Question Arithmetically, whether by Natural or Artificial Numbers, the Proportion is, As 1 to the Multiplicand, so is the Multiplier to the Product.

Example. Let the Multiplicand 8 be multiplied by 5 the Multiplier; extend the Compasses on the Line of Numbers, from 1 to the Multiplicand; the same extent being applyed the same way from the Multiplier, will cause the moveable Point to fall on the Product; for if you extend the Compasses from 1 to 8, the same extent the same way will reach from 5 to 40: And so if you would now Multiply any
Number

Number by 8, as the Compasses now stand, it is but placing one Foot in any Number given, and the moveable Point will fall on the Product, as if you place one Foot in 9, the other will fall in 72, and so from 8 it will fall in 64, and from 7 to 56, and from 6 to 48: The extent of the Compasses may be taken from 10 at the further end of the Line which you may call 1.

PROB. III. *One Number being given to be divided by another Number, to find the Quotient.*

For the Resolution of this Problem, the Proportion is thus: As the Divisor is to 1, so is the Dividend to the Quotient.

Example. Let 40 be the Dividend and let the Divisor be 8: therefore extend the Compasses on the Line of Numbers from the Divisor 8 to 1; this done, the same extent the same way shall reach from the Dividend 40 to the Quotient which is 5.

Another *Example.* Let 750 be a Number given, to be divided by 25; therefore extend the Compasses downwards from 25 to 1, then applying that extent the same way from 750, the moveable Point will fall upon 30, which is the Quotient required.

Now to know of how many Figures a Quotient ought to consist.

It will be necessary to observe how many times the Divisor may be written under the Dividend, according to the Rules of Division; for of so many Figures shall the Quotient be composed.

For *Example*: 12231 being given to be divided by 27, which said Number may be written, according to the Rules of Division, three times under the Dividend, therefore the Quotient shall consist of three Figures, and so of any other.

PROB. IV. *Three Numbers given, to find a fourth in a direct Proportion, as in the Rule of Three Direct.*

To resolve this Problem, the Proportion is thus: As the first Number given is to the second, so is the third Number to the fourth.

To perform this on the Line of Numbers, you must extend the Compasses from the first Number or Term given, to the second; which done that extent being applyed the same way from the third Term, will cause the moveable Point to fall on the fourth Term required.

Example. If the Circumference of a Circle whose Diameter is 7 Inches, be 22 Inches; what Circumference will a Circle have, whose Diameter is 14 Inches?

Therefore extend the Compasses in the Line of Numbers from 7 in the first part thereof, unto 14 in the second; this done, the same extent

† being

being apply'd the fame way from 22, will make the moveable Point to fall upon 44 Inches, the Circumference required.

Example 2 Let the Circumference of a Circle be 22 Inches, and the Diameter thereof 7 Inches, how much fhall the Diameter of a Circle be, whofe Circumference is 44 Inches?

Extend the Compaffes downwards from 22 in the fecond part of the Line, to 7 in the firft; which done, that Extent being apply'd the fame way from 44, will reach to 14, the Diameter fought.

PROB. V. *Three Numbers given, to find a Fourth in an Inverfe Proportion (or in the backward Rule of Three.)*

To refolve this Problem, the Proportion is; As the third Number is to the fecond, fo is the firft to the fourth.

Example. If 60 Men make a Trench in 45 Hours, in what time will 40 Men make fuch another?

To perform this by the Line of Numbers, extend the Compaffes from the firft of the Numbers given to the third, having both the fame Denomination: This done, if the Extent be apply'd backward from the fecond Number, the moveable Point will fall upon the fourth Number required: So that if you extend the Compaffes from 60 to 40, (thofe Terms being of the fame Denomination, *viz.* of Men) this done, the Extent being apply'd backward from 45, will reach to 67.5, the fourth Number you look for. I conclude therefore, that 40 Men will perform as much in 67 Hours and a half, as 60 Men will do in 45 Hours.

PROB. VI. *Three Numbers given, to find a 4th, in a Duplicate Proportion.*

The Ufe of this Problem is in Proportion of Lines to Superficies, or of Superficies to Lines. Now if the Denomination of the firft and fecond Terms be of Lines, then extend the Compaffes from the firft Term to the third of the fame Denomination; this done, that Extent being apply'd twice the fame way from the fecond Term, the moveable Point will ftay upon the fourth Term required.

Example 1. If the Content of a Circle whofe Diameter is 14 Inches, be 154 Inches; what will the Content of a Circle be, whofe Diameter is 28 Inches?

Here 14 and 28 having the fame Denomination, *viz.* of Lines, I extend the Compaffes from 14 to 28; then applying that Extent the fame way from 154 twice, the moveable Point will fall on 616, the fourth Proportional fought; that is, firft, from 154 to 308, and from 308 to 616.

But.

But if the firft and third Terms have the Denomination of Area's, or Contents, and the *Quæfitum* be a Line, then extend the Compaffes upon the Line of Numbers, unto half the Diftance between the firft and third Term of the fame Denomination, fo the fame extent will reach from the fecond Term given to the fourth required

Example. 2 If the Diameter of a Circle, whofe Area is 154 Inches, be 14 Inches, what Diameter will a Circle have, whofe Area is 616 Inches?

Divide the Diftance betwixt 154 and 616 into two equal parts, then fet one Foot in 14, the other fhall reach to 28, the Diameter required.

PROB VII *Three Numbers given, to find a 4th in a Triplicate Proportion.*

The Ufe of this Problem confifteth in the Proportion of Lines and Solids, &c. *coetera.*

If therefore the firft and Third Terms have the Denomination of Lines (as the Diameters of Spheres, or Sides of Solid Bodies) extend the Compaffes upon the Line of Numbers, from the firft Term to the third; this done, and that Extent apply'd three times the fame way from the fecond Term, will caufe the moveable Point to fall upon the fourth Term required

Example. 1 If an Iron Bullet, whofe Diameter is 4 Inches, weigheth 9 Pounds, what is the Weight of another Iron Bullet whofe Diameter is 8 Inches?

Therefore extend the Compaffes on the Line of Numbers from 4 to 8 ; and that extent apply'd the fame way three times from 9, the moveable Point will firft fall upon 18, then from 18 to 36; and laftly, from 36 to 72, the Weight required.

But if two given Terms be Weight or Contents of Solids, and the Diameter of a Sphere, or Side of a Cube is fought, then divide the fpace between the two given Terms of the fame Denomination into three parts, and that Diftance fhall reach from the third to the fourth Proportional.

Example 2. If an Iron Bullet that weigheth 9 Pounds be 4 Inches Diameter, what Diameter fhall the Shot of Iron be, whofe Weight is 72?

Divide the Space between 9 and 72 into three parts, and that third part fhall reach from 4 to 8, the Diameter required.

PROB. VIII *To find the Square Root of any Number under* 100000.

The Square Root of any Number is always the mean Proportional betwixt 1 and the Number propounded ; but yet with this general Caution, *viz.* If the Figures of the Number be even, that is, 2, 4, 6, 8, 10, &c. Then you muft look for the Unit, or One, at the beginning of the Line of Numbers, and the Number given in the fecond part, and
the

the Root in the firſt part; or rather reckon 10 at the end to be the Unit, and then both Root and Square will fall backwards towards the middle, in the ſecond part of the Line; but if they be odd, then the middle one will be beſt to be counted the Unit, and both Root and Square will be found from thence forward towards 10, ſo that according to this Rule, the Square Root of 9 will be found to be 3, the Square Root of 64, will be 8; the Square Root of 144, will be 12; the Square Root of 1444, to be 38; the Square Root of 57600, to be 240. And to know how many Figures any Root ought to conſiſt of, put a prick over the firſt Figure, the third, the fifth, &c. beginning from the Right Hand, and as many pricks as are noted, ſo many Figures there muſt be in the Root.

PROB IX. *To find the Cube Root of any Number under* 1000000000

The Cube Root is always the firſt of two mean Propotionals, between 1 and the Number given, and therefore will be found by dividing the Space between them into three equal Parts And to find how many Figures will be in this Root, you muſt prick over the firſt Figure, the fourth, ſeventh, &c. beginning at the Right-Hand; and ſo many pricks as you find, ſo many Figures muſt be in the Root, which Root may be eaſily found, with theſe Cautions.

1 If the laſt prick fall on the laſt Figure towards the Left-Hand, then the Unit is beſt placed at 1 in the middle of the Line, and then the Cube and Root will both fall forwards towards 10 at the end of the Line.

2. If the laſt Prick fall on the laſt Figure but one towards the Left-Hand, you may place the Unit at 1 in the beginning of the Line, and the Cube in the ſecond part of the Line, then will the Root be found in the firſt part of the Line.

If the laſt Prick fall on the laſt Figure but two, then place the Unit at 1 at the end of the Line, and then the Cube and Root will both fall backward, and be found in the ſecond part of the Line of Numbers.

Theſe Notes being obſerved, the Cube Root of 1728, will be found to be 12; and the Cube Root of 17576, will be 26; and the Cube Root of 438976, will be found 76, and the Cube Root of 8120601, will be 201; the Cube Root of 1139625, will be 225.

PROB X. *How to work a Proportion in Sines alone; or, three Sines being given, to find a fourth Proportional*

Example As Sine 22° 45′, to Sine 47° 30′, ſo is Sine 23° 15′, to a fourth Sine required;

This Problem is wrought on the Line of Sines, as the fourth Problem is on the Line of Numbers. Take the Extent from the Sine 22° 45

Z   *   on

on the Line of Sines, to the Sine 47° 30'; the fame Extent shall reach the fame way, from the Sine of 23° 15', to the Sine of 48° 50', the fourth Sine required.

PROB. XI. *How to work a Proportion in Tangents alone; or, three Tangents being given, to find a fourth Proportional.*

Example 1. As Tangent 42 deg. 40 min. to Tangent 15 deg. 20 min so is Tangent 39 deg. 8 min to the fourth Tangent required.

This Problem is wrought on the Line of Tangents, as the former Problems on the Line of Sines.

Extend the Compasses on the Line of Tangents, from the Tangent 42° 40' to the Tangent 15° 20', the fame Extent shall reach the fame way, from the Tangent 39° 8° to the Tangent 13° 35' required.

Example 2. As Tangent 14° 58', to Tangent 39° 15'; so is Tangent 47° 18', to a fourth Tangent required.

On the Line of Tangents, the Tangents above 45°, increase from 45° to 46°, 47°, 50°, 60°, &c. backwards towards the beginning of the Line: Therefore in working this Proportion, the fame Extent that reaches from 14° 58', to 39° 15', shall reach the contrary way from 47° 18', to 73° 10', the fourth Tangent required.

Example 3. As Tangent 21° 30', to Tangent 37° 20'; so is Tangent 42° 40', to a fourth Tangent required.

The Extent from the Tangent 21 deg. 30 min. to the Tangent 37° 20' if apply'd the fame way, from Tangent 42 deg. 40 min. will fall beyond 45 deg. at the end of the Line: Therefore to remedy this Inconveniency, having the distance between Tangent 21 deg. 30 min. and Tangent 37 deg. 20 min. place one point of your Compasses in the Tangent 45 deg. and let the other point fall backwards towards the beginning of the Line, and it will rest on the Tangent 27 deg. 20 min. This Point let remain fixed, and close the other Point which stands in 45 deg. to the Tangent 42 deg. 40 min. then keeping this distance, place one Point in Tangent 45 deg. the other will fall upon the Tangent 60 deg. 45 min. required.

PROB. XII. *How to Work a Proportion in Sines and Tangents together.*

Example 1. As Sine 22° 30', to Sine 37° 10'; so is Tangent 19° 40', to a fourth Tangent required.

The Extent on the Line of Sines from 22 deg. 30 min. to 37 deg. 10 min. shall reach on the Tangents from 19 deg. 40 min. to 29 deg. 25 min. required.

Example 2. As Tangent-Complement 60° 15', to Sine 56° 45'; so is the Radius to a Tangent required.

Becaufe

Becauſe there is a Tangent in the firſt place of the Proportion, and likewiſe a Tangent in the fourth, therefore this Proportion muſt be chang'd by putting Radius in the firſt Place : and inſtead of the Tangent Complement of the firſt place, take Tangent 60 deg. 15 min. (if it had been a Tangent, you muſt have taken the Tang. Comp.) and then the Proportion will remain thus :

As Radius to Sine 56° 45′; ſo is Tang. 60° 15′ to the Tang required.

The Extent from Radius, Sine 90°, to the Sine 56° 45′ on the Sines, ſhall reach from Tangent 60° 15′, to Tangent 55° 40′ required.

Example 3. As Radius to Tangent Complement 60° 15′; ſo is Tangent 55° 40′ to a Sine required.

This Proportion muſt be chang'd, becauſe there is Radius or Sine 90 deg. in the firſt Place, and a Sine required. Inſtead of the Tangent Complement 60° 15′, take the Tangent 60 deg. 15 min. and put Radius in the third Place, and ſo the Proportion follows.

As Tangent 60 deg. 15 min. to Tangent 55 deg. 40 min. ſo is Radius to the Sine ſought. Therefore the Extent from the Tangent 60 deg. 15 min to Tang. 55 deg. 40 min. ſhall reach from Radius, or Sine 90 deg. to Sine 56° 45′ required.

PROB. XIII. *How to Work Numbers and Sines together.*

Example. As 56 to 106; ſo is Sine 29° 30′ to a Sine required.

Extend the Compaſſes on the Line of Numbers, from 56 to 106, the ſame Extent ſhall reach the ſame way on the Line of Sines from 29 deg. 30 min to 68 deg. 30 min. required.

PROB. XIV. *How to Work by Numbers and Tangents together.*

Example. As 202 to 52; ſo is Tangent 73° 52′, to Tang. required.

The Extent on the Line of Numbers, from 202 to 52, ſhould reach the ſame way on the Line of Tangents from 73 deg. 52 min. to the Tangent required; but the Compaſſes ſo extended fall beyond the end of the Line, therefore this Defect muſt be remedy'd, as in the third *Example, Problem* XI. by placing the ſaid Extent in Tangent 45 deg. and letting the other Point fall backwards in the Line, which being fixed, cloſe the other Point to 73 deg. 52 min. and then placing your Compaſſes again in 45 deg. the moveable Point ſhall fall on 41 deg. 40 min. the Tangent required.

And in all Caſes in Navigation, or other Plain Triangles, where both Sides and Angles are Terms given or required; it is beſt to extend between the two given Terms that fall in one Line, (whether Numbers, Sines, or Tangents.)

Z 2

Example.

Example. In Cafe 1. of Oblique Plain Triangles, the firft and third Terms are Angles, and a Side required, but on *Gunter's* Scale it is beft to extend from Sine of ABC 45°, to Sine of BAC 33° 45'; the fame extent will reach from A C 40, to BC 31, on the Line of Numbers; which is the Side required

See the Ufe of the Meridian-line, and Equal-parts, in the Ufe of Mercator's-Chart.

SECT. III. *An Advertifement concerning the Log Line, and Half Minute Glafs.*

Seeing that the manner of keeping a Reckoning of the Ship's Way (by our *Englifh Navigators*) is commonly by the Log Line and Half-Minute Glafs, there ought to be greater care had to the truth of them, but it has been an ancient Cuftom to meafure feven Fathom between Knot and Knot upon the Log Line; which way of meafuring hath been grounded upon a meer Conjecture, that five of our Feet make a Pace and a thoufand fuch Paces make a Mile, and fixty fuch Miles make a Degree, fo that a Degree fhould contain 300000 of our Feet, and one Mile (or Minute) 5000 Feet; and becaufe an Half minute of Time is the 120th part of an Hour, the Log Line fhou'd anfwer to that Proportion, and each Knot thereof be the 120th part of a Mile, which is 41 Feet and two thirds, between each Knot on the Log Line.

But this erroneous Computation hath been fufficiently refuted by Mr. *Oughtred*, Mr *Norwood* and others

Mr *Oughtred* in his *Circles of Proportion*, p 153, doth there propofe 66 ¼ Statute Miles to anfwer to one Degree upon the Earth, each containing 5280 Feet; fo that according to this Computation, there is 349800 feet in one Degree.

And Mr. *Norwood*, in his *Seaman's Practice*, doth declare, *That (by a worthy and commendable Experiment of his) he found a Degree of the Circumference of the Earth-and the Sea to contain 367200 of our Englifh Feet* But he further confenteth, *That becaufe the Ship's Way is more than doth really appear by the Log-Line, and becaufe it is more fafe to have the Reckoning to be fomewhat before the Ship, together with the Evennefs of Numbers to allow but 360000 Feet to be one Degree, and confequently 6000 Feet to be one Minute, or the 60th part of a Degree (vulgarly called a Mile) which Number being divided by 120, giveth 50 Feet between Knot and Knot on the Log-Line, fo that upon this ground, if a Ship runneth out one of thofe Knots in a half Minute, fhe runneth one Mile (or the fixtieth part of a Degree) in an Hour, or one League and one in a mile Watch, or 4 Hours.*

Like-

Likewise Mr *Picart*, has lately measured the length of one Degree in *France*, and finds it to contain 365184 English feet, nearly agreeing with Mr. *Norwood*. But notwithstanding these Experiments, (together with the Content and Approbation of other accomplished Mathematicians in their Books of *Navigation*) have sufficiently detected this Error, yet this Truth hath not had that Entertainment, as the Excellency thereof hath deserved, because Custom hath so long prevailed against Reason.

Mr *Norwood* in his forementioned Book, hath assigned some Reasons why he supposeth this Errour hath been so long received and tolerated: I shall forbear to mention them, referring you to the Book it self But I shall assign one Reason more, which I have observed from Experience, which I hope, will in some measure help to prove the Truth of Mr. *Norwood's* Experiment, and that the Log-Line (as commonly divided) may be proved to be too short for true measure. For I have observed, that if a Half Minute Glass be made of its due length, according to the true Time, that then their Reckonings intolerably out run the Ship, and they continually complain, that those Glasses are too long· But if they have a Glass that is 5 seconds shorter than true Time, they do reasonably well agree with the Log-Line in their Reckonings; because one Errour doth ballance another, *viz.* short measure, and short time. Yet notwithstanding this Concurrence and Affinity between this Log-Line, and short Half minute Glass, it is apparent that they are both Errours, and therefore to be rejected. For I suppose it would quickly appear, that if the Log-Line were of its due length and measure, *i e* 50 foot between each Knot, and the Half minute Glass of its due length, according to true Time, there would be doubtless a greater Harmony and Concurrence of Truth, and Navigation be of more certainty than it is.

So that now it doth plainly appear, by this above mentioned Observation, that the Log-Line, as commonly divided, is too short, according to Mr. *Norwood's* Experiment, because the necessity of keeping a Concurrence in the Reckonings, is by a Glass that is too short by 5 seconds for the true time of half a minute, or 30 seconds.

But here I shall give you a Rule, to prove whether a Half-Minute Glass be of a true length or not; the way is generally approv'd to be very true, and what I have many times made Experience of, and can attest it by my own knowledge. The Experiment is mentioned by Mr. *Ph.Pips*, in his *Advancement of Navigation*, and is thus to be performed.

An easy and exact Way to measure a Half-Minute Glass, or any small Portion of Time.

Take a Bullet of any Weight whatsoever, and make fast a piece of Thread or Silk to it, being 38 ½ Inches in length, from the Center of the Bullet unto the end of the Thead, where a Noose must be made

to

to hang it on a small Pin, which is to be fastned to any Place where the Bullet may swing freely.

This *Pendulum* being thus prepared, hang its Noose on the Pin, the Thread being exactly $38\frac{1}{2}$ Inches between the Center of Gravity, and the Center of Motion each of the Swings of this Bullet (being either swift or slow) shall be a true Second of Time, so that 60 of these Swings will be the true length of a Minute, and 30 the true length of half a Minute, so by this ingenious Experiment you may know which of all your Half-Minutes is a true Glass : and if you have no Glass, you may measure any small Portion of Time by this Experiment, for half a second of Time is discovered every Time the *Pendulum* doth pass the Perpendicular, that is supposed to fall from the Pin whereon the *Pendulum* doth hang

But if it should be objected, That at Sea, when the Ship is thrown to and again by the Violence the eof, that then the *Vibrations* of the *Pendulum* may by that means be obstructed, and so the Swings to be uncertain.

A Remedy there is found against this Objection, by making the Thread 7 Inches shorter, and thereto make a small Knot, which Knot you are to hold between your Finger and Thumb, and then with the motion of your Hand, to cause the Bullet always to ascend to an Angle of 60 degree (from the Perpendicular) and so shall each Swing be e-quivalent to those before, so that if a Ship be tossed by the Violence of the Sea, yet a Man may make a shift to try this Experiment, and to measure a true Half minute of Time without the help of a Glass.

Sect. IV. *The Description and Use of the Plain-Chart.*

IN the middle is a Center, upon which there is an occult Circle described, which is divided into 32 Parts or Points ; by which are drawn several Lines quite through the Chart, representing the Rhombs or Points of the Compass, and upon these Lines are other Circles described, and Rhomb-lines drawn, Parallel to the former.

Then is the Form of the Land pourtrayed upon it, and also a Scale of Leagues to measure the Distances of Places

There is also a Meridional Line equally divided upon the Chart, which discovereth the Latitude of any Place. The several Uses follow.

1 *To find the Latitude of any Place upon the Chart.*

Take your Compasses, and set one Foot in the Place required, and ex-tend the other Foot to the nearest Distance of an East and West Line, and note where that Line doth cut the Meridian-line, (that is divided

into

into Degrees) then set one foot where it interfects the Meridian-line, and the other foot will reach upon the Meridian line, to the Latitude of the Place required.

2. *To find the Distance of one Place from another.*

If the Distance required be less then the length of the Scale, then take your Compaffes, and set one foot in one of the Places, and the other foot in the other place, then with the Extent between your Compaffes applied to your Scale of Leagues, will give the measure of the Distance of the two Places

But if the Distance between the two Places be greater then the length of the Scale, then first extend your Compaffes upon the Scale to the whole length thereof, and with that extent set one foot in one of the Places required, then direct the other foot towards the other Place by the help of a Scale or Ruler, in a Right-line, and if the Distance be great, you must turn the Distance between the Compaffes over twice, thrice, or oftner, until you come to the other place required, and if it falls out that the last extent doth fall over the second place, you must then, from the last place where the Compaffes stayed, draw in the other point, until it touch in the place required, and measure that upon the Scale of Leagues. As suppose your Scale were an hundred Leagues; and if you turn your Compaffes two or three times over, then is the Distance so many hundred Leagues, and that small Distance more, which being measured upon the Scale, it giveth the odd Leagues, and so consequently the Distance required.

3. *To find upon what Point of the Compass one Place beareth from another.*

If from the two Places propounded, there be a Rhomb-line that lieth directly from Place to Place, then there is no more trouble in it, but to look upon the small Compass upon the Chart, and see upon what Rhomb it is they bear one from another.

But in cafe a Rhomb-line doth not lie directly from one Place to the other, then extend your Compaffes from the first Place in the nearest Distance to the next Rhomb-line that you imagine in your Judgment lieth nearest a Parallel from Place to Place, and upon that Romb-line run your Compaffes along, till the other Point (being at Right-Angles with it) doth reach the other Place, and that Rhomb-line is the true Point of bearing the one from the other.

4. *To keep a Reckoning of a whole Voyage upon the Chart.*

First, It is to be understood, that you are to keep a Reckoning of every day's Work either by the Tables, or your *Instruments* (as you are before taught) or any other way necessary for such a purpose, and

and also to cast up all your Traverses for one or more Days: And then after you have so done, and brought it to the nearest Truth you can, either by Observation or otherwise, then you are to set off your Work upon your Chart, so that the Place where your Ship is, may appear to your Eye for the Satisfaction of your Mind, and for the Information of your Judgment

As suppose that you sail from the *Lizard* South-westwards, then from that very time you begin to keep your Reckoning of your several Courses, and Distances, until you have some convenient time to cast up all your Work, to find the Difference of Latitude, and your Departure from the Meridian of the *Lizard* The Difference of Latitude we will suppose to be 3°, and the Departure to be 50 Leagues, which 3°, you must subtract from the Latitude of the *Lizard*, which we suppose to be 49° 56' North, so that the Latitude the Ship is now in, is 46° 56', and 50 Leagues to the Westward

Therefore to set the place of your Ship upon your Chart you must use two pair of Plat-Compasses, with one Pair take the extent between the Latitude of 49° 56' and 46° 56', and set one Point of your Compasses in the *Lizard*, and extend the other Point towards the second place, but so that your Compasses may stand parallel to a North and South Line, which may be easily found with the other pair of Compasses, by trying whether the Legs be equi-distant from the next North and South Line This done keep one Foot of your Compasses in that Point, and with the other pair take the Departure 50 Leagues, from the Scale of Leagues, then interchange your Compasses, placing these last pair in the Point where the other pair stood, set this Departure 50 Leagues to the Westward, and so that your Compasses may stand parallel to an East and West Line, which you may try as is said before. The second Point thus found upon the Chart, is the place of the Ship (according to your Reckoning) which was required

SECT. V. *The Projection and Use of the true Chart, commonly called* Mercator's *Chart.*

Although this Chart is projected upon a Plain, and the Meridians do not incline together, and at last intersect each other as they do upon the Globe, yet (the Meridians being parallel to each other) the parallels of Latitude are contrived so at unequal Distances, that in this Projection the Rhombs are Right-lines, and the Degrees of Longitude bear the same proportion, to the Degrees of Latitude in any Parallel, that they do upon the Globe; and for the Projecting it in this manner, serves the Meridian-line, with the Line of Equal parts (the two lowest Lines upon *Gunter's* Scale) especially for a general Chart; for if you would make
a Chart

a Chart to reprefent one half of the Globe, or near it (for you cannot
go quite to the Poles, becaufe there the quantity of one Degree of Latitude is infinite) prov'de a fheet of Paper, as broad as almoft the length;
of the Scale, *viz.* that a Line drawn crofs the middle of it, may contain 180 Equal Parts; this Line fo drawn and graduated, fhall reprefent
the Æquino&ial; and thefe Divifions are 180 degrees of Longitude.
Let the length of your Paper be equal to twice its breadth, and draw
lines along each edge of it, at Right Angles with the Æquino&ial and
at each end of the 180 degrees, let thefe lines be graduated upwards and
downwards from the Æquino&ial, by the Divifions on the Meridian-
line: fo fhall you have above 85 degrees of Latitude, on each fide of
the Æquino&ial; then draw lines at every 10 degrees of thefe unequal
Divifions of Latitude parallel to the Æquino&ial, and likewife draw
Lines at each 10 Degrees of the Æquino&ial and perpendicular to it,
fo will your Meridians laft drawn interfe& the Parallels firft drawn in e-
very 10 Degrees of Latitude and Longitude: And then for laying down
any given Place, whofe Latitude and Longitude is known, take a pair of
Compaffes, and with one foot in the Latitude of the Place on the graduated Meridian, extend the other foot to the neareft Parallel or Eaft
and Weft Line, and there let them remain; then with another pair of
Compaffes, and one foot in the Longitude of the Place upon the Æqui-
no&ial, extend the other to the neareft Meridian or North and South
line, then running each pair of Compaffes along their refpe&ive lines
towards each other, the moveable Points will meet in the given Longitude and Latitude, or Point where the Place given is to be laid down,
and by two fuch Charts as thefe (which together will make a perfe&
Square) you may reprefent all the Superficies of the Earth, except a-
bout 5 Degrees of Latitude under each Pole.

But becaufe thefe Graduations are too fmall for a Chart for a particular Voyage (except at a great diftance) we fhall rather recommend
the ufe of the Table of Meridional Parts, which we fhall Illuftrate in
the following Example.

Suppofe a Ship at the *Lizard,* in Latitude 49° 55′ North, bound for
Antegoa, in Lat. 17° 00′ North, Difference of Longitude 54° 07′ Weft,
and it is required to make a *Mercator's-Chart* for this particular
Voyage. *Plate* 6.

Take a fheet of ftrong Writing-Paper, as large as you intend your
Chart fhall be, multiply your Difference of Longitude 54° by 60, and
the product 3240, is the Difference of Longitude in Minutes; and the
Meridional Difference of Latitude is 2471; then chufe fome Scale of E-
qual Parts, of which 3240 may be the breadth, and 2471 the length,
or depth; with a convenient allowance for Ruling, or what you think

A a   fit

fit to draw for Ornament about the out-side of it · then towards the North-east corner, because your Course is South Westerly, assume a Point as at L, to represent the *Lizard*, and draw L n, upon which set the Meridional Difference of Latitude from L to n, and from n draw the line n M, and thereupon set the Difference of Longitude from n to M, then is L n 2471, the Meridional Difference of Latitude, and n M 3240 the Diff Longitude, and because it will too much confuse the Draught to incert Meridians and Parallels to every Degree, we shall only draw them for every other Degree of Latitude and Longitude, and first for the Parallels of Latitude the, Meridional Diff. Latitude between *Lat* 50 and *Lat* 48 is 183, which set on the line L n from L to 48, and draw the line 48.48 parallel to n M, and thus find the Meridional Diffe-rence of Latitude between *Lat* 50 and *Lat* 46, which is 359, set that from L to 46, and draw the line 46 46, and so for the rest of the Parallels of Latitude And then for the Degrees of Longitude, which in these Charts are parallel and equi-distant, take 120 of the same Equal parts, and set from n to 2, and from 2 to 4, and from 4 to 6, *&c*. be-cause you mark but every other Degree, and draw the Meridians 2, 2. 4, 4, *&c* parallel to L n, and then if any Head-lands or Islands, *&c*. fall in this Chart you may by the Directions given in the making of a Gene-ral Chart, lay them down in their proper places.

   Example I desire to lay down the Island of St *Michael* in Latitude 38° 00' North, and Longitude 17° 18' West from the *Lizard*; I set ore foot of the Compasses in Longitude 17° 18', and extend the other to the next Meridian, which is 18°, and running one foot along the Meri-dian of 18° I observe where the other cuts the Latitude of 38° (which in this Chart is a Parallel drawn) and there is the Island of St. *Michael*, &c. and in this manner you may lay down any Island or Head-land, as *Ma-dera*, and *Teneriff*, &c. also the Capes or Principal Places on the Coast. of *Africa* may be thus found, and the form of the Land drawn from Place to Place as you may see in this *Example*.

   Now to find the Distance between any two Places, you have a Scale of *English* Leagues, fitted to all the Latitudes in the Chart, *viz*. from 15 to 50 Degrees of Latitude as you see the lines numbred up each side, the lines that go from top to bottom, intersecting the Parallels of Lati-tude at every 10 leagues; so that each Parallel contains 100 leagues in the Latitude that the Parallel is numbred with.

   Example I desire to know the Distance between the Island *Teneriff* and Cape *Bajador*, on the Coast of *Africa*; I extend the Compasses from one place to the other, and applying that extent to the Scale upon the Parallel of 28, I find it is 56 leagues.

Again

Again, if you would lay down any Courfe and Diftance or Traverfe, it's done with the fame and no more trouble then upon the Plain Chart, as for Inftance :

A Ship at the *Lizard*, bound for *Madera*, fhe fails South 52 Degrees, Weft 100 Leagues; and then S. S W. the fame diftance, and S. S. E. 100 Leagues more, and then again S. S. W. 100 Leagues. But having no Obfervation, and fuppofing himfelf to be near the Latitude of the Ifland, he fteer'd Weft 70 Leagues, but made no Land, I demand how the Ifland bears from him, and at what Diftance.

Here you fail from Latitude 49° 55', and fteer to the Southward, and may forefee that Latitude 48° will be neareft the middle Latitude you fail through (for you need not regard Minutes nor Half-degrees in this Cafe) therefore take 100 Leagues from the Parallel of 48° in the Scale, and fet from L to g South 52 deg Weft. Then from the Parallel of 45, the next middle Latitude, take 100 Leagues, and fet S.S.W. from g to h ; and from the Parallel of 40, fet 100 Leagues from h to k, and from the Parallel of 35 fet 100 Leagues from k to m, which brings the Ship to Latitude 33° neareft; therefore from the Parallel of 33 take off 70 Leagues, and fet Weft from m to d : And thus you may fee the Longitudes and Latitudes you came through, and where you are now arrived, which is in Latitude 32° 59', and Longitude Weft from the *Lizard* 12° 36', as the Chart plainly difcovers without any other Operation.

Now if you would prove the Truth hereof you may find the Difference of Latitude and Departure for the feveral Courfes, and reduce them all to one, as you are taught in the Ufe of the Traverfe-Table, and you will find the Difference of Latitude 16° 56, which fubtracted from 49°. 55' the Latitude failed from leaves 32° 59' the Latitude come to. The Meridional Difference of Latitude is 1369. Then, As Diff. Lat. 1016, To Merid. Diff. Lat. 1369.; So Departure which you will find to be 561, To Diff. Long. 756' or 12° 36', as before, and Courfe to Weft-end of *Madera* S. E. by S. ¾ S. *fere*, 16 Leagues.

How to make the Scale for the Mercator's *Chart (fuppofe of 100 Leagues, as in this* Example.)

Firft, Find the length of 100 Leagues, in the leaft Latitude (which here is 14) thus, As Sine Comp. Lat. 14°, To Radius; So is 300 Miles (the length of your Scale) To 309' or 5° 9', which taken off the graduated Line of Longitude, let it be the length of the loweft Line of the Scale P Q, upon the middle of which Line (at 50) raife the Perpendicular 50. 50. fubtract the Natural Secant of the leaft Latitude 14°, from the Natural Secant of the greateft Latitude 50°, and the Remainder

.A a 2

5251 taken from a Scale of equal Parts, set from 50 to 50 upwards upon the foresaid Perpendicular, and through 50 draw the uppermost Line
at Right Angles with the Perpendicular, and Parallel to the bottom
Line P Q, that Line represents the Parallel of 50°. Then having found
by the foregoing Proportion the length of 100 Leagues, in Lat. 50°,
which is ·467′, or 7° 47′; take half thereof, *viz* 3° 53½′ from the
graduated Line of Longitude, and set it both ways upon the foresaid
Parallel of 50 from the middle of the Line (where it is cut by the Perpendicular) to each end; so shall the distance between those two Marks
be the measure of 100 Leagues in Lat. 50°. Then from the Extremities
of the top and bottom Lines, draw the Side Lines, 50 P and 50 Q.
Now to find the intermediate Parallels, subtract the Natural Secant of
the least Lat. 14, from the Natural Secant of each greater Latitude,
as 15, 16, 17, &c to 50 the several Remainders taken in your Compasses from the same Scale of equal Parts, by which you measured the
middle Perpendicular Line, and set upon the same Line from the Line
P Q upwards shall determine the Points in that Line through which the
several Parallels must pass; therefore through these Marks draw Lines
parallel to the Line P Q, they represent the several Parallels required.
Then divide the uppermost and lowest Parallel each into 100 equal Parts,
marking them both with 10, 20, 30, &c. and between those Divisions
marked with the same Number, on each Line, draw straight Lines thro'
the Scale; these Lines will also divide each Parallel into 100 equal Parts
or Leagues, upon which you may measure your Distance in any Parallel
as before is taught.

To make it Geometrically.

Take 300 miles (the length of the Scale) off the Degrees of Longitude,
which is 5 degrees (at 60 miles to a degree, which in this Case you always allow) and with that extent sweep a half Circle, as you see in the
fourth Figure in the Use of the *Plain Scale* in this Chapter, *Sect.* 1. and
upon the end of the Diameter A B as at B, erect the Perpendicular B T;
then from the Center C, and through the given Degree of Latitude upon the Periphery of the Circle draw a Line to cut the aforesaid Perpendicular; that Line applied to the Scale shall be the length of 100
Leagues, in that Degree of Latitude through which it was drawn.
    Hence the length of any Number of Leagues in any Latitude, is no
more but the Secant of the Latitude to a Radius, consisting of the
same Quantity of Leagues taken from the Equinoctial, allowing 20 Leag.
(or 60 Miles) to a Degree. And by this Scale thus made, if you take
off 100 Leagues in the Parallel of 34° (the next whole Degree greater
than the middle Latitude of the Chart) and turn it along the pricked
                                                                    Line

Line L M, the Diſtance from the *Lizard* to *Antegoa*, will be found to be 1098 Leagues ; and the Arch a b ſhews the Courſe South 53° 10' Weſt, or South Weſt almoſt ¾ Weſt; both which are ſufficiently exact. But if you do not make your own Charts, nor cannot buy thoſe that have ſuch Scales in them, then with reſpect to the common *Mercator's* Charts, obſerve the following Directions.

1. *To find the Latitude of any Place in theſe Charts.*

This Operation upon theſe Charts is in all reſpects like that which has already been delivered for the ſame purpoſe, in the Uſe of the plain Sea-Chart; for if you ſet one Point of your Compaſſes in the place whoſe Latitude is required, and open them in the ſhorteſt Diſtance to the next Eaſt and Weſt Line, obſerving where it interſects the graduated Meridian, and then place one Point in that Interſection, turning your Compaſſes upwards or downwards, according as the Place lies, from the Eaſt and Weſt Line, and the moveable Point ſhall ſhew upon the ſaid Meridian the Latitude of the Place required.

Suppoſe the Latitude of *Uſhant* were required by this Chart.

If you take the neareſt Extent to an Eaſt and Weſt Line, and place that Diſtance from the Interſection on the graduated Meridian, as is before directed, you will find the Latitude of *Uſhant* to be 48 deg. 30 min. Northerly.

2. *To find the Longitude of a Place, and conſequently the Difference of Longitude in Degrees, between any two Places ſituate upon the Chart.*

To find the Longitude of any Place upon the Chart, ſet one Point of your Compaſſes in the ſaid Place, and take the neareſt Diſtance to the next North and South Line, and obſerve where this Line interſects the Equinoctial ; and keeping the ſame Extent in your Compaſſes, place one Point in the Interſection, and turning the Compaſſes the ſame way that the Place, whoſe Longitude is ſought, lies from the North and South Line, the moveable Point reſting in the Equinoctial, will ſhew the Longitude required.

Suppoſe the Longitude of *Barbadoes* were required.

If you place the point of your Compaſſes in the Iſland of *Barbadoes* in this Chart, and take the ſhorteſt Extent to the next North and South Line, placing the ſame at the Interſection in the Equinoctial, as is directed you will find the Longitude of *Barbadoes* to be in theſe Charts 58° 03' from *London*. But the Longitude of Places being various, according to the Place from whence it begun, ſome reckoning it from *London*, ſome from *Teneriff, &c.* the chief Buſineſs will be to find the Difference of Longitude between any two Places; which is thus to be performed.

When

When you have found the Longitude of the two Places, if they have the same Name, their Difference, but if of contrary Names, their Sum is the *Difference* of Longitude between the two Places

Suppose the two Places were the *Lizard* in the Longitude 5° 14' W. and *Barbadoes* in the Longitude 58° 03' W. subtracting 5° 14' from 58° 03', the Remainder 52° 49' is the Diff. Long.

Again, Suppose the two Places were the *Lizard*, as before, and St. *Thomas's* Isle in the Longitude 9° 58' E. Add 5° 14' to 9° 58 the Sum will be 15° 12' the Difference of Longitude between the two given Places.

3. *To know how one Place bears from another.*

For the performance of this *Problem*, lay the Edge of a Ruler from one Place to another, and with a pair of Compasses try which of the Rhomb lines the edge of the Ruler is the nearest Parallel; which being found, that sheweth the Point of the Compass the two places bear one from another.

Suppose the Bearing of *Barbadoes* from the *Lizard* were required.

Therefore lay the edge of the Ruler upon both Places, and you will find, that South West ½ a Point Westerly, is the nearest Parallel thereto, which is the bearing of *Barbadoes* from the *Lizard*, and the opposite Point North East ½ East, the bearing of the *Lizard*, from *Barbadoes*.

4. *To find the Distance of two Places upon* Mercator's Chart.

If both Places be in one and the same Latitude, take with your Compasses the length of a degree of the Meridian at that Latitude, (taking half the degree above, and half beneath the Latitude) for so oft as you shall find that length between the two Places, so many times 20 Leagues are there betwixt them; but if the Distance be great, for Expedition, you may take five times the length of that degree, and counting it for 100 Leagues, proceed as before.

Suppose the Distance were required between the Point of *Ushant* and Cape-bona-vista in *New-found-land.*

The Distance taken as before about the Latitude of 49°, you will find it to be 609 Leagues.

But if two Places have not the same Latitude, the Equinoctial not coming between them, substract the lesser Latitude out of the greater; but if the Equinoctial cometh between them, add both Latitudes together, so have you the difference of Latitude between both Places.

Now if both Places have the same Longitude, so many degrees as there are in the difference of Latitude, so many times 20 Leagues is the Distance.   But

But if the Places differ both in Latitude and Longitude, then look how many degrees the Difference of Latitude contains, so many degrees of the Equinoctial take between your Compasses; then lay a Ruler to both Places whose distance you seek, and observe where the Ruler crosses the Equinoctial, or some other East and West Line, (or Parallel of Latitude) and leading one foot on the Equinoctial or other Parallel, move forwards the other also Parallel-wise, keeping always that distance, till it cross the Rhomb of those two Places, in such sort, that one foot resting by the Edg of the Ruler, the other carried about, may but only touch the Equinoctial, or other Parallel cut by the Edge of the Ruler; then take with your Compasses the Segment, or part of that Rhomb between that place and the crossing of the Equinoctial or Parallel, which measure in the Equinoctial, and see how many degrees are contained betwixt them, so many times 20 Leagues is the distance of those two Places.

Or, if that Segment of the said Rhomb be greater than can well be taken with the Compasses, take the length of 5 degrees of the Equinoctial between your Compasses, and look how oft you can find that length in the Segment of the Rhomb aforesaid, for so many hundred leagues is the Distance of those two Places

If the Distance from the *Lizard* to *Barbadoes* were required, the difference of Latitude between those Places is 3 5° 45′ therefore take 36° 46′ from the Equinoctial, and laying a Ruler over both places, until it will cross some Parallel of Latitude; then keeping this distance of degrees in your Compasses, apply one Point to the edg of the Ruler, so that the other Point may but just touch the Parallel crossed by the Ruler; the Segment of the Rhomb between the Point where the Compasses stay, and the Intersection by the Ruler and Parallel of Latitude; measured by the degrees of the Equinoctial, gives the distance about 1140 Leagues, which was required: But if your Chart have such a Scale to it as we have just now Described, you may save all this trouble and take off your Distance at one extent, as you are already taught:

There is nothing else that will be of any Difficulty in the common Use of this Chart, if these Plain Directions be understood.

SECT. VI. *The Description and Use of the* Globes.

OF *Globes* there are two forts, one is *Terrestrial,* and the other *Cælestial.*

The *Terrestrial* hath on the *Superficies* of the Body pourtrayed and described the whole Form and Fashion of the Earth and Sea, with the Circles of the Sphere, as Colures, Equinoctial, Tropicks, &c.   The

The *Cœlestial Globe* hath on it Surface the Conftellations of all the known Stars in the Heavens, placed in their Latitudes and Longitudes, Right Afcenfions, and Declinations, drawn into feveral Images and Figures, according to the Fictions of the Ancients, with the Circles of the Sphere, as in the *Terreftrial Globe.*

Geographical Definitions neceffary to be underftood.

Defin. I The Globe of the Earth is a Spherical Body, compofed of Earth and Water, and is divided into Continents, Iflands and Seas.

II A *Continent* is a great quantity of Land, not divided nor feperated by the Sea, wherein are many Kingdoms and Principalities; as *Europe, Afia,* and *Africa,* are one Continent, and *America* is another.

III. An Ifland is fuch a part of the Earth that is environed round with Water, as the Ifland of *England* and *Scotland,* and alfo *Ireland,* the Ifle of *Wight, Barbadoes, &c*

IV. A *Peninfula* is fuch a part of Land as is almoft encompaffed about with Water, and is only joined with the Land by an *Ifthmus* ; fuch is that great part of Land in *America,* called *Peruviana,* and *Morea* in the *Levant.*

V. An *Ifthmus* is a narrow Neck of Land, which joineth the *Peninfula* to the Continent.

VI A *Promontory* is fome high Mountain, or great Cape of Land, that fhooteth it felf into the Sea; as *Cape Bon Efperance,* or *Cape de Verde* in *Africa.*

VII. The *Ocean* is a general Collection of the Waters, which (except where the Land lies above it) environeth the Earth on every fide.

VIII. The *Sea* is part of the Ocean, to which we cannot come but through fome Strait, as the *Mediterranean* and *Baltick* Sea.

IX A *Strait* is a part of the *Ocean,* reftrained within narrow Bounds, and opening a way to the Sea; as the *Straits* of *Gibralter* that leadeth into the *Mediterranean,* and the *Sound* that leadeth into the *Baltick* Sea.

X. A *Creek* is a fmall narrow part of the Sea, or Rivers that go up but little way into the Land.

XI. A *Bay* is a great Inlet of the Land, as the Bay of *Bifcay,* and the Bay of *Mexico.*

XII. A *Gulph* is a great Inlet of the Land, deeper than a Bay; fuch is the Gulph of *Venice,* and the Gulph of *Florida.*

XIII. A *Climate* is a certain fpace of Earth and Sea, that is included within the fpace of two Parallels; and of them there have been anciently accounted feven.

1. *Dia Meroes.* 2. *Dia Syenes.* 3. *Dia Alexandria.* 4. *Dia Rhodes.* 5. *Dia Rhomes.* 6. *Dia Boriftthenes.* 7. *Dia Ripheos.* But now there are

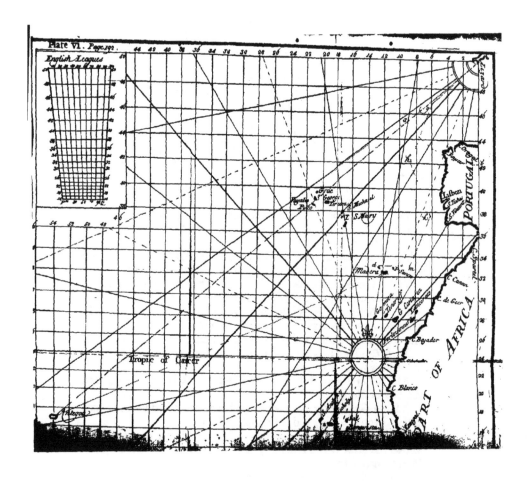

Plate VI. Page 192.

English Leagues

PORTUGAL

PART OF AFRICA

Tropic of Cancer

Lisbon

Madera

C. Canar

C. de Geer

C. Bojador

C. Blanco

S. Mary

are 24 on each side of the Equator being limited by every half Hours Increase of the Day, Beginning at the Equator, and ending where the longest Day is 24 Hours.

XIV. A *Zone* is a certain space of the Earth, contained between certain Circles of the Sphere, and are thus divided:

The Earth is divided into five *Zones*, viz. one Torrid or Burning *Zone*, two Temperate, and two Frozen *Zones*

The Torrid *Zone* is that which is on each side the Equinoctial, bounded by the Tropicks of *Cancer* and *Capricorn*

The two Temperate *Zones* are contained between each Tropick, and the Polar Circles.

The two Frigid or Frozen *Zones*, are contained between each Polar Circle and their respective Poles

The *Globe* of the Earth is divided into these four Parts, *Viz.*

EUROPE,	AFRICA,
ASIA,	AMERICA,

EUROPE, is bounded from *Africa* by the *Mediterranean Sea*, on the East with the River *Tanais*, and on the West with the Western Ocean; and containeth these Provinces.

Germany,	Spain,	Sweedland,	Hungary,
Italy,	Denmark,	Muscovy,	Sclavony,
France,	Norway,	Poland,	Greece,
Portugal,	Romania	P. of Tartary,	Dalmatia,

The Principal Islands are,

Great Britain,	Candia,	Sardina,	Cyprus,
Ireland,	Sicily,	Corsica,	

ASIA is bounded on the North with the Northern Ocean, and on the South with the Red-Sea; on the East with the East Indian Ocean, and on the West with the Flood *Tanais*.

The Principal Regions are,

Anatolia,	Armenia,	Assyria,	Persia,	China,
Syria,	Arabia,	Mesopotamia,	Mogul,	India, and the
Palestine;	Georgia,	Chaldea,	Tartaria,	Islands thereof.

AFRICA, is bounded on the East with the Red-Sea, on the West with the *Atlantick* Ocean, on the South with the Southern Ocean, and on the North with the *Mediterranean Sea*.

The Provinces are,

Egypt,	Barbary,	Æthiopia,
Abyssines,	Monomotapa,	Nubia,

The Principal Islands are,

Madagascar, or St. Laurence,	St. Thomas,	Cape de Verde.
The Canary Islands,	The Madera Islands,	Islands.

B b

AME-

A M E R I C A is bounded on the East with the *Atlantick* Ocean, on the West with the *Pacifick* South Sea, on the North with the Northern Ocean, and on the South with the *Magellanick Sea.*

It confifts of two, *viz.* North and South *America.*

The Provinces of North *America* are,

New France,	*New Jerfey,*	*Carolina*
New England,	*Maryland,*	*Terra Florida,*
Penfylvania,	*Virginia,*	*Mexico, or New Spain,*

And *Groenland,* not yet fully difcovered.

The Chief Iflands are,

Ifeland,	*Hifpaniola,*	*Jamaica,*
Greenland,	*Cuba,*	*New-found-land.*
California,	*Porto Rico,*	*Barbadoes,* and the reft of the *Caribbe* Iflands.

The Provinces of South *America* are,

Brazil,	*Chili,*	*Amazones,*	*Magellanick-Land.*
Terra Firma,	*Peru,*	*Paragua,*	*Guianea,*

One Ifland, *Terra del Fuego.*

The Names of the Seas in feveral Parts of the World.

Mar del Nort, Narrow Sea, Mediterranean Sea, Mare Majore, Mare Pacificum, Mare Cafpium, Eaft-Indian Sea, Perfian Sea, Red Sea.

The Names and Numbers of the Stars of each Conftellation on the Cœleftial Globe.

Northern Conftellations are 23, *viz.*

1 *Urfa Major,*	7	13 *Serpentarius,*	24
2 *Urfa Minor,*	27	14 *Serpens,*	18
3 *Draco,*	31	15 *Sagitta,*	5
4 *Cepheus*	11	16 *Aquila,*	9
5 *Bootes*	22	17 *Antinous,*	7
6 *Corona Borealis*	8	18 *Delphinus,*	10
7 *Engonafes, or Hercules,*	29	19 *Equiculus,*	4
8 *Lyra*	10	20 *Pegafus,*	20
9 *Olor, or Cygnus,*	17	21 *Andromeda,*	23
10 *Caffiopeia,*	13	22 *Triangulum,*	4
11 *Perfeus,*	26	23 *Coma Berenices.*	14
12 *Auriga,*	14		

Zodiack

Zodiack Conftellations, 12, viz.

1 *Aries,*	13	7 *Libra,*	8
2 *Taurus,*	23	8 *Scorpio,*	21
3 *Gemini,*	18	9 *Sagitarius,*	31
4 *Cancer,*	9	10 *Capricornus,*	28
5 *Leo,*	26	11 *Aquarius,*	42
6 *Virgo,*	27	12 *Pifces.*	34

Southern Conftellations, 27.

1 *Cetus,*	22	15 *Pifces Auftrius,*	11
2 *Orion,*	31	16 *Grus,*	13
3 *Flumen Eridanus,*	34	17 *Phænix,*	15
4 *Lepus,*	12	18 *Indus,*	12
5 *Canis Major,*	18	19 *Pavo,*	20
6 *Canis, Minor,*	2	20 *Apus avis Indica,*	11
7 *Argo Navis,*	41	21 *Apis Mufca,*	4
8 *Hydra,*	25	22 *Camelion,*	10
9 *Crater,*	7	23 *Triangulum Aufter,*	5
10 *Corvus,*	7	24 *Pifcis volans,*	7
11 *Centaurus,*	37	25 *Dorado,*	7
12 *Fera, aut Lupus,*	19	26 *Toucan,*	8
13 *Ara,*	7	27 *Hydrus.*	21
14 *Corona Auft.*	10		

The Globes are compofed of thefe Parts.

Firft, *The Body or Globe it felf.*
Secondly, *The Brazen-Meridian.*
Thirdly, *The Quadrant of Altitude.*
Fourthly, *The Hour-Circle and Index.*
Fifthly, *The Wooden-Frame in which it Stands,* called the *Horizon.*

The *Globe* doth reprefent the natural Situation and Pofition of the Earth and Heavens, and performs Problems of the Sphere, either in *Aftronomy* or *Geography.*

1. The *Brazen-Meridian* is divided into 4 Parts or Quadrants, each being divided into 90°; within this Meridian the Body of the Globe turneth upon the Axis, being two ftrong Wires.

2. The *Hour-Circle* is a flat Ring of Brafs, fastned upon the North-part of the Meridian, and is divided into the 24 Hours of a natural Day; and each of thefe Hours is fubdivided into Halves and Quarters.

3. The *Quadrant of Altitude* is a long and thin Slip of Brafs divided into 90°, and is to move up and down upon the Surface of the Globe to

any

any Pofition required : and when placed in the *Zenith*, the Edge thereof reprefenteth an *Azimuth*, and the Divifions fhew the *Almicanters*, or Circles of Altitude

4. The *Horizon* is a flat and round Frame of *Wood*, in which the *Brazen-Meridian*, and confequently the whole Globe doth move, being divided into a *Kalender*, fhewing the Day of the Month, the Place of the Sun, the Rhombs, *&c.*

PROB. I. *How to fet the Globe to the Latitude of a Place*

You have next the Edge of the Wooden-Frame, which Reprefents the *Horizon*, the 32 Points of the Compafs, by which you know which is the North and which is the South part of the *Horizon*, therefore put the North Pole of the Globe to the North, and the South Pole to the South part of the Frame, and if you are in the North Latitude draw up the North Pole (but if in South Latitude the South Pole) of the Globe till the given Degree of Latitude upon the *Brazen-Meridian* under the Elevated Pole juft cut the *Horizon*, and then is the Globe fet to the Latitude of the place and fit for ufe.

The Use of the Terreftrial Globe.

PROB. II. *To find the Latitude of any Place upon the Globe.*

Firft find the place required upon the Globe, then turn the Globe about, until the Place whofe Latitude is required be juft under the *Brazen-Meridian*, then note what Degree ftands againft it on the Meridian ; that is the Latitude of the Place which was required.

Example. Let it be required to find the Latitude of *Rome* : Turn the Body of the Globe about till *Rome* be juft under the Brafs Meridian, and you will fee 41° 51' to be right againft it, which is the Latitude of *Rome*.

PROB. III. *To find the Longitude of any Place upon the Globe.*

Turn the Body of the Globe about, till the Place whofe Longitude you require, comes under the Meridian : then obferve what Degree of the Equinoctial is cut by the Brafs-Meridian, and the Number of thofe Degrees is the Longitude of a place you feek for.

Example. Let it be required to find the Longitude of *Rome*, as before, therefore bring *Rome* under the Meridian, which being done, the Meridian will cut the Equinoctial in 36°½, the Longitude of Rome required, if you ufe Globes that begin Longitude at the Ifland of St. Michaels ; but of late the Globes frequently begin to Reckon Longitude from the Meridian of *London*, and then if you turn the Globe as before, you will find *Rome* in Longitude 11° 38' Eaft from *London*, &c.

PROB.

PROB. IV. *To find the Diſtance of any two places on the Globe.*

To perform this, lay the beginning of a Deg. on the *Quadr.* of *Altitude* upon one of the Places required, and note how many Deg there are contained between them; which is the diſtance between the ſaʼd places.

Example. Let it be required to find the Diſtance between *London* and *Rome*, therefore ſay the Quadrant of Altitude from one Place to another, and you will find 13° to be intercepted between the aforeſaid Places, which is the Diſtance between *London* and *Rome*

PROB. V. *To find the Poſition of Places one from another.*

Firſt ſet the Globe to the Lat. of one of the Places, and bring the ſame Place under the Meridian, and extend the Quadr of Altitude, being fixed over the firſt Place to the other Place, and the end of the Quadr ſhall point out on the Horizon the Poſition that one Place hath from the other.

Ex. Let it be required to know the Poſition of *Rome*, from *London*, therefore bring *London* under the Meridian, and there fit the Quadr. of Altitude, and lay the edge thereof upon *Rome*, and the end of the Quadr. of Altitude will point to 53°, which is the Poſition of *Rome* from *London*.

The Uſe of the Cæleſtial Globe.

PROB. VI. *The Day of the Month being given, to find what Sign and Degree the Sun is in.*

Firſt find the day of the Month in the Kalender, on the Horizon, and right againſt it you ſhall find the Sign and Degree in which the Sun is.

Example. Let it be required to find the Sun's Place on the fifth of *May*. You muſt find the fifth of *May* in the Kalender, and right againſt it you will find 25 degrees in *Taurus*, which is the Sun's Place that Day.

PROB. VII. *How to place the Index of the Hour Circle for any Day in the Year.*

The Place of the Sun found (as in the laſt Propoſition) you muſt find that degree on the Ecliptick line of the Globe, and bring that degree to the Brazen-Meridian; then ſtaying the Globe there, turn about the Index of the Hour-Circle till it points juſt upon the upper Line of XII in the Hour-Circle, which being done, the Hour-Circle is rectified for that Day.

PROB. VIII. *To find the Time of the Sun's Riſing and Setting.*

The Hour Circle being rectified, and the Globe ſet to the Latitude, then turn the Globe about till the degree of the Ecliptick in which the Sun is, cut the Eaſt ſide of the Horizon; and then caſting your Eye upon.

on the Hour Circle, the Index will shew you the Time of the Sun's-Rising. And the Globe being turned about till the degree of the Sun cut the West-side of the *Horizon,* the Index will shew you the Time of the Sun's Setting

Ex Let it be required to find the Sun's Rising and Setting the fifth day of *May,* in the Lat of *London,* the Sun being then in 25° of *Taurus.*

First, find the 25th deg. of *Taurus* in the Ecliptick-line, which being turned to the East part of the Horizon, you will find the Index point to a quarter after four of the Clock, the same Point of the Ecliptick being turned to the West part of the Horizon, you will find the Hour Index point to 3 quarters past 7, the Time of Sun-setting.

Having the time of the Sun's Rising and Setting, you may find the Length of the Day and Night, for the Time of the Sun's Rising being doubled, gives the Length of the Night, and the Time of Sun setting doubled, the length of the Day.

Example. The fifth of *May,* the Sun riseth a quarter past 4 of the Clock which being doubled, is 8 Hours and a half, the length of the Night; and the Sun-setting, which is at 7 a Clock and three quarters, being doubled, is 15½ Hours, the Length of the Day.

PROB. IX. *To find the Sun's Amplitude.*

The Amplitude of the Sun is an Arch intercepted between the East or West-points, and that part of the Horizon where the Sun riseth or setteth.

The finding of the Amplitude differeth little from the last Proposition: For having brought the Degree of the Sun's Place to the Horizon, you count how many Degrees of the Horizon are intercepted between the East or West-point, and that part of the Horizon where the Sun either riseth or setteth

Example The fifth of *May,* I desire to know the Sun's Amplitude in the Latitude of *London,* therefore bring the Place of the Sun that Day to the Horizon, and you find $31°\frac{1}{4}$ intercepted between the Point of the Horizon, and the East-point, which is the Sun's Amplitude Northerly.

PROB X *How to find the Sun's Declination any Day of the Year.*

The Declination of the Sun is an Arch of the Meridian, intercepted between the Sun's Place and the Equinoctial; to find which, you must bring the Degree in which the Sun is, to the Brazen Meridian, and there stay it, and count how many Degrees of the Meridian are contained between the Equinoctial and the Sun's Place, and that is the Declination.

Example. I would know what Declination the Sun hath the fifth of *May,* the Sun being 25° in *Taurus,* which being brought to the Meridi-

an

an, you will find 19°intercepted between that Point and the Equinoctial on the Brazen Meridian, which is the Declination required.

PROB. XI. *To find the Meridian Altitude of the Sun any Day of the Year.*

The Meridian Altitude of the Sun is an Arch of the Meridian, intercepted between the Horizon, and the Degree in which the Sun is. To
perform which, turn the Globe about till the Degree of the Sun be juft
under the Brafs Meridian Then ftaying the Globe there, count how many Degrees are contained between the Place of the Sun under the Meridian, and the Horizon; and that is the Meridian Altitude.

Example On the fifth of *May* it is required to find the Meridian Altitude, of the Sun that Day in the Latitude of *London*, the Sun's Place
in the Ecliptick is 25° in *Taurus*, therefore bring that Degree under
the Brafs Meridian, and you will find 57° and a half to be intercepted
upon the Brafs Meridian, between the Place of the Sun and the Horizon; that is the Meridian Altitude of the Sun that Day.

PROB. XII. *How to know what Altitude the Sun fhall have any Hour of
the Day, on any Day of the Year*

Having found the Sun's Place, and rectified the Globe to the Latitude,
and the Index of the Hour Circle for the Day propofed, turn the Globe
about till the Index of the Hour Circle be juft upon the Time when you
fhould know the Altitude, then ftaying the Body of the Globe here, bring
the Quadrant of Altitude, being fcrœd on the Zenith, and lay it over
the Sun's Place: Then the Number of Degrees contained betwixt
the Horizon and the Sun's Place, counted on the Quadrant of Altitude,
is the Altitude of the Sun at that Hour.

Example Let the Time given be the tenth Day of *April*, in the Lati-
tude of *London*, at which time (by the fixth Propofition) I find that the
Sun is in the beginning of *Taurus*, and I would know what Altitude the
Sun will have at nine of the Clock in the Morning. The Index of the
Hour-Circle being rectified for that Day, turn the Body of the Globe
about till the Index of the Hour-Circle lies juft upon 9 of the Clock;
then ftaying the Globe there, lay the Quadrant of Altitude on the Sun's
Place and the number of Degrees between the Horizon and the Sun's
Place (counted upon the Quadrant of Altitude) is the Height of the Sun,
which here I find to be 36° at that time, or at three in the Afternoon;
for the Sun hath the fame Altitude (nearly) at 9, 8, 7, 6, &c. in the
Morning, as it hath 3, 4, 5, 6, &c. in the Evening.

PROB

PROB XIII *How to find the Hour of the Day by the Globe.*

This Proposition cannot be performed conveniently by the Globe only, but the Altitude of the Sun must be first taken by some Instrument, and then this is but the Converse of the former Proposition which it performs thus The Globe being set to the Latitude, and the Index of the Hour Circle rectified, turn the Globe about till the Degree of the Sun's Place meet with the Altitude, taken by the Instrument, upon the Quadrant of Altitude, and then will the Index on the Hour-Circle shew you the Hour of the Day , do the like by a Star to find the Hour of the Night.

PROB. XIV *To find both the Right and Oblique Ascension, and Oblique Descension of the Sun*

The Globe being set to your Latitude, bring the Degree of the Sun to the *Brazen-Meridian*, there staying it ; see what degree of the *Equinoctial* is cut by the said *Brazen-Meridian*, and that is the *Right Ascension* of the Sun that Day.   So the Sun being in the beginning of *Taurus*, his *Right Ascension* will be found to be about 28° , and bringing the Sun's Place to the East-part of the *Horizon*, in the Latitude of *London*, the *Horizon* will cut the *Equinoctial* in 13°; which is the Oblique Ascension, and bringing the Sun's Place to the West part of the Horizon, the Horizon will cut the Equinoctial in 42³, the Oblique Descension.

PROB. XV. *To find the Meridian Altitude of a Star, or the Altitude of a Star at any time.*

To find the Meridian Altitude, let the Globe be set to your Latitude and then turn the Body of the Globe about, till the Star be under the Brazen Meridian, and then the Number of Degrees of the Meridian intercepted between the Star, and the North or South-part of the Horizon, according as the Star is situated, is the Meridian Altitude thereof.

Now to find the Altitude at any other Hour, turn about the Globe till the Index of the Hour-Circle be at the Hour you would know the Altitude of the Star (the Index of the Hour-Circle being first rectified to the Sun's Place) and then apply the Quadrant of Altitude to the Star, and the Degree of the Quadrant cut by the Star, is the Altitude, at that Time.

PROB. XVI. *To know at any time of the Day or Night, what Stars be above the Horizon.*

This is no other than to place the Globe in a true Position at that Time : Which is easily performed by turning the Globe (the Index first rectified to the Sun's Place) till the Hour-Index point to the Hour of the Day or Night ; and staying the Globe there, you will see all the Stars that are above the Horizon at that Time

PROB.

PROB. XVII. *How to know the Rising, Culminating, and Setting of any Fixed Star; also what part of the Horizon he riseth and setteth in.*

Having rectified the Index of the Hour-Circle, and placed the Globe according to the Latitude, then bring the Star, whose Rising, Culminating or setting you desire, to the East-side of the Horizon; then will the Index of the Hour-Circle shew you the time of his Rising; then bring the same Star under the Brazen Meridian, and there staying the Globe, the Index will shew you at what Hour the said Star comes to the Meridian; Lastly, bring the same Star to the Western part of the Horizon, and then the Index of the Hour-Circle will shew you at what Hour the said Star setteth, and by the Horizon you may know the Amplitude, as of the Sun.

SECT. VII. *Of the Properties of the* Loadstone.

The *Magnet* or *Loadstone* (though seemingly mean and contemptible, yet) for its wonderful secret Properties, and for its real Usefulness to Mankind, and the great improvements that have been made in Navigation by the help thereof, may justly be admired amongst the choicest Miracles of Nature, and valued above all the Gems and precious Stones in the spacious Universe

These Stones as they are found in divers parts of the World, and are of different Colure, Weight, and Force; so they have different degrees of Attractive and Directive Power and Virtue; but differ not in Property, for they all have the same Direction, but some more weak, and some more vigorus and strong, amongst the rest those that are found about *China,* and *Bengall* in the *East-Indies* are reckoned the best. But there are others also found in *Arabia,* some at *Porto Feraro* in the *Levant;* some there are also found in *High Germany, Norway, Spain,* and *Bohemia;* and some in the *West* of *England,* and most commonly in Iron Mines, being supposed by some to be of the Iron Oar, or to participate of the very nature of Iron it self; as appears by its Sympathetick affection to Iron or Steel in drawing it to it self, as soon as it comes within the Orb of its Attraction; for if you apply a piece of Iron to either of the Poles, it will there hold it, and at a Distance draw a small piece of Iron, with more or less vigour according to the strength of the Stone, which may be Artificially augmented by capping each Pole of the Stone with a smooth and bright piece of Iron or Steel, into which, as into a Center; the virtue of each Pole (which before was more diffused) will be contracted and united, and thereby the same Stone rendred more vigorus and powerful.

C c

Of

Of the Sympathetical and Antipathetical Property of the Loadstone.

When a Needle is touched upon a Loadstone, the North and South-ends of this Needle will apply themselves respectively to those Poles from whence they received their Magnetical Life, to wit, the North-end of the Needle to the North-end of the Stone, which denotes their mutual Sympathy, but putting the North-end of the Stone to the South-end of the Needle, when it is upon a Pin, the South-end of the Needle will immediately fly away; and if you put the South-end of the Stone to the North-end of the Needle, it will also discover its Antipathetical Nature, and fly away from it.

But a contrary Operation there is yet in the two Needles to that of the Loadstone; for if one of the Needles be hung upon a Pin, that you apply the North-end of the Needle to the North-end of that upon the Pin, it shall immediately fly away, which denoteth a contrary Operation in the Needle to that of the Loadstone, and the South-end of one will immediately come to the North end of the other.

The same Property of Sympathetical Coition, and Antipathetical Repulsion, is also discovered by two Loadstones, floating in two little Boats in a great Bason of Water, the two Poles of either Stone being disposed parallel to the Plain of the Horizon; and if you put both the South-poles together, they shall avoid the Contact of one another by a natural Antipathy; but if the North-pole of the one be directed to the South-pole of the other, they will immediately manifest their natural Sympathy one to another, and will cleave together by a strong Attraction.

If a Loadstone be confusedly broken into many Pieces, each of the Pieces shall be an entire Loadstone, having both its Poles distinctly of it self, with all the other Properties that were in the Stone before it was broken.

But if a Loadstone be divided in the midst between the two Poles, in the Equinoctial, then it is absolutely two entire Loadstones, and those Parts which were the Equinoctials before are now become two Poles, and the two Poles that were Poles before, do continue the same.

But if a Stone be cut Meridionally quite thro' the two Poles, so that one Axis is now converted into two, it is also become two entire Loadstones, the Axis of either of them will retire into the Gravity of either Piece, and if you join these two pieces together again, the two Axis will again become one, which is most admirable to behold.

But if you cut off a piece of the Stone at the very Pole, in a parallel Section, the virtue of that piece will immediately retire from it unto the main Stone, and will scarcely have any Virtue at all therein, but applying this small Piece that was cut off to the same Place again, the Stone will forthwith impart the same Virtue as was before, into this Piece so cut off, so long as it doth abide in that Place.   Of

Or, if you apply a weak Stone to the Poles of a ſtrong one, the ſtrong Stone will impart of its Virtue to the weak Stone, making it to be as ſtrong as its ſelf, but when this weak Magnet deſerts this neighbourly Propinquity, the ſtrong Magnet will draw its Virtue to its ſelf again, and will truſt it no further than the power of its recal.

To find the Poles of a Stone

THere are ſeveral Ways for the Performance of this Experiment. Firſt you may have a thin piece of Steel about an Inch in length, and half of an Inch broad, which being bent circular and laid on the Stone, will immediately lie parallel to the *Axis* of the Stone, and direct which way the Poles do lie. Which being diſcovered near where they lie, you may find them more exactly by a ſmall piece of ſewing Needle; which being laid on the Stone, if it be near either of the Poles, will elevate one end thereof; then move it farther and farther, till it doth erect it ſelf Perpendicular, and that very Point will be the Pole of the Stone.

Now to know which Pole it is, you may apply a ſmall Needle of a Dial to it, and if the Pole draw the North-end of the Needle, then is that the North Pole of the Stone; and the contrary.

Or otherwiſe you may find the Pole by a ſewing Needle and Thread, by hanging it over the Stone where you ſuppoſe the Pole to be, and keep it a little ſhort from the Stone, and the end of the Needle will directly point to the Pole of the Stone.

To Infuſe Magnetical Virtue into a Needle, without the help of a Loadſtone.

IRon being a Mineral of the Earth, and having a Sympathetical Quality with the *Loadſtone*, acquiring this Verticity from the Magnetiſm of the Earth, being diſperſed according to the various Poſitions thereof; for all Iron, whoſe Poſition is parallel to the *Axis* of the World, or if it be perpendicular to the Horizon, the upper part thereof ſhall have North, and the lower part South Virtue; as Bars in Windows, Caſments, Tongs, and Fire-Forks, and all ſuch Things; which Virtue they acquire in a very little time, as I experienced by a Fire-Fork, which within 10 days after it was firſt made, (being kept in a perpendicular poſture) its upper end did very ſenſibly draw the North point of the Compaſs, and the lower end the South point; but the longer any ſuch piece of Iron continues in that Poſition, the ſtronger Virtue it doth contract; ſo that I once made an Experiment upon a ſmooth piece of Iron, which had for ſeveral Years been in a perpendicular Poſture, and I filed the upper end thereof bright, and touched a ſmall new Needle thereon, the South end I touched upon the North or upper part of the Iron, and the North end upon the South or lower end; and I found the Needle to play indifferently well, and to conform it ſelf to the Magnetical Meridian.

Here followeth ſeveral neceſſary T A B L E S, with their Uſe and Application in the Art of Navigation.

A

M.		D.	H.	M.		D.	H.
January.	Full moon	05	08A	*July.*	Full moon.	01	10A
	Laſt quart.	12	01A		Laſt quart.	09	04A
	New moon.	20	01A		New moon.	16	05A
	Firſt quart.	28	01A		Firſt quart.	23	08M
					Full moon.	31	04M
February.	Full moon.	04	06M				
	Laſt quart.	11	04M	*Auguſt.*	Laſt quart.	08	06M
	New moon	19	07M		New moon.	15	01M
	Firſt quart.	26	12A		Firſt quart.	21	07A
					Full moon.	29	08A
March.	Full moon	05	03A				
	Laſt quart.	11	08A	*September.*	Laſt quart.	06	06A
	New moon.	20	11A		New moon.	13	08M
	Firſt quart.	28	09M		Firſt quart.	20	09M
					Full moon.	29	00N
April.	Full moon.	04	01M				
	Laſt quart.	11	02A	*October.*	Laſt quart.	06	02M
	New moon.	19	02A		New moon.	12	06A
	Firſt quart	26	04A		Firſt quart.	20	01M
					Full moon.	28	05M
May.	Full moon.	03	00N				
	Laſt quart.	11	08M	*November.*	Laſt quart.	04	11M
	New moon.	19	01M		New moon.	11	06M
	Firſt quart.	25	09A		Firſt quart.	18	10A
					Full moon.	26	09A
June.	Full moon.	01	12A				
	Laſt quart.	09	10A	*December.*	Laſt quart.	03	07A
	New moon.	17	10M		New mooſi.	10	08A
	Firſt quart.	24	02M		Firſt quart.	18	08A
					Full moon.	26	10M

The Year 1718 *hath* 4 *Eclipſes,* 2 *of the Sun, and* 2 *of the Moon.*

The firſt will be a Solar Defect on *Feb.* 19*th* Day, but not viſible to us.
The ſecond will be an inviſible Eclipſe of the Moon, on *March* the 5*th* day.
The third will be an Eclipſe of the Sun, on *Auguſt* the 14*th* day inviſible to us.
The fourth will be a *Lunar Deliquium,* or *Aug.* 29*th* day, about 8 in the Evening viſible and total

M.		D	H.		M.		D	H.
January.	Laſt quart.	02	04M		July.	New moon.	06	08M
	New moon.	09	01A			Firſt quart.	13	04M
	Firſt quart.	17	05A			Full moon.	20	07M
	Full moon.	24	10A			Laſt quart.	28	09M
	Laſt quàrt.	31	02A					
Februa.	New moon.	08	07M		Auguſt.	New moon.	04	05A
	Firſt quart.	16	11M			Firſt quart.	11	09M
	Full moon.	23	08M			Full moon.	18	09A
						Laſt quart.	27	01M
March.	Laſt quart.	02	01M		September.	New moon.	03	02M
	New moon	10	01M			Firſt quart.	09	06A
	Firſt quart.	17	12A			Full moon.	17	01A
	Full moon.	24	06A			Laſt quart.	25	04A
	Laſt quart.	31	02A					
April.	New moon.	08	09A		Octob̄er.	New moon.	01	11M
	Firſt quart.	15	06A			Firſt quart.	09	05M
	Full moon.	2	02M			Full moon.	17	07M
	Laſt quart.	30	06M			Laſt quart.	25	04M
						New moon.	31	09A
May.	New moon.	08	09M		November.	Firſt quart.	07	08A
	Firſt quart	15	06A			Full moon.	16	03M
	Full moon	22	10M			Laſt quart.	23	04A
	Laſt quart.	29	11A			New moon.	30	07M
June.	New moon.	06	10A		December.	Firſt quart.	07	04A
	Firſt quart.	13	11A			Full moon.	15	07A
	Full moon.	20	07A			Laſt quart.	23	01M
	Laſt quart.	28	03A			New moon.	29	08A

The Year 1719 hath three Eclipſes, two of the Sun and one of the Moon.
The firſt is ot the Sun, Feb 8. about 7 in the Morning.
The ſecond will be an Eclipſe of the Sun, Auguſt 4th, Inviſible.
The third will be on Auguſt 18th, about 9 in the Evening, where-
in the Moon will be Eclipſed Viſible 5 Digits.

M		D	H		M		D	H
January	First quart.	06	02 A		July	First quart.	02	01 M
	Full moon.	14	10 M			Full moon.	08	04 A
	Last quart	21	09 M			Last quart.	16	05 M
	New moon.	28	10 M			New moon.	24	05 M
						First quart.	31	05 M
February	First quart.	05	10 M		August	Full moon.	07	02 M
	Full moon	12	11 A			Last quart.	14	10 A
	Last quart	19	05 A			New moon.	22	03 A
	New moon	27	02 M			First quart.	29	11 M
March	First quart.	06	06 M		September	Full moon.	05	03 A
	Full moon	13	09 M			Last quart.	13	05 A
	Last quart.	20	02 M			New moon.	21	07 M
	New moon.	27	06 A			First quart.	27	06 A
April	First quart.	04	09 A		October	Full moon.	05	07 A
	Full moon	11	06 A			Last quart.	13	11 M
	Last quart	18	10 M			New moon.	20	01 A
	New moon.	26	11 M			First quart.	27	04 M
May	First quart.	04	09 M		November	Full moon.	04	01 M
	Full moon.	11	01 M			Last quart.	12	02 M
	Last quart.	17	10 A			New moon.	18	10 A
	New moon.	26	02 M			First quart.	25	04 A
June	First quart.	02	06 A		December	Full moon.	03	07 A
	Full moon.	09	08 M			Last quart.	11	05 A
	Last quart.	16	01 A			New moon.	18	08 M
	New moon.	24	03 A			First quart.	25	10 M

The Year 1720 hath two Eclipses, and both of the Sun.

The first will be a *Solar* Eclipse on *January* 28th, Invisible.

The second will be a *Solar* Eclipse on *July* 24 Invisible.

		D.	H.		M.		D.	H.
January.	Full moon.	02	03A	July	Last quart.		05	06M
	Last quart.	10	04M		New moon.		13	09M
	New moon.	16	08A		First quart.		21	02M
	First quart.	24	06M		Full moon.		27	04A
February	Full moon.	01	08M	August	Last quart.		03	08A
	Last quart.	08	01A		New moon.		11	11A
	New moon	15	09M		First quart.		19	08M
	First quart.	23	04M		Full moon.		26	01M
March.	Full moon.	02	10A	September.	Last quart.		02	01A
	Last quart.	09	08A		New moon.		10	01A
	New moon.	16	10A		First quart.		17	03A
	First quart.	24	09A		Full moon.		24	00N
April	Full moon.	01	10M	October.	Last quart.		02	09M
	Last quart.	08	02M		New moon.		10	03M
	New moon.	15	00N		First quart.		16	09A
	First quart.	23	03A		Full moon.		24	03M
	Full moon.	30	07A					
May.	Last quart.	07	10M	November.	Last quart.		01	06M
	New moon.	15	03M		New moon.		08	02A
	First quart.	23	05M		First quart.		15	06M
	Full moon.	30	02M		Full moon.		22	08A
					Last quart.		30	04A
June.	Last quart.	05	07A	December	New moon.		08	01M
	New moon.	13	06A		First quart.		14	05A
	First quart.	21	06A		Full moon.		22	02A
	Full moon.	28	08M		Last quart.		30	05M

The Year 1721 hath six Eclipses, 3 of the Sun, and 3 of the Moon.
The first will be an Eclipse of the Moon *Jan* the 2d. Day, invisible.
The second will be of the Sun, on *Jan.* 16th invisible.
The third will be of the Moon, on *June* 28th, invisible.
The fourth will be on *July* the 13th about 9 in the Morning, wherein the Sun will be Eclipsed visible 3 Digits.
The fifth will be of the Sun, on *December* the 7th, invisible.
The sixth will be of the Moon, on *December* 22d, part visible.

M.	New/quarter	D	H.	M.	New/quarter	D	H.
January	New-moon.	06	11M	July	New moon.	02	10M
	First quart.	13	07M		First quart.	10	01A
	Full moon.	21	01M		Full moon.	17	09M
	Last quart.	29	06M		Last quart.	24	01M
February	New moon.	04	09A	August	New moon.	01	02M
	First quart.	11	11A		First quart.	08	11A
	Full moon.	20	04M		Full moon.	15	05A
	Last quart.	27	04A		Last quart.	22	01A
					New moon.	30	05A
March	New moon.	06	08M	September	First quart.	07	10M
	First quart.	13	06A		Full moon.	14	01M
	Full moon.	21	08A		Last quart	21	06M
	Last quart.	28	11A		New moon.	29	09M
April	New moon.	04	07A	October	First quart.	06	06A
	First quart.	12	01A		Full moon.	13	11M
	Full moon.	20	08M		Last quart.	21	01M
	Last quart.	27	05M		New moon.	28	12A
May	New moon.	04	06M	November	First quart.	05	01M
	First quart.	12	08M		Full moon.	11	12A
	Full moon.	19	06A		Last quart.	19	11A
	Last quart.	26	10M		New moon.	27	04A
June	New moon.	02	08A	December	First quart.	04	09M
	First quart.	10	12A		Full moon.	11	04A
	Full moon.	18	02M		Last quart.	19	07A
	Last quart.	24	04A		New moon.	27	03M

The Year 1722 hath four Eclipses, 2 of the Sun, and 2 of the Moon.

The first will be an Eclipse of the Sun, June the 2d. invisible.

The second will be on June the 18th about two in the Morning, wherein the Moon will be Eclipsed visible 13 Digits.

The third will be on November the 27th, about 4 in the Afternoon, wherein the Sun will be Eclipsed (partly visible) 6 Digits.

The fourth will be on December the 11th, wherein the Rising Moon will be Eclipsed, part visible 7 Digits.

M.		D.	H.	M.		D.	H.
January.	First quart.	02	06A	July.	Full moon	07	01M
	Full moon.	09	09M		Last quart.	13	06A
	Last quart.	18	10A		New moon.	21	02M
	New moon	25	02A		First quart.	29	06M
February.	First quart.	01	06M	August.	Full moon.	05	09M
	Full moon.	09	03M		Last quart.	12	01M
	Last quart.	17	05M		New moon.	19	05A
	New moon.	23	11M		First quart.	27	09A
March.	First quart.	02	07A	September.	Full moon.	03	06A
	Full moon.	10	10A		Last quart	10	10M
	Last quart.	18	06A		New moon.	18	10M
	New moon.	25	09M		First quart.	26	09M
April.	First quart.	01	11M	October.	Full moon.	03	02M
	Full moon.	09	03A		Last quart.	09	11A
	Last quart.	17	02M		New moon.	18	03M
	New moon.	23	07A		First quart.	25	08A
May	First quart.	01	02M	November.	Full moon.	01	00N
	Full moon.	09	05M		Last quart.	08	04A
	Last quart.	16	08M		New moon.	16	09A
	New moon.	23	04M		First quart.	24	06M
	First quart.	30	10A		Full moon.	30	12A
June.	Full moon.	07	04A	December.	Last quart.	08	01A
	Last quart.	14	01A		New moon.	16	02A
	New moon.	21	02A		First quart	23	03A
	First quart.	29	02A		Full moon	30	02A

In this Year there will happen two Eclipses only, and both of the Sun.

The first will happen on *May* the 23d Day. }
The second on *November* the 16th Day } Both Invisible.

D d

A Tide-Table for the Sea Coasts of Great Britain, Ireland, Norway, Holland, Flanders, France, Biscay, *&c. Shewing what Moon makes Full-Sea, upon the Full and Change-days, at the Places following, in an Alphabetical Order.*

A

Place	H	M
AT *Army,* N.N E. and S S.W	01	30
At *Amsterdam,* and *Armentars,* N E. and S.W.	03	00
At *Abarwarck,* E. N. E. and W.S.W.	04	30
At *Abermoruck,* and *Antwerp,* East and West	06	00
At *Alborough,* S. E. by S. and N. W. by N.	09	45

B

Place	H	M
At *Beachy* and *Blacktail,* and before the *Race* of *Blanquet,* N. and S.	12	00
Thwart of *Beachy* in the *Offing* N by E. and S. by W.	12	45
At *Blacknefs* in *Blues,* at *Bell Isle* N N.E. and S.S.W	01	30
Without *Blues,* and at *Berwick,* N.E by N. and S W. by S	02	15
The River of *Bourdeaux* the South Coast of *Britagn,* the Coast of *Biscay* and at *Boeknefs,* N.E. and S. W.	03	00
At *Brest,* before the *Bass,* the River of *Bourdeaux* within the Haven N. E. by E. and S. W. by W.	03	45
In the *Braefound, Bley, Baltimore* E. N. E and W.S.W.	04	30
Before *Bremen,* and at *Blackney* and in the Channel before *Bourdeaux,* East and West.	06	00
At *Briffol* Key, E. by S. and W. by N.	06	45
At *Bridgwater,* E. S. E. and W. N. W.	07	30
Bulleys-deep, S.S.E. and N N.W.	10	30

C

Place	H	M
In the *Condado,* N. and S	12	00
In the *Chamber* of *Rye.* N. by E. and S by W.	12	45

Place	H	M
Without *Calice,* at *Corpus Christi* Point, before and at *Camfer,* N.N.E and S S.W.	01	30
Between *Calice* and *Dover* before *Conquet,* and at the *North Cape* N.E. and S.W	03	00
At *Cork, Calice, Cape Clear,* and in the *Creek,* E N E & W S W.	04	30
At *Caldy,* and in the Bay of *Carnarvan,* E. by N and W by S	05	15
At *Concale,* East and West.	06	00
Without the *Caskets,* in the Channel S E by E and N W by W	08	15
Between *Guernsey* and the *Caskets,* before *Cromer,* before the *Caskets* and *Guernsey,* at *Sevenclifts* and at *Catnefs,* S E. and NeW	09	00
At the *Caskets,* and at *Chambernefs,* S E by S & N W. by N.	09	45
At *Cows,* in the Fofs of *Caen,* in *Calice* Road, and in *Chambernefs* Road S S.E. and NNW.	10	30
Before the Haven of *Caen,* in in *Chamber,* between *Cripple-Sand,* and the *Creyl,* and at *Culbot,* S. by E. and N. by W	11	15

D

Place	H	M
At *Dover-Peer,* and before *Dunkirk* North and South.	12	00
At *Dembigö* and *Dawns* in the Road, N E. by N. & S W. by S	02	15
At *Dort,* N. E. and S W.	03	00
At *Dungarvan,* E. N E. and W. S W	04	30
At *Dartmouth* East and West.	06	00
At *Dublin,* S. E. by E. and N W. by W	08	15
At *Dunbar,* S E. and N.W.	09	00
At *Dungenefs* and *Dunnofe,* S.E. by S. and N.W. by N.	09	45

At

	H.	M.
At *Dover*, *Diep*, and in the *Downs* a shoar, S.S.E. and N.N. W.	10	30
E		
At *Emden*, before the *Elve* before the *Eydes*, and before *Enchusan*, North and South.	12	00
At *Edams* N.N.E. and S S.W.	04	30
Before the Eastern and Western *Emes*, and at *Egmonds* S. E. and N. W.	09	00
F		
On the Coast of *Flanders* N. and S.	12	00
At *Flusbing*, N. by E. and S. by W.	12	45
Before the *Few*, in the Channel, N.N.E and S.S W.	01	30
Without *Fountney*, N.E. by N. and S W. by S	02	15
Without the Banks of *Flanders*, N.E. and S. W.	03	00
At *Flamborough* and *Bridlington*, E.N.E. and W.S. W.	04	30
At the *Forn*, in *Foy*, at *Falmorth*, E. by N. and W. by S.	05	15
Between *Foy* and *Falmouth*, in the Channel, and at *Foulnefs*, E. by S. and W. by N.	06	45
Before the Coast of *Frizeland* and the *Fly*, E.S.E. and W.N. W.	07	30
Without the *Fly*, S. E. by E. and N.W. by W.	08	15
At *Frize*, and *Farr-Ifles*, N.W. and S.E.	09	00
In the *Firth*, and at the *South-Foreland*, S. S E. and N. N. W.	10	30
In *Fair-Ifle* Roads, and at the *North-Foreland*, South by East and North by West.	11	15
G		
In the Road of *Gibralter*, at *Graveling*, and before *Cherbury* North and South.	12	00
Before *Goree* at *Guernfey*, and		

	H.	M.
at *Gravefend*, N.N.E and S. S. W.	01	30
At *Groy*, at *Gafcoign*, and the Coast of *Galicia*, North East and South West.	03	00
Between *Guernfey* and *Caskets*, SouthEast and NorthWest.	09	00
Thwart of *Guernfey*, in the Channel, S E. by S. and N.W. by N	09	45
In the *Chamber* and *Goree-end* S. by E and N. by W.	11	15
H		
Before the *Hever*, before *Horn*, and at *Hampton-Key*, N and S.	12	00
Under *Holy Ifland*, and at *Horn*, N.N.E and S.S.W.	01	30
Before *Hartlepool*, N.E. and S. W.	03	00
At *Huntcliff-foot*, N.E. by E. and S. W. by W.	03	45
At *Humber*, E. by N. & W. by S.	05	15
Before *Hamborough*, at *Hull*, at the *Holms*, and before *Humber's*, Mouth East and West.	06	00
At *Harlem*, *Havre de Grace*, and *Home-head*, S. E. and N.W.	09	00
At St *Hellens*, at *Harwich*, and without the Banks of *Harwich* S.S.E. and N.N.W.	10	30
At *Harwich*, within, S. by E. and N. by W.	11	15
I		
At *Jutland Iflands*, N. and S	12	00
On the West Coast of *Ireland*, N.E. and S.W.	03	00
In all the Havens on the South Coast of *Ireland*, E. by N. and W. by S.	05	15
K		
Kentifh Knock, N. and S.	12	00
At *Kellerrs*, N. E. and S.W.	02	00
At *Kingfale*, E. N. E. and W. S.W.	04	30
At *Kildwyn*, E. S E. & W N W.	07	30
At *Kildrve*, S E. and N. W.	09	00

At

L

	H.	M
At Leith, North and South	12	00
At Lisbon, N E. by N. and S W. by S,	02	15
At London, N. E. and S. W.	03	00
Thwart of Londey, and before Lin, E by N and W. by S.	05	15
At Lin, half Tide at Londey, East and West	06	00
At Lin, East by South and and West by North	06	45
At the Lizard by the Land, E S E and W N W	07	30
At Lambay, S E by E. and N. W by W	08	15
At Leystaff, and thwart of it without the Banks, S. E. by S and N. W by N.	09	45
In Leystaff Road, and at Long-sand-head, S S E. and N. N. W.	10	30

M

	H.	M
Within the Maes, at Maldon, N by E. and S by W	12	45
Before the Maes, N. N. E and S.S. W.	01	30
At the Maes, and before St Matthews Point, N E by E. and S W by W	03	45
In Mousehole, at St Matthews, and within Mounts-bay E N E and W S W	04	30
In Milford, at Moonless, at St. M. or E by N and W by S.	05	15
Between Mousehole and Falmouth, and in Milford-Haven, E S. E. and W. N. W.	07	30
In St. Magnes-sound, and at Magne's-Castle, S. E. by E. and N. W by W.	08	15
At the Isle of Man, S. E. and N W	09	00
Before Margate, South by East and North by West	11	15

N

	H.	M
At Newport, Half-Tide North and South	12	00
At the West-end of the Nowre, N. by E. and S. by W.	12	45

	H.	M
Before the River of Nantz, North East and South West	03	00
At Newcastle, East by North and West by South	05	15
Before St. Nicholas, East by South and West by North	06	45
At the Needles, at the Isle of Wight, S E by E. & N. W. by W	08	15
All the Coast of Normandy, and Picardy, S. S. E and N N. W	10	30
Between the Naze and Warbear of Loner, South by East and North by West	11	15

O

	H.	M
At Orkness, N. E. and S. W.	03	00
At Orkney, S E and N.W.	09	00
At Orfordness, S. E. by S. and N. W. by N.	09	45
At Orfordness, without the Bank, and between Orford and Orwell-Waves, S. S. E. and N. N. W.	10	30
At Orfordness, within the Sands, S by E. and N. by W.	11	15

P

	H.	M
At Portsmouth, Half-Tide, North and South	12	00
At the Pens, Portbus, and Poustu, North East and South West	03	00
On the Coast of Portugal, N. E. by E. and S. W. by W.	03	45
In Plymouth, and before St. Pauls, E. by N. and W. by S.	05	15
At St. Pauls in the Haven, East and West	06	00
Before Podessemsk, East by South and West by North	06	45
Thwart of Plymouth, E. S E. and W. N. W.	07	30
At the Race of Portland, S. E. and N. W.	09	00

Q

	H.	M
At Quinborough, N. and S.	12	00

R

	H.	M
At Rochester, N. by E and S by W.	12	45
At Ramkins, N.N.E. and S.S.W	01	30
At Rotterdam, in Robin-Hood's Bay		

	H	M		H	M
Bay, and from the Race to the Pole-head, N.E. and S W ———	03	00	**U** Before U*ek*, N. and S. ———	12	00
At *Rouen*, and before *Rochel*, N.E by E. and S.W by W. —	03	45	At U*se*, N.E. and S.W. ———	03	00
In R*amsey*,E. by N. & W.by S.	05	15	Between U*shant* and the Main, N.E. by E. and S.W. by W.	03	45
S In the *Sleve*, between U*shant* and *Scilly*, at the *Shoe*, at the *Spits*, at *South-Hampton*, and along the *Swim*, N. and S. ———	12	00	In the *Yourd*, at the Bay, within U*shant*, E. N E. and W.S.W.	04	30
			Without U*shant*, E. and W.	06	00
Upon the Coaft of *Spain*, and in *Shetland*, N.E. and S W. —	03	00	St. *Vallery*, S.S.E. and N.N.W.	10	30
At *Scilly*,in the*Sound*,*Scarborough*, & at *Staples*,N.E.byE. S W.byW.	03	45	**W** At *Winchelsey*, N.byE.&S.byW.	12	45
At 7 *Isles*, without the Haven in the broad *Sound*, E. N E. & W S. W. ———	04	30	At the *Weilings*, and from the Weft-end of the *Wight*, N.N.E. and S.S. W. ———	01	30
At the Mouth of *Severn*,between *Scilly* and the *Lizard*, at the *Spurn*, & *Stockton*, E. by N.& W. by S.	05	15	Before the *Weilings*, N. E. by N. and S.W. by S.———	02	15
.Without *Scilly*. in the Channel and at *Salcomb*, E. and W	06	00	At *Whitby*, N.E. and S. W.	03	00
			In the Sea of *Wales*, and Se*vern*, E N E. and W.S.W.	04	30
At *Sedmouth*, and at the *Start*, E. by S and W by N.	06	45	In *Wales*, E. by N. & W. by S.	05	15
Off the *Start*, in the Channel, E.S E and W N.W ———	07	30	At *Wells*, at *Weymouth*, and at *Waterford*, Eaft and Weft——	06	00
Within the *Seyn*, and before *Schelberg*,& at 7 *Clifts*, S E &N.W.	09	00	At *Weymouth-Key* E. by S. and W. by N.———	06	45
At *Shoram*,S.E.byS. &N.W.byN	09	45	At the *Ness*, by *Wieringhen*, at *Wintertou*, E.S E and W N.W.	07	30
At *Seyn-head*, S S.E. & N.N.W	10	30	Thwart of the *Isle of Wight*, in the Channel, all within the *Isle of Wight*, between the *Isle of Wight*, and *Beachy*, by the fhore, S. E. by E. N. W. by W. —	08	15
T Within *Tervere*, N. by E and S by W. ———	12	45			
Before *Tervere*, before the River of *Thames*, and at *Tinmouth*, N. N E. and S.S. W. ———	01	30	At the Eaft-end of the *Wight*, and on *Wieringhen* Flats, S. E. and N. W. ———	09	00
Before the *Tees* and *Tinmouth*, before the Bay of *Tinmouth*, N.E. and S W. ———	03	00	**Y** Before *Yarmouth*, N. N. E. & S S. W. ———	01	30
At the Clifts of the *Texel*, E. N. E. and W..S.W. ———	04	30	At *Youghall*, E.N.E. & W.S.W.	04	30
In *Torbay* and before the *Texel*, Eaft and Weft ———	06	00	At *Yarmouth*, S. E. by E. and N. W. by W. ———	08	15
In the Road of the *Texel*, E.S E and W.N. W. ———	07	30	In *Yarmouth-Road*, in *Yarmouth* Haven, S.S.E. and N.N W.	10	30
At *Tergon*, S.E. by S. and N. W by N. ———	09	45	**Z** On the Coaft of *Zealand*, N.N.E. and S.S. W.———	01	30
			In the *Zerick-sea*, N. E.&S. W.	03	00

A

Days	Jan ⊙ Right Ascen. H. M.		Feb. ⊙ Right Ascen. H. M.		March. ⊙ Right Ascen. H. M.		April. ⊙ Right Ascen. H. M.		May. ⊙ Right Ascen. H. M.		June. ⊙ Right Ascen. H. M.	
1	19	36	21	43	23	29	01	22	03	15	05	20
2	19	40	21	47	23	33	01	26	03	19	05	24
3	19	44	21	51	23	37	01	30	03	23	05	28
4	19	49	21	55	23	40	01	34	03	27	05	32
5	19	53	21	59	23	44	01	37	03	31	05	37
6	19	57	22	03	23	47	01	41	03	35	05	41
7	20	01	22	07	23	51	01	45	03	39	05	45
8	20	05	22	11	23	54	01	48	03	43	05	49
9	20	09	22	15	23	58	01	52	03	47	05	53
10	20	14	22	18	00	02	01	55	03	51	05	57
11	20	18	22	22	00	06	01	59	03	55	06	01
12	20	23	22	26	00	09	02	03	03	59	06	05
13	20	27	22	30	00	13	02	07	04	03	06	09
14	20	31	22	34	00	16	02	11	04	07	06	13
15	20	35	22	37	00	20	02	14	04	11	06	18
16	20	39	22	41	00	24	02	18	04	15	06	22
17	20	43	22	45	00	27	02	22	04	19	06	27
18	20	47	22	49	00	31	02	26	04	23	06	30
19	20	51	22	53	00	34	02	30	04	27	06	34
20	20	55	22	56	00	38	02	33	04	31	06	39
21	20	59	23	00	00	42	02	37	04	35	06	43
22	21	04	23	04	00	45	02	41	04	39	06	47
23	21	08	23	07	00	49	02	45	04	43	06	51
24	21	12	23	11	00	53	02	49	04	47	06	55
25	21	16	23	14	00	56	02	52	04	51	06	59
26	21	20	23	18	01	00	02	56	04	55	07	03
27	21	24	23	22	01	04	03	00	04	59	07	07
28	21	28	23	26	01	07	03	04	05	03	07	11
29	21	32			01	11	03	08	05	07	07	15
30	21	36			01	15	03	11	05	12	07	20
31	21	39			01	18			05	16		

A

Days	July. ⊙ Right Afcen.		August. ⊙ Right Afcen.		Septem. ⊙ Right Afcen.		October. ⊙ Right Afcen.		Novem. ⊙ Right Afcen.		Decem. ⊙ Right Afcen.	
	H.	M.	H.	M.	H.	M.	H.	M.	H.	M.	H.	M.
1	07	24	09	26	11	20	13	09	15	08	17	16
2	07	28	09	30	11	24	13	13	15	12	17	21
3	07	32	09	34	11	27	13	16	15	16	17	26
4	07	36	09	38	11	31	13	20	15	20	17	30
5	07	40	09	41	11	34	13	23	15	24	17	35
6	07	44	09	45	11	37	13	27	15	28	17	39
7	07	48	09	49	11	42	13	31	15	32	17	43
8	07	52	09	52	11	45	13	35	15	37	17	48
9	07	56	09	56	11	49	13	39	15	41	17	52
10	08	00	09	59	11	52	13	42	15	46	17	57
11	08	04	10	03	11	56	13	46	15	50	18	01
12	08	08	10	07	12	00	13	50	15	54	18	06
13	08	12	10	11	12	03	13	54	15	59	18	10
14	08	16	10	15	12	07	13	58	16	03	18	15
15	08	20	10	18	12	10	14	01	16	08	18	20
16	08	24	10	22	12	14	14	05	16	12	18	24
17	08	28	10	26	12	18	14	09	16	16	18	29
18	08	32	10	29	12	21	14	13	16	20	18	34
19	08	36	10	33	12	25	14	17	16	24	18	38
20	08	40	10	36	12	28	14	21	16	29	18	42
21	08	44	10	40	12	32	14	25	16	33	18	46
22	08	48	10	44	12	36	14	29	16	37	18	50
23	08	52	10	48	12	39	14	33	16	41	18	55
24	08	56	10	51	12	43	14	37	16	45	18	59
25	08	59	10	54	12	46	14	40	16	50	19	04
26	09	03	10	58	12	50	14	44	16	54	19	08
27	09	07	11	02	12	54	14	48	16	58	19	12
28	09	11	11	05	12	58	14	52	17	03	19	17
29	09	15	11	09	13	02	14	56	17	07	19	21
30	09	18	11	12	13	06	15	00	17	12	19	26
31	09	22	11	16			15	04			19	31

A

A Table ſhewing the Right Aſcenſion, Declination and Magnitude of the Principal Fixed Stars.

Names of the Stars	Magnit.	Right Aſcenſ. H. M.		Decli- nation D. M.	
Pole Star	2	00	32	87	33 N
Girdle ſ Andromeda	2	00	50	33	50 N
Achenar, or laſt in Eridanus	1	01	28	58	55 S
Brighteſt Star ſ Aries	2	01	51	22	04 N
Meduſas Head	2	02	49	39	48 N
Bright Side of Perſeus	2	03	04	04	48 N
Brighteſt of the ſeven Stars	3	03	29	22	55 N
Aldebaran, or Bull's-Eye	1	04	18	5	50 N
Capella, or the Goat	1	04	55	45	38 N
Bright Foot of Orion	1	05	01	08	37 S
Middle Star in Orion's Belt	3	05	20	01	26 S
Orion's Right Shoulder	1	05	39	07	18 N
Auriga's Right Shoulder	2	05	44	44	56 N
Bright Foot of Gemini	2	06	19	16	38 N
Sirius, or the Great Dog	1	06	32	16	20 S
Caſtor, or Apollo	2	07	16	32	29 N
Procyon the Little Dog	2	07	24	05	57 N
Pollux or Hercules	2	07	25	28	46 N
South Arm of the Crab	3	08	40	13	48 N
Hydra's Heart	1	09	12	07	10 S
Lyon's Heart, or Baſiliſk	1	09	51	13	36 N
The Lower of the Pointers	2	10	41	58	08 N
The Upper of the Pointers	2	10	43	63	32 N
Lyon's Tail	1	11	31	16	12 N
Upper of 2 laſt in □ of Great Bear	2	12	00	58	51 N
Laſt but 2 in the Great Bear's Tail	2	12	40	57	47 N
Virgin's Spike	1	13	10	09	31 S
Laſt but one in the Great Bear's Tail	2	13	10	56	41 N
Laſt in the Great Bear's Tail	2	13	34	51	00 N
Dragon's Tail	2	13	59	65	56 N
Arcturus	1	14	02	20	54 N
South Ballance	2	14	32	14	33 S
Foremoſt Guard	2	14	51	75	36 N
Brighteſt of the Crown	2	15	21	27	43 N
Brighteſt in the Serpents Neck	2	15	33	16	30 N
Antares, the Scorpion's Heart	1	16	12	25	46 S
Head of Hercules	3	17	02	14	45 N
Ophineus, or Serpent's Head	3	17	22	12	48 N
Lyra, or the Harp	1	18	27	38	33 N
Swan's Bill	3	19	17	27	18 N
Vulture, or Eagles Heart	2	19	34	08	00 N

Hand

Hand of Antinous	3	19 56	01	39	S
Swan's Tayl	2	20 30	44	05	N
Mouth of Pegasus	3	21 27	08	19	N
Fomelhaut	1	22 41	31	51	S
Marchab, or Pegasus Wing	2	22 48	13	28	N
Scheat, or Pegasus Leg	2	22 56	26	50	N
Cephus's Knee	3	23 20	76	05	N
Andromeda's Head	2	23 53	27	28	N
End of Pegasus Wing	2	23 57	13	20	N

The Explanation and Use of the TABLE of the Sun's Right Ascension, and of the Table of the Star's Right Ascension and Declination.

IN the Table of the Sun's Right Ascension, the first Page contains the first six Months of the Year ; the next Page the other six Months. At the Head of the Table are the Months, in the first Column towards the Left Hand are the Days of the Month, and in the opposite Column is the Right Ascension in Hours and Minutes.

In the Table of the Fixed Stars, there are four Columns; in the first towards the Left Hand, are the Names of the Stars; in the second, the Stars Magnitude; in the third, the Right Ascension in Hours and Minutes, in the 4th, their Declination in Degrees and Minutes, N. or S.

First, To find the Time of the Stars coming upon the Meridian.

The Rule. Look the Right Ascension of the Sun and Star, and subtract the Right Ascension of the Sun from the Right Ascension of the Star, but if the Star's Right Ascension be less than the Sun's add thereto 24 hours, and then subtract ; the Remainder after Substraction, is the time of the Star's coming upon the Meridian from Noon. But if the Remainder exceed 12 hours, subtract 12 hours therefrom, and then the Remainder is the time from Midnight.

Example 1. Suppose the time that Fomelhaut comes upon the Meridian on the 10th of October were required.

I find in the Table the Star's Right Ascension to be 22 hours 41 min. and the Sun's to be 13 hours 42 min. which subtracted from the Star's Right Ascension, leaves 8 hours, 59 min. the time of the Star's coming upon the Meridian, Afternoon.

Secondly, The time being given, to find what Star will come to the Meridian about the same time.

The Rule. To the Sun's Right Ascension, add the time from Noon, at which the Star's coming to the Meridian is desired, the Sum is the Right Ascension of the Star that will come to the Meridian at that time; with which enter the Table of the Star's Right Ascension and Declination, where look what Star's Right Ascension agrees with the Right Ascension before found, or nearest thereto, and that is the Star sought for.

Example Suppose March the 27th, I desire to know what Star will come upon the Meridian about 8 at Night.

The Sun's Right Ascension is 1 hour 4 minutes: the time from Noon is 8 hours, which added to the Sun's Right Ascension, makes 9 hours 4 minutes: the nearest in the Table is Hydra's Heart, whose Right Ascension is 9 hours 12 minutes, and therefore Souths at 8 hours 8 minutes, and so in others.

E e

Direct.

A Table of the Latitude and Longitude of the Principal Harbours Headlands, and Iſlands in the World, Corrected by the lateſt ard beſt Obſervations, accounting the Longitude from the Meridian of LONDON

Note, When the Latitude and Longitude of an Iſland is given, the middle of the Iſland is meant, except ſome particular Part of it be expreſſed

Places Names	Latitude D M	Longit D M	Places Names	Latitude D. M.	Longit D M
The C of England			S ctland S. Point	59 52	01 30 W
			Bucheneſs	57 55	01 20
BErwick	55 50	01 59 W	Aberdeen	57 24	01 37
Newcaſtle	54 58	01 20 W	Dundee	56 30	02 36
Stockton	54 55	01 25 W	Edenburgh	55 57	02 46
Spurn	55 35	00 20 E			
Yarmouth	2 45	01 40 E	The Coaſt of Ireland		
LONDON	51 22	00 00	Dublin	53 20	07 00
North-Foreland	51 28	01 10 E	Wexford	52 13	07 16
Beachy	50 48	00 25 E	Waterford	52 07	07 52 W
Dunnoſe Iſle Wight	50 58	01 23	Cork	51 49	09 30
Portland	50 30	02 48	Cape Clear	51 10	10 30
Start Point	50 09	02 45	Limrick	52 22	09 48
Lizard	49 55	05 14	Galway	53 10	10 03
Lands end	50 06	06 00	Slint Head	53 20	11 15
St Mary's Scilly	49 57	06 15	London derry	54 55	08 00
Hartland-point	51 05	04 35	Belfaſt	54 36	06 50
Lundy Iſle	51 20	04 40	The Coaſt of Holland and Flanders		
Briſtol	51 52	02 35	Scaw	57 46	10 10
St David's-head	51 55	05 22	Helighland	54 28	08 35
Barſey Iſle	52 46	04 58	Hambrough	53 41	10 24 E
Holy head	53 23	04 40	Emden	53 05	08 00
Liverpool	53 20	02 58	The Fly	53 18	05 35
Ware-Haven	54 25	03 15	The Texel	53 10	04 59
Carliſle	54 45	02 25	Amſterdam	52 21	04 51
The Coaſt of Scotland.			Rotterdam	51 55	04 41
Glaſcow	55 53	4 05	The Brill	51 56	04 10
N part of Sky Iſland	57 50	05 21	Sluyce	51 19	03 50
N.part of Lewis-Iſla	58 20	07 15	Calice	50 57	02 00
St. Kilda	58 02	10 05	The Coaſt of France and Portugal;		
Farra-head	58 23	05 05	Diep	49 56 N	01 06 E
Northermoſt Iſles of Orkney	59 15	03 30	Cape de Hague	49 46 N	02 06 W
					Caskets

Places Names.	Latitude D. M.	Longit. D. M.	Places Names.	Latitude D. M.	Longit. D. M.
Caskets	49 50	02 32	Athens	38 00	24 29
Guernsey	49 36	02 40	Cape Martelo S ⎱ P of Negropont ⎰	38 00	25 45
Morlaix	48 37	03 50	Cape Monte Sancto	40 05	26 05
Ushant	48 30	05 05	Gallipoli	40 30	27 58
Brest	48 23	04 24	Constantinople	41 07	30 00
Penmark	47 48	04 15	Smyrna	38 30	27 27
Bell-Isle	47 20	03 10	Ephesus	37 54	27 15
Nantz	47 14	01 49	Antiochetta	36 40	31 37
Island Dieu	46 40	02 15	Scanderoon	36 00	35 58
Island Ree	46 13	01 30	Tripoli	34 40	35 50
Rochel	46 10	01 14	Alexandria	31 07	30 42
Bourdeaux	44 50	00 24	Cape Rusato	33 15	21 55
Bilboa	43 30	03 00	Cape Misorato	32 43	16 23
Cape Ortegal	44 02	07 40	Tripoli	32 55	13 00
Cape Finister	43 06	10 00	Cape Bona	37 08	10 35
Port a Port	41 18	09 20	Bona	37 00	07 33
Burlings	39 39	10 25	Algier	36 40	03 05
Rock of Lisbon	38 54	10 20	Cape de Tres Forcas	35 34	01 25 W
Cape St. Vincent	37 06	09 32	Tetuan	35 28	05 52 W
Cadiz	36 26	06 06	Seuta	35 55	05 47 W
Cape Trefalger	36 10	05 56	Tangier	35 55	06 14 W

(North Latitude / West Longitude — left; North Latitude / East Longitude — right)

The Coast on the Main Continent within the Straits

Islands within the Straits

Places Names.	Latitude D. M.	Longit. D. M.	Places Names.	Latitude D. M.	Longit. D. M.
Gibralter	36 11	05 13 W	Alboran	36 10	03 00 W
Cape de Gat	37 03	01 33 W	Formentaria	38 44	01 31
Cape Paul	37 58	00 10 W	Yvica	39 05	01 30
Cape Martin	39 00	00 28	Majorca City	39 48	02 49
Barcelona	41 30	02 21	Port Maun Minorca	40 02	04 25
Marseilles	43 20	05 15	Gallitta	37 40	08 34
Toulon	43 06	05 40	Sardinia S. end	39 12	08 34
Genoa	44 25	08 40	Corsica N. end	42 57	09 45
Leghorn	43 18	10 29	Gorgona	43 34	09 38
Rome	41 51	12 28	Capraia	43 06	09 40
Naples	41 05	14 28	Lilboa	42 44	10 05
Cape Spartavento	38 00	16 11	Messina	38 22	15 45
Cape Collone	39 10	17 16	Maritimo	38 12	11 55
Gallipoli	40 08	18 05	Cape Passero	36 48	15 08
Cape St. Mary	39 56	18 31	Malta	36 10	14 49
Ancona	43 31	14 30	Corfu	39 45	20 42
Venice	45 18	13 10	Chefalonia	38 15	21 49
Lepanto	38 20	21 55	Zant	37 47	22 10
Cape Matapan	36 35	22 20	Modon on Morea	36 52	21 32
Cape St. Angelo	36 41	23 10	Lemnos	39 50	25 27

Scio

Places Names.	Latitude D. M.	Longitude D. M.
Scio	38 20	23 31
Cape St. John, West end of Candy	35 20	23 27
Cape Solomon, East end of Candy	35 25	26 31
Rhodes City	36 40	28 00
West end of Cyprus	35 21	31 35
East end of Cyprus	35 35	34 25

N. Lat. — E. Long.

The Coast of Barbary and Guiney.

Places Names.	Latitude D. M.	Longitude D. M.
Cape Spartel	35 46	5 55
Salle	33 43	6 30
Cape Cantin	32 16	9 20
Cape de Geer	30 4	10 10
Cape Bajador	26 12	14 30
Cape Olorado	23 41	15 50
Cape Blanco	20 35	16 55
Senegal	15 15	15 40
Cape de Verde	14 30	16 25
River Gambia	13 16	15 20
Serralion	8 36	12 15
Monferado	6 05	9 20
Cape Palmos	4 3	5 36
Jaque Jaque	4 16	2 30
Affene	4 15	1 0
Cape 3 Points	4 13	0 45
River Volto	5 40	3 30
River Formosa	7 0	7 40
Cape Formosa	4 40	8 0
New Callabar	4 12	10 25
Old Callabar	4 18	11 32
River Camerones	4 2	13 10
River de Angra	0 49	13 15
Lopas	1 5	12 20
River Congo	5 45	15 25
Angola	8 51	15 55
Cape Negro	16 8	14 46
Cape St. Thomas	23 10	14 23
Secos	28 56	15 32
Cape Bona Esperance	34 25	17 25

North Latitude. — West Longitude. — East Longitude. — South Lat.

Western Islands.

Places Names.	Latitude D. M.	Longitude D. M.
Corvo	40 5	29 55
Flores	39 40	29 50
Fyal	38 53	27 16
Pico	38 32	26 31
St. George	38 56	26 10
Tercera	38 53	24 42
St Michael	38 0	22 32
St. Maryes	37 0	22 17

North Latitude. — West Longitude.

The Canary Islands

Places Names	Latitude D. M.	Longit. D. M.
Ferro	28 0	18 12
Palma	28 50	18 0
Gomero	28 8	17 26
Tenarif	28 20	16 45
Madera West end	32 17	17 00
Porto Sancto	32 50	15 34
Canaria	27 56	15 30
Fortavertura	27 54	13 24
Lancerota	28 32	12 54

North Latitude. — West Longitude.

Cape de Verde Islands.

Places Names	Latitude D. M.	Longit. D. M.
St. Antonio	17 10	25 20
St. Vincent	16 55	25 10
St. Lucia	16 45	24 58
St. Nicholas	16 40	24 22
Brava	14 35	24 38
Fuogo	14 42	24 00
Java	15 20	23 10
Isle of May	15 10	22 12
Isle Sal	16 45	22 02
Bonavista	16 05	21 55

North Latitude. — West Longitude.

Southern Islands

Places Names	Latitude D. M.	Longit. D. M.
St. Mathews	1 40S	3 55W
Afcenfion	8 10S	12 35W
St. Hellena	16 6S	5 40W
Farnandepo	2 35N	11 55E
Princeps	1 25N	11 0E
St. Thomas	0 0	9 58E
Annabona	1 22S	9 28E

The Coast of the Main Continent in the East Indies

Places Names	Latitude D. M.	Longit. D. M.
Cape Bona Esperance	34 25S	17 25
Cape Lagulas	35 35S	18 40
Cape Corintes	23 52S	35 35
Mosambique	15 5S	40 30
River de Fugos	0 0	41 15
Cape Baffos	4 0	49 50
Cape Guardafoy	11 50	52 30
Cape Rosulgat	22 27	60 45
Cape Muca	26 56	57 10
Buffera	30	49 5
Surrat	21 8	73 25
Goa	15 22	74 37
Calecute	11 17	75 54
Cochin	9 58	76 45
Cape Comarine	7 50	78 25
Fort St. George	13 8	81 42

North Latitude. — East Longitude.

Dew

Places Names.	Latitude D. M.	Longitud D. M.
Dew Point	15 50	82 05
Visegapatam	7 40	85 07
Cape Palmeris	20 45	88 10
Bengal	22 27	91 49
Cape Negrais	16 23	93 05
Malacca	02 21	101 20
Siam Entrance	13 10	101 01
Cambodia Entrance	10 30	105 20
Cochin	18 25	103 58
Cantam	23 30	113 20
Amoy' or Quemoy	24 35	116 55
Lampo	30 10	120 25
Nanquim	32 55	120 05

(North Latitude — East Longitude)

Islands in the East-Indies.

Places Names.	Latitude D. M.	Longitud D. M.
Madagasc. or S. end	26 06	46 20
St. Laurence N. end	12 10	50 10
Mayetta	13 10	45 45
Mohilla	12 15	43 41
Comero	11 50	43 44
St. Juan de Nova	17 30	42 35
Mauritias	20 05	55 05
Digo Roves	19 45	61 35
Romiras de Castelamos	29 05	66 56
Amsterdam	39 50	74 24
St. Brandon	16 38	64 30
Digo Gratiosa	08 42	69 05
Quabella	03 49	52 39
Ballos de Chagos	05 05	70 25
Yas de Digo Rays	00 00	72 05
Maldivia N. end	07 05	73 05
Maldivia S. end	01 00	76 15
Malique	09 00	73 15
Saccatra	12 28	55 37
Abdeleur	12 10	54 23
Cape Gallo in Zelean	06 07	80 45
Yas de Amber	00 00	52 30
Andaman	13 00	91 25
Nicobor	07 05	92 55
Sumatra N. W. end	05 28	93 45
Verkins Island	02 22	94 07
Nassau Island	02 44	98 32
Bencola	03 50	101 13
Sumatra S. E. end	05 42	104 04
Engano	05 40	100 53
Selam	08 20	102 13
Princes Island	06 30	104 02
Bantam on Java	05 47	105 11
Batavia	05 37	106 27

(South Latitude — North Lat — East Longitude — South Latitude)

Places Names.	Latitude D. M.	Longitud D. M.
Java East-end	8 35	112 27
Straits of Sundy	5 52	104 18
Banca S. end	3 25	106 37
Borneo S. point	4 14	112 52
Bandy Isl s	5 5	126 37
Celebes { South end	6 0	117 27
Celebes { North end	1 40	121 30
Mindano W. point	6 30	118 35
Borneo N. point	7 10	112 45
Luconio { S. point	12 30	120 50
Luconio { N.E point	18 35	119 5
Anain { W. point	19 30	108 6
Anain { E. point	19 55	111 16
Formosa { S. point	22 0	119 30
Formosa { N point	25 32	120 25
Piscadore Isles	23 30	117 35
Island Chusan	30 38	120 35
Japan { S E. point	39 50	135 15
Japan { S W point	39 10	126 55

(South Latitude — North Latitude — East Longitude)

The Coast of America in the South Sea, from California to Cape Horn.

Places Names.	Latitude D. M.	Longitud D. M.
Cape St. Sebastian	42 40	129 55
Cape St. Luca	23 25	111 56
Cape Corientes	19 40	110 30
Aquapulco	17 0	106 28
Aquatulco	15 27	101 3
Guatimala	14 25	96 0
Panama	8 56	82 18
Bay Bonaventura	3 28	80 6
Islands of Gallopega	0 0	90 10
Cape del Agujo	16 38	83 50
Lima	12 30	78 30
Arica	18 12	74 10
La Serena	24 40	76 32
Island Juan Fernando	33 20	86 48
Baldivia	39 35	81 20
Port Steven	46 50	82 36
Cape Victory	52 15	83 20
Cape Horn	57 58	79 55

(North Lat — South Latitude — West Longitude)

The Coast of Brazile in South America, from Cape Horn to Cape Roque.

Places Names.	Latitude D. M.	Longitud D. M.
Magellan E. entrance	51 58	75 30
River Julian	48 40	74 32
Cape Blanco near }	46 50	72 5
River Camarones }		
Buenas Aires R. Plata	36 10	57 30
River Grand	31 55	51 40
St. Katharines	28 0	47 50

(South Latitude — West Longitude — Cape)

Places Names.	Latitude D. M.	Longitud D. M.	
Cape Frio	23 10	42 45	West Longitude.
Spir to Sancto	19 58	42 0	
P. Segura	16 22	40 55	
Bay Todos Sanctus	13 25		
R. St. Francisco	11 55	37 4	
Cape St. Augustine	5 5	35 20	
C. de R.	5 0	35 52	
Tr. de le Cur.	57 5	35 33	
The Cita	23 40	100 0	

The Coast of the Main Continent in the West Indies.

	Latitude	Longitude	
A. Amazones Entr.	0 0	49 0	West Longitude.
North Cape	2 5	49 55	
Surinam	6 0	56 55	
Oronoque	8 15	59 5	
C. Coquibaca	12 50	70 40	
Cartagena	10 50	75 50	
Scots Settlement	8 30	78 45	
Nicaragua Entrance	11 15	85 58	
Cape Catocha	21 22	88 55	
Campeche	19 20	93 05	
La vera Cruz	19 15	100 25	
Escondide	28 20	99 00	
Cape Florida	24 48	81 55	

The Caribbe Islands.

	Latitude	Longitude	
Trinadada	0 05	60 05	
Tobago	11 10	59 20	
Granada	12 07	60 30	
Barbadoes	13 10	58 03	
St. Vincent	13 12	59 22	
St. Lucia	13 52	59 17	
Martinico	14 48	58 25	
Domnico	5 35	58 27	
Mangalante	15 53	58 20	
Guardalupa	16 15	59 23	North Latitude. West Longitude.
Monserat	16 40	59 35	
Antegoa	17 00	59 21	
Nevis	17 06	60 18	
St. Christophers	17 22	60 35	
Barbuda	17 43	59 25	
St. Bartholomew	17 54	60 45	
St. Martins	18 05	60 49	
Anguilla	18 13	60 55	
Virgins	18 23	62 22	
St. Cruz	17 38	62 35	
Bieque	18 00	63 15	
Port Rico St. Johns	18 33	64 20	
St. Domingo Hispan.	18 15	68 50	

Places Names.	Latitude D. M.	Longitud D. M.	
Port Royal Jamaica	18 00	77 53	West Long.
East end of Cuba	20 20	74 25	N. Latit.
Havana	22 50	83 30	
Bay Hondy	22 35	84 40	
Cape St. Antoi	21 50	86 30	

Bahama Islands.

	Latitude	Longitude	
Bermudas	32 30	61 30	
Bahama Bank N. Point	28 22	78 15	
Bahama Island	27 05	78 58	
Abacoa S. Point	25 50	77 20	
Harbour Island	25 40	76 35	
Andros N. Point	25 15	79 00	
Providence	25 00	77 45	
Ilathera S. Point	24 30	76 12	
Cat Island	24 25	75 20	North Latitude. West Longitude.
Watling Iland	24 07	74 50	
Rum Key	23 45	75 05	
Exuma	23 25	76 07	
Crooked Isle N. Point	23 03	74 00	
Athins Key	22 00	74 15	
Merapervouz	21 57	74 40	
Atwoods key	23 09	73 30	
French Keys	22 40	73 35	
Nasaguina	22 35	73 00	
Hogstyes	21 15	73 50	
Hyneago	20 57	73 20	
Caicos bank N. Point	21 50	71 15	
Turks Island	21 35	70 08	
Abrolho N. Point	21 40	68 40	
Plate wrack	20 30	68 10	

The Coast of Carolina, Virginia, Mary Land, Pensilvania, New England, and Newfoundland.

	Latitude	Longitude	
Charles Town upon Ashly River	32 40	78 50	
Cape Hateras	35 10	74 25	
Cape Henry	37 00	74 30	
Cape Charles	37 14	74	North Latitude. West Longitude.
Cape Hinloper	39 04	73 25	
Long Island	40 50	70 40	
New York	41 00	72 05	
Cape Cod	42 10	57 45	
Boston	42 35	58 50	
Cape Sable	43 45	53 25	
Island Sable	44 30	59 5	
Cape Britain	46 20	58 15	
Quebeck	47 15	58 10	
Bay of Brest	52 10	55 0	

Bell

Places Names.	Latitude D. M.	Longitude D. M.	Places Names	Latitude D. M	Longit. D. M
Bell Island —	52 5	4 10	Whales head —	77 15	21 30
Cape St. John —	50 9	52 35	Hope Island —	76 22	22 0
Cape Bonavista —	49 11	2 3	Cherry or Bear Isl. —	74 35	8 5
Trinity Bay —	48 27	2 0	Admiralty Island —	75 5	19 50
Conception Bay —	47 53	2 0	Fretum Borrough —	9 55	52 5
St Johns Harbour —	47 25	1 25	Cape Candenose —	69 27	42 30
Bay of Bulls —	47 40	1 6	Catinose —	55 43	35 14
Cape Raze —	46 35	1 25	Archangel Bar —	55 5	35 30
Cape St Mary —	47 10	3 20	Cross Island —	56 31	36 33
Placentia —	47 57	53 0	Sweetnose —	68 8	34 42
Cape Roy —	48 21	7 15	Kiduyn —	29 32	30 15

The Coast of Hudson's Bay and Straits

Places Names	Latitude D. M.	Longitude D. M.	Places Names	Latitude D. M	Longit. D. M
Buttons Isle —	60 5	66 50	North Cape —	71 25	22 0
Cape Charles —	62 33	75 20	Surroy —	71 5	18 40
Cape Walsingham —	63 15	77 40	Tronsound —	70 18	16 0
Mansfield I. —	62 20	80 50	Loefort S. W. point —	57 47	9 35
Cape Jones —	55 03	79 15	Dronton —	54 0	10 40
Ruperts River —	51 16	79 55	Stadland —	52 10	4 38
Albans River —	52 32	84 7	North-bergen —	50 16	5 40
The Cubbs —	54 15	82 0	Naze of Norway —	57 50	7 22
C. Henriet. Maria —	55 5	84 2			
Port Nelson —	57 5	92 47			
Cape Churchil —	59 0	92 57			

Sea Coast in the Sound, and Baltick Sea.

Places Names	Latitude D. M.	Longitude D. M.	Places Names	Latitude D. M	Longit. D. M
Cape Southampton —	61 57	88 30	Mardou —	58 25	9 5
Shark Point —	64 27	83 20	Larwick —	58 54	9 20
Nottingham I. —	63 38	79 47	Christiana —	59 10	9 45
Q. Anns Foreland —	63 32	73 57	Maesterland —	57 58	11 45
Resolution I. —	61 55	65 50	Gottenberg —	57 33	12 25
Cape Farewell —	59 10	46 35	Elsinor —	56 00	12 32
			Copenhagen —	55 44	12 35
			Valsterborn —	55 20	12 55

The Coast of Iceland, Greenland, Nova Zembla, and the Northern Isles

Places Names	Latitude D. M.	Longitude D. M.	Places Names	Latitude D. M	Longit. D. M
Sound Royal —	66 22	14 15	Kalmer —	56 40	16 40
Bargazar Point —	66 30	11 12	Stockholm —	59 20	18 25
Whales Back —	65 27	10 05	Wyborg —	50 20	29 25
Merch. Foreland —	63 20	14 05	Petersberg —	59 25	29 50
Hallsford —	64 30	24 15	Narve —	58 39	29 14
Fair Foreland —	65 10	26 45	Revel —	59 00	24 45
Grims Island —	66 51	17 45	Riga —	56 52	24 50
Westmania Isles —	63 55	18 10	Derwanda —	57 20	22 00
Isles of Fero —	62 6	5 0	Conningsberg —	55 00	20 20
Beerenberg or John? Mains I. —	71 45	4 30	Dantzick —	54 22	19 00
Point Look-out —	76 40	16 25	Wishuy in Gotland —	57 37	18 50
Horn Sound —	77 23	14 20	Bornholm —	55 27	14 53
Fair Foreland —	79 18	10 50	Straelsound —	54 45	13 20
Hacluits Headland —	79 55	12 0	Lubeck —	54 25	11 5
Helies Sound —	79 15	12 50	Anout —	56 42	10 58
Lees Foreland —	78 5	23 25	Lesou —	57 5	10 40
			Scaw —	57 26	10 10

M	d	1d	2d	3d	4d	5d	6d	7d	8d	9d	10d	11d	12d	13d	M
0	0	60	120	180	240	300	361	421	481	542	603	664	725	787	0
1	1	61	121	181	241	301	362	422	482	543	604	665	726	788	1
2	2	62	122	182	242	302	363	423	483	544	605	666	727	789	2
3	3	63	123	183	243	303	364	424	484	545	606	667	728	790	3
4	4	64	124	184	244	304	365	425	485	546	607	668	729	791	4
5	5	65	125	185	245	305	366	426	486	547	608	669	730	792	5
6	6	66	126	186	246	306	367	427	488	548	609	670	731	793	6
7	7	67	127	187	247	307	368	428	489	549	610	671	732	794	7
8	8	68	128	188	248	308	369	429	490	550	611	672	733	795	8
9	9	69	129	189	249	309	370	430	491	551	612	673	734	796	9
10	10	70	130	190	250	310	371	431	492	552	613	674	735	797	10
11	11	71	131	191	251	311	372	432	493	553	614	675	736	798	11
12	12	72	132	192	252	312	373	433	494	554	615	676	737	799	12
13	13	73	133	193	253	313	374	434	495	555	616	677	738	800	13
14	14	74	134	194	254	314	375	435	496	556	617	678	740	801	14
15	15	75	135	195	255	315	376	436	497	557	618	679	741	802	15
16	16	76	136	196	256	316	377	437	498	558	619	680	742	803	16
17	17	77	137	197	257	317	378	438	499	559	620	681	743	804	17
18	18	78	138	198	258	318	379	439	500	560	621	682	744	805	18
19	19	79	139	199	259	319	380	440	501	561	622	683	745	806	19
20	20	80	140	200	260	320	381	441	502	562	623	684	746	807	20
21	21	81	141	201	261	321	382	442	503	563	624	685	747	808	21
22	22	82	142	202	262	322	383	443	504	564	625	686	748	809	22
23	23	83	143	203	263	323	384	444	505	565	626	687	749	810	23
24	24	84	144	204	264	324	385	445	506	566	627	688	750	811	24
25	25	85	145	205	265	325	386	446	507	567	628	689	751	812	25
26	26	86	146	206	266	326	387	447	508	568	629	690	752	813	26
27	27	87	147	207	267	327	388	448	509	569	630	691	753	814	27
28	28	88	148	208	268	328	389	449	510	570	631	692	754	815	28
29	29	89	149	209	269	329	390	450	511	571	632	694	755	816	29
30	30	90	150	210	270	330	391	451	512	572	633	695	756	817	30
31	31	91	151	211	271	331	392	452	513	574	634	696	757	819	31
32	32	92	152	212	272	332	393	453	514	575	635	697	758	820	32
33	33	93	153	213	273	333	394	454	515	576	636	698	759	821	33
34	34	94	154	214	274	334	395	455	516	577	638	699	760	822	34
35	35	95	155	215	275	335	396	456	517	578	639	700	61	823	35
36	36	96	156	216	276	336	397	457	518	579	640	701	762	824	36
37	37	97	157	217	277	337	398	458	519	580	641	702	763	825	37
38	38	98	158	218	278	338	399	459	520	581	642	703	764	826	38
39	39	99	159	219	279	339	400	460	521	582	643	704	765	827	39
40	40	100	160	220	280	340	401	461	522	583	644	705	766	828	40
41	41	101	161	221	281	341	402	462	523	584	645	706	767	829	41
42	42	102	162	222	282	342	403	463	524	585	646	707	768	830	42
43	43	103	163	223	283	343	404	464	525	586	647	708	769	831	43
44	44	104	164	224	284	344	405	465	526	587	648	709	770	832	44
45	45	105	165	225	285	345	406	466	527	588	649	710	771	833	45
46	46	106	166	226	286	346	407	467	528	589	650	711	772	834	46
47	47	107	167	227	287	347	408	468	529	590	651	712	773	835	47
48	48	108	168	228	288	348	409	469	530	591	652	713	774	836	48
49	49	109	169	229	289	349	410	470	531	592	653	714	775	837	49
50	50	110	170	230	290	350	411	471	532	593	654	715	776	838	50
51	51	111	171	231	291	351	412	472	533	594	655	716	777	839	51
52	52	112	172	232	292	352	413	473	534	595	656	717	778	840	52
53	53	113	173	233	293	353	414	474	535	596	657	718	779	841	53
54	54	114	174	234	294	354	415	475	536	597	658	719	780	842	54
55	55	115	175	235	295	355	416	476	537	598	659	720	782	843	55
56	56	116	176	236	296	356	417	477	538	599	660	721	783	844	56
57	57	117	177	237	297	357	418	477	539	600	661	722	784	845	57
58	58	118	178	238	298	358	419	478	540	601	662	723	785	846	58
59	59	119	179	239	299	360	420	480	541	602	663	724	786	847	59

month days	Week days	Remarkable days, & southing of stars at midnight	First Year 1717 1725 ⊙ pla. ♎	1721 1729 ⊙ dec. South.	Second Year 1718 1726 ⊙ pla ♎	1722 1730 ⊙ dec. South.	Third Year 1719 1727 ⊙ pla ♎	1723 1731 ⊙ dec South.	Leap 1720 1728 ⊙ pla. ♎	Year 1724 1732 ⊙ dec South.
			D. M.	D. M.	D. M.	D. M.	D. M.	D. M.	D. M.	D. M.
1	A	Sun r. 6. 38.	18 56	07 25	18 42	07 20	18 27	07 14	19 12	07 32
2	B		19 56	07 48	19 41	07 42	19 27	07 37	20 12	07 54
3	C		20 55	08 10	20 41	08 05	20 27	08 00	21 12	08 14
4	D		21 55	08 33	21 41	08 27	21 26	08 22	22 11	08 39
5	E		22 55	08 55	22 40	08 50	22 26	08 44	23 11	09 01
6	f		23 55	09 17	23 40	09 12	23 26	09 06	24 11	09 23
7	G		24 54	09 39	24 40	09 34	24 25	09 28	25 11	09 45
8	A		25 54	10 01	25 40	09 56	25 25	09 50	26 11	10 07
9	B		26 54	10 23	26 40	10 17	26 25	10 12	27 10	10 29
10	C		27 54	10 44	27 39	10 39	27 25	10 34	28 10	10 50
11	D	Andromeda's	28 54	11 06	28 39	11 00	28 25	10 55	29 10	11 11
12	E	southermoft Foot.	29 54	11 27	29 39	11 22	29 25	11 17	♏ 10	11 33
13	f	Sun r. 7. 4	♏ 54	11 48	♏ 39	11 43	♏ 25	11 38	01 10	11 54
14	G		01 54	12 09	01 39	12 03	01 25	11 59	02 10	12 14
15	A		02 54	12 29	02 39	12 24	02 25	12 19	03 10	12 35
16	B		03 54	12 50	03 39	12 45	03 25	12 40	04 10	12 55
17	C		04 54	13 10	04 40	13 05	04 25	13 00	05 10	13 16
18	D	Luke Evan.	05 54	13 30	05 40	13 25	05 26	13 20	06 11	13 36
19	E		06 54	13 50	06 40	13 45	06 25	13 40	07 11	13 55
20	f		07 55	14 10	07 40	14 05	07 25	14 00	08 11	14 15
21	G		08 55	14 29	08 40	14 24	08 26	14 20	09 11	14 34
22	A		09 55	14 48	09 41	14 44	09 26	14 39	10 12	14 54
23	B		10 56	15 07	10 41	15 03	10 26	14 58	11 12	15 12
24	C		11 56	15 26	11 41	15 21	11 27	15 17	12 12	15 31
25	D	Sun r. 7. 24.	12 56	15 44	12 42	15 40	12 27	15 35	13 13	15 49
26	E		13 57	16 02	13 42	15 58	13 27	15 54	14 13	16 07
27	f		14 57	16 20	14 42	16 16	14 28	16 12	15 14	16 25
28	G	Sim. & Jude.	15 58	16 38	15 43	16 34	15 28	16 29	16 14	16 43
29	A		16 58	16 55	16 43	16 51	16 29	16 47	17 15	17 01
30	B		17 59	17 13	17 44	17 08	17 29	17 04	18 15	17 17
31	C	Sun r. 7. 33.	18 59	17 33	18 45	17 25	18 30	17 21	19 16	17 34

Month days	Week days	Remarkable days, and southing of stars at midnight.	First Year. 1717. 1721. 1725. 1729. ☉ pla. D. M.	☉ dec. D. M.	Second Year. 1718. 1722. 1726. 1730. ☉ pla. D. M.	☉ dec. D. M.	Third Year. 1719. 1723. 1727. 1731. ☉ pla. D. M.	☉ dec. D. M.	Leap-Year. 1720. 1724. 1728. 1732. ☉ pla. D. M.	☉ dec. D. M.
			♏ south.		♏ south.		♏ south.		♏ south.	
1	D	All Saints.	20 00	17 47	19 45	17 42	19 30	17 38	20 16	17 51
2	E	Sun r. 7.36.	21 00	18 03	20 46	17 59	20 31	17 55	21 17	18 07
3	F		22 01	18 18	21 46	18 15	21 32	18 11	22 18	18 22
4	G	K. W. Nat.	23 02	18 34	22 47	18 30	22 32	18 27	23 18	18 37
5	A	Pow. plot.	24 02	18 49	23 48	18 46	23 33	18 42	24 19	18 52
6	B		25 03	19 04	24 48	19 00	24 34	18 57	25 20	19 07
7	C		26 04	19 18	25 49	19 15	25 35	19 12	26 20	19 22
8	D		27 05	19 32	26 50	19 29	26 35	19 26	27 21	19 38
9	E		28 05	19 46	27 51	19 43	27 36	19 40	28 22	19 50
10	F	Mart n B.	29 06	19 55	28 51	19 56	28 37	19 53	29 23	20 03
11	G		♐ 07	20 12	29 52	20 09	29 38	20 06	♐ 24	20 16
12	A		01 08	20 25	♐ 53	20 22	♐ 38	20 19	01 24	20 28
13	B	Sun r. 7.53.	02 09	20 37	01 54	20 3?	01 39	20 31	02 25	20 40
14	C		03 10	20 49	02 55	20 46	02 40	20 43	03 26	20 52
15	D		04 11	21 01	03 56	20 58	03 41	20 55	04 27	21 03
16	E	Aldebaran.	05 12	21 12	04 57	21 09	04 42	21 06	05 28	21 15
17	F		06 13	21 22	05 58	21 20	05 43	21 17	06 29	21 25
18	G		07 14	21 33	06 59	21 30	06 44	21 28	07 30	21 35
19	A		08 15	21 43	08 00	21 40	07 45	21 38	08 31	21 45
20	B		09 16	21 52	09 01	21 50	08 46	21 48	09 32	21 54
21	C		10 17	22 01	10 02	21 59	09 47	21 57	10 33	22 03
22	D		11 18	22 10	11 03	22 08	10 48	22 06	11 34	22 12
23	E		12 19	22 13	12 04	22 16	11 49	22 14	12 35	22 20
24	F	Sun r. 8.5.	13 20	22 26	13 05	22 2?	12 50	22 22	13 37	22 28
25	G	Capella, or	14 21	22 34	14 06	22 32	13 51	22 30	14 38	22 35
26	A	the Goat.	15 22	22 41	15 07	22 35	14 53	22 37	15 39	22 42
27	B	Orion's Left	16 23	22 47	16 08	22 46	15 54	22 44	16 40	22 48
28	C	Foot	17 25	22 53	17 10	22 52	16 55	22 50	17 41	22 54
29	D	Bulls Hor.	18 26	22 58	18 11	22 57	17 56	22 56	18 42	23 00
30	E	Andr. Ap.	19 27	23 03	19 12	23 02	18 57	23 01	19 43	23 05

Month Days	Week Days	Remarkable days, and southing of stars at midnight.	First Year 1717. 1721. 1725.				Second Year 1718. 1722. 1726. 1729. 1730.				Third Year 1719. 1722. 1723. 1727. 1730. 1731.				Leap Year 1720. 1724. 1728. 1732.			
			☉ pla. ♐ South.		☉ dec.		☉ pla. ♐ South.		☉ dec.		☉ pla ♐ South.		☉ dec.		☉ pla ♐ South.		☉ dec.	
			D.	M.	D.	M.	D.	M.	D.	M.	D.	M.	D.	M.	D.	M.	D.	M.
1	f	First in Ori-	20	28	23	07	20	13	23	07	19	58	23	06	20	45	23	09
2	B	on's Belt.	21	29	23	12	21	14	23	11	21	00	23	10	21	46	23	11
3	A	Last in Orion's	22	31	23	16	22	16	23	15	22	01	23	14	22	47	23	17
4	B	Belt.	23	22	23	19	23	17	23	19	23	02	23	18	23	48	23	26
5	C	Orion's right	24	33	23	22	24	18	23	22	24	03	23	21	24	50	23	23
6	D	shoulder, and	25	34	23	24	25	19	23	24	25	04	23	23	25	51	23	25
7	E	Auriga's	26	35	23	26	26	21	23	26	26	06	23	25	26	52	23	26
8	f	right should.	27	37	23	28	27	22	23	28	27	07	23	27	27	53	23	28
9	B		28	38	23	29	28	23	23	28	28	08	23	28	28	55	23	29
10	A		29	39	23	29	29	24	23	29	29	09	23	29	29	56	23	29
11	B	Shortest day	♑	41	23	29	♑	26	23	29	♑	11	23	29	♑	57	23	29
12	C		01	42	23	29	01	27	23	29	01	12	23	29	01	58	23	29
13	D	Foot of the	02	43	23	28	02	28	23	28	02	13	23	28	03	00	23	28
14	E	great Dog.	03	44	23	26	03	30	23	27	03	15	23	27	04	01	23	26
15	f	Bright Foot	04	46	23	24	04	31	23	25	04	16	23	25	05	02	23	24
16	f	of Gemini.	05	47	23	22	05	32	23	22	05	17	23	23	06	03	23	21
17	A	Sun r. 8. 12.	06	48	23	19	06	33	23	19	06	19	23	20	07	05	23	18
18	B	Mouth of	07	50	23	16	07	35	23	16	07	20	23	17	08	06	23	15
19	C	great Dog,	08	51	23	12	08	36	23	12	08	21	23	14	09	07	23	11
20	D	or Syrius.	09	52	23	07	09	37	23	09	09	22	23	10	10	09	23	06
21	E	Thomas Ap.	10	53	23	02	10	39	23	04	10	24	23	05	11	10	23	00
22	f		11	55	22	57	11	40	22	59	11	25	23	00	12	11	22	55
23	A	Sun r. 8. 8.	12	56	22	51	12	41	22	53	12	26	22	54	13	13	22	49
24	A		13	57	22	45	13	42	22	47	13	28	22	48	14	14	22	43
25	B	Nat. Christ.	14	59	22	38	14	44	22	41	14	29	22	42	15	15	22	36
26	C	St. Stephen.	16	00	22	31	15	45	22	34	15	30	22	35	16	16	22	29
27	D	John Evan.	17	01	22	24	16	46	22	27	16	31	22	27	17	18	22	22
28	E	Innocents.	18	02	22	16	17	47	22	19	17	33	22	20	18	19	22	14
29	f	Castor.	19	04	22	08	18	49	22	11	18	34	22	12	19	20	22	05
30	B	Pollux.	20	05	21	59	19	50	22	02	19	35	22	03	20	21	21	56
31	A	Sun r. 8. 1.	21	06	21	50	20	51	21	53	20	36	21	54	21	23	21	47

A Table of the Variation of the Sun's Declination, to every 15 Degrees of Longitude from the Meridian of *London*.

Degrees of Longitude from the Meridian of London.

Diurn. Variat min.	D 15 m.	D 30 m.	D 45 m.	D 60 m.	D 75 m.	D 90 m.	D 105 m.	D 120 m.	D 135 m.	D 150 m.	D 165 m.	D 180 m.
2	00	00	00	00	00	00	01	01	01	01	01	01
3	00	00	00	00	01	01	01	01	01	01	01	01
4	00	00	00	01	01	01	01	01	01	02	02	02
5	00	00	01	01	01	01	01	02	02	02	02	02
6	00	00	01	01	01	01	02	02	02	02	03	03
7	00	01	01	01	01	02	02	03	03	03	03	03
8	00	01	01	01	02	02	02	03	03	03	04	04
9	00	01	01	01	02	02	03	03	03	04	04	04
10	00	01	01	02	02	02	03	03	04	04	05	05
11	00	01	01	02	02	03	03	04	04	05	05	05
12	00	01	01	02	02	03	03	04	04	05	05	06
13	01	01	02	02	03	03	04	04	05	05	06	06
14	01	01	02	02	03	03	04	05	05	06	06	07
15	01	01	02	02	03	04	04	05	06	06	07	07
16	01	01	02	03	03	04	05	05	06	07	07	08
17	01	01	02	03	04	04	05	06	06	07	08	08
18	01	01	02	03	04	04	05	06	07	07	08	09
19	01	02	02	03	04	05	06	06	07	08	09	09
20	01	02	02	03	04	05	06	06	07	08	09	10
21	01	02	03	03	04	05	06	07	08	09	10	10
22	01	02	03	04	05	05	06	07	08	09	10	11
23	01	02	03	04	05	06	07	08	09	10	11	11
24	01	02	03	04	05	06	07	08	09	10	11	12

In each Page there are Eleven Columns; The Firſt ſheweth the Day of the Month, The ſecond the Day of the Week, The third ſome Remarkable Days and Southing of ſeveral Stars at Midnight; as you will find againſt *April* the fourth, there ſtands, *The laſt in the Great Bear's Tail,* which ſhews that the ſaid Star comes to the Meridian the fourth of *April* at midnight; The fourth Column ſhews the place of the Sun for the firſt Year after Leap-Year, as againſt the ſaid fourth of *April* in the fourth Column, which is under firſt Year, you find the SunsPlace in ♈ 25° 28' The Fifth Column ſhews the Suns Dec. for the firſt after Leap-Year, ſo on the aforeſaid fourth of *April* under Firſt Year, and ☉ Dec. you find the Suns Declination 9° 51' North. After the ſame Manner under-ſtand all the other Columns, where to avoid the trouble of Reckoning whe-ther it be firſt, Second, Third or Leap-Year, you may find the Year at the Top of the Table (under the Title of the Month) and under that againſt the Day of the Month you have the Suns Place and Declination ti'l *Anno* 1732; thus *July,* 1 1730 the Suns Place is 19° 35' of *Cancer.* his Declination 22° 3' North.

For the Declination of the Sun out of the Meridian of London.

Anno 1721, *April* 11, at ſix of the Clock Afternoon, I would know the Sun's Declination. The 11th day at Noon, I find it in the Table 12° 17' North, and the 12th day 12° 37'; therefore ſubtracting the leſſer Declination 12° 17' out of the greater, 12° 37'; the Reſidue 20' is the daily encreaſe. Then in the Table of Variation in Hours, &c. under 6 Hours or 90° in the Head, and againſt 20' on the Left-hand, I find 5m. the proportional Part; which (becauſe the Hour was Afternoon, and Declination encreaſing) added to the fore-found 12° 17' the Sum is 12° 22' North, the Declination: but if it had been 6 hours before Noon *viz.* at 6 in the Morning the Proportional part muſt have been ſubtracted, &c.

Here follows

A Table of Difference of *Latitude* and *Departure* to every Point and Quarter-Point of the Compaſs.

With the Uſe thereof in Working of a *Traverſe,* and keeping a *Sea-Reckoning.*

Diſt	¼ Points		½ Point		¾ Point		1 Point		1¼ Point		1½ Point		Diſt
	Lat	Dep	Lat	Dep	Lat	Dep	Lat	Dep	Lat	Dep	Lat	Dep	
1	00.99	00.06	00.29	00.12	00 99	00 15	00.98	00 20	00.97	00 24	00.96	00 29	1
2	01 99	00.10	01 99	00 20	01 98	00 2)	01 96	00 39	01 94	00.47	01.91	00 58	2
3	02 99	00.15	02.97	00.2X	02.97	00 44	02 94	00 59	02.91	00 72	02 87	00.87	3
4	03 99	00.20	03 98	00.3X	03 96	00 59	03 92	00 78	03 88	00 97	03.8	01 16	4
5	04.99	00.24	04.96	00 39	04.95	00.73	04 90	00 98	04 85	01 22	04.79	01 46	5
6	05 99	00.29	05 97	00.59	05 94	00 88	05 89	01.17	05 82	01 46	05.74	01 74	6
7	06 99	00.34	06 97	00.69	06 92	01 03	06.87	01 37	06 79	01 70	06.70	02 03	7
8	07 99	00.39	07 96	00 78	07 91	01 17	07 85	01 56	07 76	01 94	07 66	02 32	8
9	08 99	00.4.	08 96	00.88	08 90	01 32	08 83	01.76	08 73	02 19	08.62	02.61	9
10	09 99	00.49	09.95	00.98	09 89	01 47	09 81	01 95	09 70	02.43	09 57	02.90	10
11	10.98	00.54	10.95	01 08	10.88	01 62	10.79	02 15	10.67	02.67	10.53	03.19	11
12	11 98	00.59	11 94	0. 18	11 87	0. 76	11 77	02 34	11 64	02.92	11.48	03.48	12
13	12.98	00.64	12.94	01.28	12 85	01 91	12.75	02.54	12 61	03 16	12.44	03 77	13
14	13 98	00.69	13 93	01 3	13 35	02 06	13 73	02.73	13 58	03.40	13 40	04.06	14
15	14 98	00.73	14 93	01.47	14 84	02 20	14 71	02.93	14 55	03 65	14 36	04 36	15
16	15 98	00.78	15 92	01 57	15 83	02 35	15 70	03 12	15 52	03 89	15 31	04 64	16
17	16.98	00.83	16 92	01 67	16 81	02.49	16 68	03 3	16 49	04 11	16.27	04 93	17
18	17 98	00.89	17 91	01 76	17 80	02 64	17 66	03.57	17 46	04 37	17 23	05.21	18
19	18 98	00.93	18 7	01 86	18 79	02.79	18.64	03 71	18.43	04.62	18 19	05 51	19
20	19 93	00.98	19 90	01 96	19 73	02.93	19.62	03 90	19 40	04 86	19 14	05 81	20
21	20 97	01.03	20 90	02 06	20 77	03 08	20.60	04 10	20.37	05.10	20.10	06 10	21
22	21 97	01 08	21 89	02 16	21 76	03 22	21.58	04.29	21.34	05 35	21 05	06 39	22
23	22 97	01 13	22 89	02 26	22 75	03 37	22.56	04.49	22.31	05 5	22 01	06 68	23
24	23 97	01 18	23 88	02 3	23 74	03 52	23 54	04.68	23 28	05 83	22 97	06 97	24
25	24.97	01 23	24.88	02.45	24 73	03 66	24 52	04.88	24 25	06.06	23.93	07.27	25
26	25 97	01 27	25 87	02 55	25 72	03.81	25 51	05.0	25 22	06 31	24 88	07 55	26
27	26.97	01 32	26.87	02 65	26 70	03.96	26 49	05 27	26.19	06 56	25 84	07 84	27
28	27 96	01.37	27.86	02.74	27 69	04.10	27.47	05.46	27 16	06 80	26 80	08.13	28
29	28.96	01 42	28 86	02.84	28 68	04.25	28.45	05 66	28.13	07 05	27.76	08.42	29
30	29 96	01.47	29 85	02.94	29 67	04.40	29 42	05.85	29 10	07 29	28 71	08.71	30
31	30 96	01 52	30.85	03 24	30.66	04.55	30.40	06.05	30.07	07 53	29.67	09 00	31
32	31 96	01 57	31 84	03 14	31 65	04 69	31.38	06 24	31.04	07 78	30.62	09.29	32
33	32 96	01.62	32 84	03 24	32.64	04 84	32.36	06 44	32 01	08 02	31 58	09.58	33
34	33 95	01 67	33 83	03 33	33.63	04.99	33 34	06 63	32.98	08 26	32 54	09.87	34
35	34 95	01.71	34.83	03 43	34.62	05 13	34.32	06 83	33.95	08.51	33 50	10 17	35
36	35 95	01 76	35.82	03 53	35.61	05 28	35 31	07 02	34.92	08.75	34.45	10.45	36
37	36.95	01 81	36.82	03 62	36.59	05.43	36.29	07.22	35 89	08 9	35 41	10.74	37
38	37 95	01.86	37.81	03 72	37 58	05 57	37 27	07 41	36.86	09.23	36.37	11.03	38
39	38 95	01 91	38 81	03.82	38.57	05 72	38.25	07 61	37 83	09 46	37 33	11.32	39
40	39 95	01 96	39.81	03.92	39.57	05 87	39 23	07.80	38 80	09.72	38 28	11.61	40
41	40.94	02.01	40 80	04.01	40 56	06.02	40 21	08.00	39 77	09.96	39 24	11 90	41
42	41 94	02.06	41 80	04 11	41 55	06.16	41 19	08 19	40.74	10 21	40.19	12 19	42
43	42.94	02.11	42.80	04.21	42.54	06 31	42.17	08 39	41 71	10.45	41.15	12.48	43
44	43 94	02.16	43.79	04.31	43 53	06.46	43 15	08 58	42.68	10.69	42 11	12.77	44
45	44.94	02 22	44.79	04.41	44.52	06.60	44.13	08 78	43.65	10.94	43.07	13.07	45
46	45 94	02.25	45 78	04 51	45 51	06 75	45 12	08 97	44.62	11 18	44.03	13 35	46
47	46 94	02.30	46 78	04.61	46.49	06 90	46 10	09 17	45 59	11 42	44.98	13.64	47
48	47.94	02 35	47 77	04.70	47 48	07.04	47.08	09 36	46.56	11 66	45 94	13.93	48
49	48 94	02.40	48 77	04.80	48 47	07 19	48.06	09 56	47 53	11 91	46 90	14 22	49
50	49.94	02.45	49 76	04.90	49 46	07 34	49 04	09.76	48.50	12 15	47 85	14.51	50
Diſt	Dep	Lat	Dep	Lat	Dep	Lat	Dep	Lat	Dep	Lat	Dep	Lat	Diſt
	7¾ Points		7½ Point		7¼ Point		7 Point		6¾ Point		6½ Point		

Dist	¼ Point		½ Point		¾ Point.		1 Point.		1¼ Point		1½ Point		Dist
	Lat.	Dep	Lat.	Dep	Lat.	Dep	Lat.	Dep.	Lat	Dep	Lat	Dep	
51	50 93	02.50	50 75	05.00	50.45	07 49	50.02	09 96	49·47	12 33	48 81	14 ·5	51
52	51 93	02·55	51 75	05·10	51 44	07.63	51.00	10·15	50·44	12.64	49·76	15.09	52
53	52 93	02 60	52 75	05·19	52·43	07 76	51 98	10·35	51·41	12.88	50·72	15 30	53
54	53 93	02.65	53 74	05 29	53 42	07 93	52·96	10·55	52 36	13 13	51.68	15.67	54
55	54 93	02.69	54·74	05 39	54 41	08 07	53·94	10·74	53·35	13·37	52.64	15 97	55
56	55·93	02·74	55 73	05 49	55·40	08.22	54 93	10 94	54 32	13 61	53·59	16.25	56
57	56 93	02 79	56 73	05·59	56 38	08 37	55·91	11.13	55 29	13 85	54 5ᶜ	16 54	57
58	57 93	02 84	57 72	05 68	57 37	08 51	56 89	11 33	56 2ᶜ	14 09	55 51	16.83	58
59	58 93	02·89	58 72	05 78	58 36	08.66	57.87	11.52	57 23	14.34	56·47	17.12	59
60	59·93	02 94	59 71	05 88	59 35	08.80	58 85	11 71	58 20	14·58	57 42	17 42	60
61	60 92	02 99	60 71	05 98	60 34	08 95	59 83	11.91	59 17	14 82	58 38	17 71	61
62	61 92	03 04	61.70	06 ·8	61 3ᶜ	09.09	60.81	12.10	60 14	15 07	59 33	18.00	62
63	62.92	03 09	62 70	06 17	62 32	09.24	61.79	12 30	61.11	15 31	60.29	18.29	63
64	63.92	03 14	63 69	06 27	63 31	09 39	62 77	12 49	62.08	15 55	61 25	18 58	64
65	64·92	03 18	64 69	06 37	64.30	09 53	63 75	12 69	63 05	15 80	62 21	18 88	65
66	65 92	03·23	65 68	06.47	65 29	09 68	64·74	12.88	64 02	16 04	63 16	19·16	66
67	66 92	03 28	66 68	06.57	66.27	09 83	65·72	13 08	64 99	16.28	64 12	19 45	67
68	67 92	03 33	67·67	06 66	67 26	09 97	66 70	13 27	65 96	16 53	65 08	19 74	68
69	68 92	03 38	68.67	06 76	68 25	10.12	67.68	13 47	66 93	16 77	66.04	20 03	69
70	69 92	03·43	69 66	06 8ᶜ	69 24	10.27	68 66	13 66	67 90	17 01	66 98	10.32	70
71	70 91	03 48	70 66	06 9ᶜ	70 23	10.42	69 64	13 86	68 87	17 25	67 94	20·61	71
72	71·91	03 53	71 65	07 05	71 22	10 56	70·62	14·05	69 8.	17 50	68 89	20.90	72
73	72 91	03 58	72 65	07 15	72 21	10 71	71·60	14·25	70·81	17 74	69 85	21 19	73
74	73 91	03·63	73 64	07 25	73 20	10.86	72 58	14 45	71 78	17.98	70 81	21.48	74
75	74·91	03 67	74.64	07 35	74 19	11 00	73 56	14 64	72·75	18 23	71·77	21 78	75
76	75 91	03 72	75 63	07·45	75 18	11 15	74·55	14.84	73 72	18 47	72 72	22.06	76
77	76 9ᶜ	03·77	76.63	07 54	76 16	11.30	75·53	15 03	74 69	18 71	73 68	22.35	77
78	77 90	03 82	77 62	07 64	77 15	11.44	76·51	15 23	75 66	18 95	74 64	22.64	78
79	78·90	03 87	78 62	07 74	78 14	11.59	77·49	15 42	76 63	19.20	75 60	22.93	79
80	79·90	03·92	79·61	07 84	79·13	11.74	78.46	15 61	77.60	19.44	76 56	23.22	80
81	80.90	03 97	70·61	07.94	80 12	11.89	79.44	15 81	78 57	19.68	77 52	23.51	81
82	81.90	04.02	81 60	08 04	81 11	12.03	80.42	16 00	79 54	19 93	78 47	23 80	82
83	82.89	04.07	82.60	08.13	82 10	12 18	81.40	16 20	80 51	20.27	79·43	24.09	83
84	83 89	04.12	83 59	08.23	83 09	12.33	82.38	16 39	81·48	20.41	80.39	24.38	84
85	84 89	04 16	84 59	08 33	84 08	12.47	83 36	16.59	82 45	20.66	81 35	24.68	85
86	85·89	04.21	85·58	08.43	85 0ᶜ	12.62	84 35	16 78	83 42	20.90	82 30	24.96	86
87	86.89	04.26	86·58	08 53	86.06	12.77	85.33	16 98	84 39	21.14	83.26	25 25	87
88	87.89	04.31	87 57	08.62	87.05	12.91	86.31	17.17	85·36	21 38	84 22	25.54	88
89	88.89	04.36	88 57	08 72	88.04	13.06	87·29	17.37	86.33	21 63	85 18	25 83	89
90	89.89	04.42	89·57	08.82	89 03	13 21	88.27	17 56	87 30	21 87	86.13	26.13	90
91	90.88	04.47	90.56	08.92	90.02	13 36	89·25	17 76	88 27	22 11	87.09	26.42	91
92	91.88	04.52	91·56	09.02	91 01	13 50	90.13	17 95	89 24	22 36	88.04	26 71	92
93	92.88	04.57	92.56	09.11	92.00	13.65	91 21	18.15	90.21	22.60	89.00	27 00	93
94	93.88	04.62	93 55	09.21	92 99	13.80	92.19	18.35	91.18	22.84	89.96	27.29	94
95	94.88	04.66	94·55	09.31	93 98	13 94	93.17	18 54	92·15	23 09	90.92	27.59	95
96	95 88	04.71	95·54	09.41	94·97	14.09	94.15	18.74	93 12	23 33	91.87	27 87	96
97	96.88	04.76	96.54	09.51	95 95	14.24	95.14	18.93	94 09	23.57	92.83	28 16	97
98	97.88	04.81	97 53	09.60	96 94	14.38	96.12	19 13	95 06	23.81	93·79	28.45	98
99	98.88	04.86	98 53	09.70	97 93	14 53	37 10	19.32	96.03	24.06	94.75	28 74	99
100	99.88	04 91	99.52	09.80	98.92	14.67	98·08	19 51	97 00	24.30	95.69	29 03	100
Dist	Dep.	Lat.	Dep	Lat	Dep.	Lat	Dep.	Lat	Dep	Lat	Dep	Lat	Dist
	7¾ Point.		7½ Point		7¼ Point		7 Point.		6¾ Point		6½ Point		

Dist.	1¾ Points		2 Point		2¼ Point		2½ Point		2¾ Point		3 Point		Dist.
	Lat.	*Dep*	*Lat.*	*Dep*	*Lat*	*Dep*	*Lat*	*Dep*	*Lat*	*Dep*	*Lat*	*Dep*	
1	00.94	00.34	00.92	00.38	00.90	00.43	00.83	00.47	00.86	00 51	00.83	00.56	1
2	01.88	00.68	01 85	00 77	01 81	00.86	01.76	00.94	01 72	01 03	01 66	01 11	2
3	02.83	[illegible]	02.77	01 15	02.71	01 25	02.65	01 41	02.57	01 54	02 49	01.67	3
4	03 77	01 35	03 70	[illegible]	03 62	01 71	03 53	01 89	03 43	02.06	03 33	02 22	4
5	04 71	01 6[illegible]	04 62	0. 91	04.52	02.14	04.41	02.36	04.29	02 57	04.16	02 78	5
6	05.65	02.02	05 54	02 3[illegible]	05 42	02 57	05.29	02.83	05 15	03 08	05.99	03 33	6
7	06.59	02 36	06.47	02.68	06 33	02 97	06 17	03 30	06.00	03.60	05.82	03 89	7
8	07 53	02.70	07 39	03 06	07 23	03 42	07.05	03 77	06.86	04 11	06 65	04.44	8
9	08.47	03.03	08 32	03.44	08.14	03 85	07 94	04.24	07 72	04.63	07 48	05, 00	9
10	09.42	03.37	09.24	03.83	09.04	04.28	08 82	04 71	08 58	05 14	08 31	05 56	10
11	10.36	03 71	10.16	04.21	09 94	04.71	09 70	05 18	09 44	05 65	09 14	05 12	11
12	11 30	04.04	11.09	04 60	10.85	05 14	10.58	05 65	10.30	06 1,	09 9,	06 67	12
13	12.25	04.38	12.01	04.98	11.75	05 56	11.47	06 12	11.15	06 68	10 80	07 23	13
14	13 19	04.72	12.94	05.36	12.66	05 99	12.35	06.60	12.01	07 20	11 64	07 78	14
15	14.13	05.06	13.86	05.74	13.56	06.42	13 23	07 07	12.87	07 71	12.4,	08 34	15
16	15.07	05.39	14.78	06.13	14.46	06.65	14.11	07.54	13.73	08.22	13 30	08 89	16
17	16 01	05 73	15 71	06 51	15 37	07.27	14.93	08 01	14.58	08 7	14.13	09 45	17
18	16 95	06.07	16 63	06 89	16 27	07 70	15.83	08 48	15.44	09.25	14.96	10.00	18
19	17 89	06.40	17.56	07 27	17 18	08.13	16 76	08 95	16 30	09.77	15.79	10.56	19
20	18.83	06 74	18.48	07.65	18.08	08 55	17 64	09 43	17 15	10.2[illegible]	16 63	11.11	20
21	19 77	07.0[illegible]	19.40	08.03	18 98	08.98	18 52	09 90	18.01	10 79	17.46	11.67	21
22	20.71	07.41	20.34	08.42	19 89	09.41	19 40	10.37	18.87	11.31	18.29	12 22	22
23	21.66	07.75	21.25	08 80	20.79	09.83	20.29	10.84	19.72	11 82	19.12	12 78	23
24	22.60	08 09	22.18	09.18	21.70	10.26	21.17	11.32	20.58	12.34	19 96	13.33	24
25	23.54	08.43	23.10	09.56	22.60	10.69	22.05	11.79	21.44	12.85	20.79	13 89	25
26	24.48	08 76	24.02	09 95	23 50	11.12	22.93	12.26	22.30	13 36	21 62	14.44	26
27	25.42	09 10	24.95	10.33	24.41	11.54	23 81	12.73	23 15	13.88	22 45	15 00	27
28	26.36	09.44	25.87	10.71	25 31	11 97	24 70	13 20	24.01	14 39	23 28	15.55	28
29	27 30	09 77	26.80	11.09	26 22	12.40	25 58	13 67	24.87	14.9	24 11	16 11	29
30	28.25	10.11	27.72	11 48	27 12	12.83	26 46	14.14	25 73	15 42	24.94	16 67	30
31	29.19	10.45	28.64	11.86	28 0-	13 26	27 34	14 61	26.59	15 93	25.77	17 23	31
32	30.13	10.78	29 57	12.25	28 93	13 69	28 22	15 08	27 45	16.45	26.60	17 78	32
33	31.08	11.12	30.49	12 63	29.83	14.11	29.11	15.55	28.30	16.96	27 43	18 34	33
34	32.02	11 46	31.42	13.01	30.74	14.54	29 99	16.03	29 16	17.48	28 27	18 89	34
35	32.96	11 80	32.34	13.39	31 64	14.97	30.87	16.90	30.02	17.99	29.10	19 45	35
36	33 90	12.13	33.26	13.78	32.54	15.40	31 75	16.97	30.88	18 50	29 93	20.00	36
37	34.84	12.47	34.19	14.16	33 45	15.82	32.63	17 [illegible]	31 73	19.02	30.76	20 56	37
38	35 78	12.81	35.11	14.54	34.35	16.25	33 52	17 91	32.59	19.53	31 59	21 11	38
39	36 72	13 14	36.04	14.92	35 26	16.68	34.40	18 38	33 45	20.05	32.42	21.67	39
40	37 66	13.48	36.95	15 31	36.16	17 10	35 27	18.86	34.31	20.56	33 26	22 22	40
41	38.60	13.82	37.87	15.69	37.06	17 53	36.15	19 33	35.17	21.07	34.09	22.78	41
42	39 54	14.15	38.80	16.08	37.97	17 96	37 03	19 80	36.02	21.59	34.92	23.33	42
43	40.49	14.49	39.73	16.46	38 87	18 38	37 92	20.27	36.88	22.10	35 76	23.89	43
44	41.43	14 84	40.65	16 84	39.78	18 81	38.80	20 75	37.74	22.62	36.59	24.45	44
45	42.37	15 17	41 57	17.22	40.68	19.24	39.68	21 22	38.60	23.13	37.42	25 00	45
46	43 31	15 50	42.49	17 61	41 58	19.67	40.56	21 69	39.45	23.64	38 25	25 55	46
47	44 25	15.84	43.42	17 99	42.49	20.09	41.44	22.16	40.31	24.36	39 08	26 11	47
48	45.19	16.18	44.34	18 37	43.39	20.52	42.32	22.63	41.17	24.67	39 91	26.66	48
49	46.13	16.51	45 26	18.75	44.30	20.95	43 21	23 10	42.03	25 19	40.74	27.22	49
50	47.08	16.85	46 19	19 14	45 20	21.38	44.10	23 57	42.89	25.71	41 57	27 78	50
Dist.	*Dep.*	*Lat.*	*Dep.*	*Lat*	*Dep*	*Lat*	*Dep*	*Lat*	*Dep*	*Lat*	*Dep*	*Lat*	Dist.
	6¾ Points		6 Point		5¾ Point		5½ Point		5¼ Point		5 Point		

Dist.	1¾ Point Lat	1¾ Point Dep	2 Points Lat	2 Points Dep	2¼ Point Lat	2¼ Point Dep	2½ Point Lat	2½ Point Dep	2¾ Point Lat	2¾ Point Dep	3 Point Lat	3 Point Dp	Dist.
51	48.02	17 19	47.11	19.52	46.10	21 81	44 98	24 04	43 7	26 21	42 20	28 36	51
52	48 96	17 52	48 04	19 91	47 01	22 24	45 8	24 51	44 61	26 74	43 2	28 89	52
53	49 91	17.86	48 96	22.2	47 71	22 66	46 76	24 9	45 4	27 26	44 0	29 45	53
54	50 85	18 20	49 89	20.67	48 82	23 09	47.6	25 4	41 32	27 7	44 9	30.00	54
55	51 79	18 54	50 81	21 05	49 72	23.52	48 5	25 7	47 1	28 25	45 7	30 5	55
56	52 73	18.87	51 73	21 44	50 62	23 95	49 39	26 40	48 0	28 7	46 5	31.11	56
57	53 67	19.21	52 68	21 82	51 53	24 37	50.2	26 87	48 8	29 31	47 30	31 67	57
58	54 61	19 55	53 58	22 20	52 43	24.80	51 1	27 3	49 75	29 82	48 2	32 22	58
59	55 55	19 88	54 51	22.57	53 34	25 23	52.04	27 81	50.61	30 34	49.0	32 78	59
60	56 49	20 21	55 43	22.9	54 24	25 65	52.91	28 28	51.4	30 85	49.8	33 33	60
61	57 43	20.55	56.35	23 34	55 14	26 07	53 79	28.75	52 3	31 36	50 72	33 89	61
62	58 37	20 88	57 28	23 73	56 05	26.51	54 67	29 22	53 18	31 88	51.55	34 44	62
63	59 32	21 22	58 20	24 11	56 95	26 93	55 5	29 69	54.0	32.39	52.3	35 00	63
64	60.26	21 56	59 13	24.49	57 86	27 36	56 44	30 17	54 8	32 91	53.22	35 55	64
65	61 20	21 90	60.05	24.87	58 76	27 79	57 32	30 54	55 75	33.42	54.05	36 11	65
66	62.14	22 23	60.97	25 26	59 66	28 22	58.20	31 11	56 6	33 93	54.8	36 66	66
67	63 08	22 57	61 90	25 64	60.57	28 64	59 08	31.58	57 36	34 45	55 71	37 22	67
68	64.02	22 91	62.82	26 02	61 47	29 07	59 97	32.05	58.3	34.9	56.5	37 77	68
69	64 96	23 24	63.74	26 40	62 38	29 50	60 85	32.52	59.1	35 48	57.3	38 33	69
70	65 91	23 58	64.67	26.79	63 28	29 93	61 73	33 00	60.0	35 99	58.20	38 89	70
71	66 85	23.92	65.59	27.17	64.18	30 36	62.61	33 47	60 9	36.50	59.0	39.45	71
72	67 79	24.25	66 52	27 5	65 09	30 79	63 49	33 94	61.7	37 02	59 8	40.00	72
73	68 74	24.59	67.44	27 94	65.99	31 22	64 38	34.41	62.61	37.5	60.6	40.56	73
74	69 68	24 93	68 37	28.32	66.90	31 64	65 26	34.89	63 47	38 05	61.5	41.11	74
75	70 62	25 27	69.29	28 70	67 80	32 07	66 14	35 36	64.33	38.5	62.3	41.67	75
76	71.56	25.60	70.21	29 09	68 70	32.48	67.02	35 83	65.1	39 07	63.1	42.22	76
77	72.50	25 94	71 14	29.47	69.61	32.92	67.90	36 30	56.c	39.5	64.02	42.78	77
78	73 44	26 28	72.06	29 85	70.51	33.35	68 79	36 77	66 9c	40.10	64.8	43.33	78
79	74 38	26.61	72.99	30.23	71 42	33 78	69.67	37 2	67 7	40 62	65.67	43.89	79
80	75.32	26 95	73.91	30.62	72.32	34 21	70.55	37 71	68 62	41 3	66.52	44.45	80
81	76 26	27 29	74.83	31.00	73.22	34.64	71 43	38 18	59.48	41.64	67.35	45 00	81
82	77 20	27 62	75.76	31 39	74.13	35 07	72.31	38 65	70.3	42.16	58 18	45.55	82
83	78 15	27 96	76.68	31.77	75.03	35 49	73 20	39 12	71 1	42.67	68 95	46 11	83
84	79.09	28.30	77.61	32.15	75 94	35.92	74 0	39 60	72.05	43 1	69.8	46.66	84
85	80.08	28.64	78 58	32.53	76 84	36.35	74 96	40.07	72.91	43.7	70.68	47 22	85
86	80.97	28 97	79.45	32.92	77 74	36 78	75 84	40.54	73.77	44 21	71.51	47.77	86
87	81 91	29 31	80.38	33.30	78 65	37.20	76 72	41 02	74.62	44.71	72.34	48 33	87
88	82 85	29.65	81.30	33 68	79.55	37 63	77 61	41.48	75.48	45 26	73 17	48.88	88
89	83.79	29.98	82.23	34.06	80.46	38 0	78 49	41.95	76.34	45.76	74.00	49.44	89
90	84.74	30 32	83 15	34 44	81.36	38 48	79 37	42.42	77.20	46 27	74.8	50.00	90
91	85.68	30 66	84.07	34 82	82 26	38.91	80 25	42.89	78 06	46.78	75 6	50.56	91
92	86 62	30.99	85 00	35 2	83 17	39.34	81.1	43 36	78 92	47 30	76.46	51.11	92
93	87.57	31.33	85.92	35.59	84.07	39 76	82.02	43 8	79.77	47 8	77.32	51 67	93
94	88 51	31.67	86.85	35.97	84.98	40.19	82 90	44.31	80.63	48.31	78.1c	52.22	94
95	89 45	32.01	87 77	36.35	85 88	40.61	83 78	44 78	81.49	48.84	78 99	52.78	95
96	90.39	32 34	88 69	36.74	86 78	41.05	84.66	45 25	82.35	49 35	79.82	53.33	96
97	91 33	32.68	89.62	37 12	87 69	41 47	85 54	45.72	83 20	49.8	50.65	53 89	97
98	92 27	33.02	90.54	37 50	88.59	41.90	86.4	46.19	84.06	50 3	81.4	54.44	98
99	93 21	33 35	91 47	37 88	89 50	42.33	87 3	46.66	84 92	50 9	82.3	55 00	99
100	94 16	33 69	92.39	38.27	90.40	42.16	88 1	47 14	85.77	51 41	83.15	55 56	100

Dist.	Dep	Lat	Dep	Lat	Dep	Lat	Dep	Lat	Dep	Lat	Dep	Lat	Dist.
	6¼ Point		6 Points		5¾ Point		5½ Point		5¼ Point		5 Point		

Ii

Diff.	3¼ Point Lat	3¼ Point Dep	3½ Point Lat	3½ Point Dep	3¾ Point Lat	3¾ Point Dep	4 Point Lat	4 Point Dep	Diff.
1	00.50	00.60	00.77	00.63	00.74	00.67	00.71	00.71	1
2	01.61	01.19	01.55	01.27	01.48	01.34	01.41	01.41	2
3	02.41	01.79	02.32	01.90	02.22	02.01	02.12	02.12	3
4	03.21	02.38	03.09	02.54	02.96	02.69	02.83	02.83	4
5	04.02	02.98	03.86	03.17	03.70	03.36	03.53	03.53	5
6	04.82	03.57	04.64	03.81	04.45	04.03	04.24	04.24	6
7	05.62	04.17	05.41	04.44	05.19	04.70	04.95	04.95	7
8	06.43	04.77	06.18	05.07	05.93	05.37	05.66	05.66	8
9	07.23	05.36	06.96	05.71	06.67	06.04	06.36	06.36	9
10	08.03	05.96	07.73	06.34	07.41	06.72	07.07	07.07	10
11	08.83	06.56	08.50	06.97	08.15	07.39	07.78	07.78	11
12	09.64	07.15	09.28	07.61	08.89	08.06	08.48	08.48	12
13	10.44	07.75	10.05	08.24	09.63	08.73	09.19	09.19	13
14	11.24	08.34	10.82	08.88	10.37	09.41	09.90	09.90	14
15	12.05	08.94	11.59	09.51	11.11	10.08	10.60	10.60	15
16	12.85	09.53	12.37	10.15	11.86	10.75	11.31	11.31	16
17	13.65	10.13	13.14	10.78	12.60	11.42	12.02	12.02	17
18	14.46	10.73	13.91	11.41	13.34	12.09	12.73	12.73	18
19	15.26	11.32	14.69	12.05	14.08	12.76	13.43	13.43	19
20	16.05	11.91	15.46	12.69	14.82	13.43	14.14	14.14	20
21	16.86	12.51	16.23	13.32	15.56	14.10	14.85	14.85	21
22	17.6?	13.10	17.01	13.96	16.30	14.77	15.55	15.55	22
23	18.47	13.70	17.78	14.59	17.04	15.44	16.26	16.26	23
24	19.27	14.29	18.55	15.23	17.78	16.12	16.97	16.97	24
25	20.08	14.89	19.2	15.86	18.52	16.79	17.67	17.67	25
26	20.88	15.48	20.10	16.50	19.27	17.45	18.38	18.38	26
27	21.68	16.08	20.87	17.13	20.01	18.13	19.09	19.09	27
28	22.48	16.68	21.64	17.76	20.75	18.80	19.80	19.80	28
29	23.28	17.27	22.42	18.40	21.49	19.47	20.50	20.50	29
30	24.10	17.87	23.19	19.03	22.23	20.15	21.21	21.21	30
31	24.89	18.47	23.96	19.66	22.97	20.82	21.92	21.92	31
32	25.70	19.06	24.74	20.30	23.71	21.49	22.62	22.62	32
33	26.50	19.66	25.51	20.93	24.45	22.16	23.33	23.33	33
34	27.30	20.25	26.28	21.57	25.19	22.84	24.04	24.04	34
35	28.11	20.85	27.05	22.20	25.93	23.51	24.74	24.74	35
36	28.91	21.44	27.83	22.84	26.68	24.18	25.45	25.45	36
37	29.71	22.04	28.60	23.47	27.42	24.85	26.16	26.16	37
38	30.51	22.64	29.37	24.10	28.16	25.52	26.87	26.87	38
39	31.31	23.23	30.15	24.74	28.90	26.19	27.57	27.57	39
40	32.12	23.83	30.92	25.38	29.64	26.86	28.28	28.28	40
41	32.92	24.43	31.69	26.01	30.38	27.53	28.99	28.99	41
42	33.73	25.02	32.47	26.65	31.12	28.20	29.69	29.69	42
43	34.53	25.62	33.24	27.28	31.86	28.87	30.40	30.40	43
44	35.33	26.21	34.01	27.92	32.60	29.55	31.11	31.11	44
45	36.13	26.81	34.78	28.55	33.34	30.22	31.81	31.81	45
46	36.94	27.40	35.56	29.19	34.09	30.88	32.52	32.52	46
47	37.74	28.00	36.33	29.82	34.83	31.56	33.23	33.23	47
48	38.54	28.60	37.10	30.45	35.57	32.23	33.94	33.94	48
49	39.34	29.19	37.88	31.09	36.31	32.90	34.64	34.64	49
50	40.10	29.78	38.65	31.72	37.05	33.58	35.35	35.35	50
	ep	at	Dep	Lat	Dep	Lat	Dep	Lat	

Dist.	3¼ Point. Lat.	3¼ Point. Dep.	3½ Point. Lat	3½ Point. Dep	3¾ Point Lat.	3¾ Point Dep.	4 Point. Lat.	4 Point. Dep.	Dist.
51	40.96	30.38	39 42	32.35	37 79	34.25	36.06	36.06	51
52	41.77	30.97	40 20	32.99	38 53	34.92	36.76	36 75	52
53	42.57	31.57	40.97	33.62	39 27	35.59	37.46	37.46	53
54	43.37	32.16	41 74	34 26	40.01	36.27	38.18	38.18	54
55	44.18	32.76	42 51	34.89	40.75	36.94	38.88	38 88	55
56	44.98	33.35	43 29	35.53	41 50	37.61	39.59	39.59	56
57	45.78	33.95	44.06	36.16	42.24	38 28	40.30	40.30	57
58	46.58	34.55	44.83	36.79	42 97	38.95	41.01	41 01	58
59	47.39	35.14	45 61	37.43	43.72	39.62	41.71	41.71	59
60	48.19	35.74	46.38	38.06	44.46	40.29	42.43	42.43	60
61	48.99	36.34	47 15	38.69	45 20	40.96	43.14	43.14	61
62	49.80	36.93	47.93	39.33	45.94	41 63	43.84	43.84	62
63	50.60	37.53	48.70	39.96	46.68	42.30	44 55	44 55	63
64	51.40	38 12	49.47	40.60	47 42	42.98	45.26	45 26	64
65	52.21	38.72	50.24	41.23	48 16	43.65	45.96	45.96	65
66	53.01	39 31	51.02	41.87	48.91	44.29	46.67	46.67	66
67	53.81	39.91	51.79	42.50	49 65	44.99	47.38	47 38	67
68	54.62	40.51	52.56	43.13	50.39	45.66	48.09	48 09	68
69	55.42	41.10	53 34	43.77	51.13	46.33	48.79	48.79	69
70	56.23	41.70	54.11	44.41	51.8	47 01	49.50	49 50	70
71	57.03	42.30	54.88	45.04	52.61	47 68	50.21	50.21	71
72	57 84	42.89	55.66	45 68	53.35	48.35	50.91	50.91	72
73	58.64	43 49	56.43	46 31	54.09	49.02	51.62	51.62	73
74	59.44	44.08	57.20	46.95	54.83	49.70	52.33	52.33	74
75	60.25	44.68	57.97	47.58	55.57	50.37	53.03	53 03	75
76	61.05	45.27	58.75	48.22	56.32	51.04	53.74	53 74	76
77	61.85	45.87	59.52	48.85	57 06	51.71	54.45	54.45	77
78	62.66	46.47	60.29	49.48	57.80	52 38	55.16	55.16	78
79	63.46	47.06	61.07	50.12	58.54	53.05	55.86	55.86	79
80	64.26	47.66	61 84	50.75	59.28	53.72	56.57	56 57	80
81	65.06	48.26	62.61	51.38	60 02	54.39	57.28	57.28	81
82	65.87	48 85	63.39	52.02	60.76	55.06	57.98	57.98	82
83	66.67	49.45	64.16	52.65	61.50	55.73	58.69	58 69	83
84	67.47	50.04	64.93	53 29	62 24	56.41	59.40	59.40	84
85	68.28	50.64	65.70	53.92	62.98	57.08	60.10	60 10	85
86	69.08	51.23	66.48	54.56	63.73	57 72	60.81	60.81	86
87	69.88	51.83	67.25	55.19	64.47	58.42	61.52	61.52	87
88	70.69	52.43	68.02	55 82	65.21	59.09	62.23	62 23	88
89	71.49	53.02	68.80	56.46	65.95	59.76	62.93	62.93	89
90	72.29	53.61	69 57	57.10	66.69	60.44	63.64	63.64	90
91	73.09	54.21	70.34	57.73	67.43	61.11	64.35	64.35	91
92	73.90	54.80	71 12	58 37	68 17	61.78	65.05	65.05	92
93	74.70	55.40	71.89	59.00	68.91	62.45	65.76	65.76	93
94	75.50	55.99	72.66	59.64	69.65	63.13	66.47	66.47	94
95	76.31	56 59	73.43	60.27	70 39	63 80	67.17	67.17	95
96	77.11	57.18	74.21	60.91	71.14	64.47	67.88	67.88	96
97	77.91	57.78	74.98	61.54	71.88	65.14	68.59	68 59	97
98	78.72	58 38	75 75	62 17	72.62	65.81	69.30	69.30	98
99	79.52	58.97	76 53	62.81	73.36	66.48	70.00	70.00	99
100	80.32	59 57	77.30	63.44	74.10	67.16	70.71	70.71	100
Dist.	Dep.	Lat.	Dep.	Lat.	Dep.	Lat	Dep.	Lat.	Dist.
	4¾ Point.		4½ Point.		4¼ Point		4 Point.		

The Use of the preceeding Table of Difference of Latitude and Departure

THis is a large Table, giving the Difference of Latitude and Departure to any Diſtance not exceeding 10000, and to every Quarter-Point of the Compaſs.

The Courſe ſtands at the Head and Foot of the Table , at the Head it begins at ¼ Point, ſo ½ Point, ¾ Point, increaſing to 4 Points ; at the Foot it begins at 4 Points, ſo 4 ¼ Points, 4 ½ Points, increaſing backwards to 7 ¾ Points, The Diſtance is placed in the two outermoſt Columns of each Page, under the word *Diſt* on the Left hand Page, beginning at 1, and increaſing to 50 ; on the Right-hand Page, beginning at 51, and increaſing to 100. The Difference of Latitude and Departure ſtands under the Courſe at the Head of the Table, and over the Courſe at the Foot thereof, diſtinguiſhed by the words, *Lat.* and *Dep.*

1 In this Table, if your Diſtance exceed not 100 Miles or Leagues the Difference of Latitude and Departure will be given in Miles or Leagues, and 100 Parts of a Mile or League . But it may ſuffice, if the Difference of Latitude and Departure be taken only to Miles or Leagues, and tenth Parts of a Mile or League, with this Allowance, that if the Parts be 16 or more, inſtead thereof ſet down 2 Tenths, (which is 20 hundred parts,) if 26, or more, 3 Tenths; if 36, or more, 4 Tenths, if 46, or more, 5 Tenths, if 56, or more, 6 Tenths; if 66, or more, 7 Tenths ; if 76, or more, 8 Tenths, if 86, or more, 9 Tenths; if 96, or more, then make the Miles or Leagues of Difference of Latitude or Departure, 1 more then they are in the Table : As for inſtance, inſtead of 19. 16, ſet down 19 2 Tenths , for 27 27 place 27.3 ; for 49.59, place 49.6 ; for for 52 78, place 52 8 ; for 76 96, place 77 , for 78 96, place 79 Miles or Leagues.

2 If the Diſtance be above 100, and not exceeding 1000, this Table gives the Difference of Latitude and Departure in Miles or Leagues, and tenth Parts, being taken out at twice.

3. If the Diſtance be more than 1000, and exceeds not 10000, the Difference of Latitude and Departure is given in Miles or Leagues, as ſhall be explained by what follows.

This Table is very uſeful in the reſolving theſe 6 *Problems* in Navigation following; provided, in the 5 laſt *Problems,* the Diſtance either given or required exceeds not 100 Miles or Leagues.

Problem I *The Courſe and Diſtance given ; to find the Difference of Latitude and Departure.*

Example 1 *A Ship ſails W. S. W. ½ Weſt,* 50 *Miles ; to find the Difference of Latitude, and the Departure.*

On the Left-hand Page of the Table, over 6 ½ Points, and right againſt 50 Miles diſtance, you will find over the word *Lat.* 14 51, and over *Dep.* 47.85 ; which being contracted according to the firſt Rule foregoing, ſhews your Diff. of Lat. to be 14.5 Tenths, and your Departure 47.8 Tenths, as was required.

Example 2 *A Ship ſails E by N. half Eaſt,* 125 *Miles ; to find the Difference of Latitude and Departure.*

This muſt be taken out of the Table at twice, after this following manner.

To

To perform this, you muſt account . 1 at the beginning of the Table to be 10; and 2 to be 20; 3, 30; 4, 40; 5, 50 And ſo 10 to be 100, 11, 110; 12, 120, and 20 to be 200, 30, 300, 40, 400; 50, 500; 60, 600, 70, 700, 80, 800, 90, 900, and 100 at the end, to be 1000.

According to this Direction, againſt 12 (which ſtands for 120) on the Left-hand Page, over 7 ¼ Points, ſtands 1. 18 over *Lat.* and 11.94 over *Dep* which done, according to the ſecond Rule before given, your Difference of Latitude is 11.8, and your Departure 119 4   Then take out the Diff. of Lat. and Dep for the Remainder, which is 5, according to the firſt Rule aforegoing, and after the manner of the firſt Example of this *Problem*, ſo you will find Difference of Latitude to be 0.5, and your Departure 5.0· This done, ſet them down, and add them together after this manner

Drſt.	Lat.	Dep.
120	11.8	119.4
5	0.5	5 0
125	12 3	124 4

So that your Difference of Latitude for the whole Diſtance 125 Miles is 12.3 Tenths, and your Departure 124.4 Tenths.

Example 3. *A Ship ſails NW. by N. ¼ Weſt,* 976 *Miles; to find the Difference of Latitude and Departure.*

Under 3 ¼ Points, and againſt 97 (taken for 970) ſtands 77 91, and 57.78, that is the Difference of Latitude 779.1 Tenth, the Departure 577 8 Tenths. againſt 6 ſtands 4 82, and 3.57 that is, the Difference of Latitude 4 8 Tenths; the Departure 3.6 Tenths; which added together, makes the whole Difference of Latitude 783.9, and the Departure 581.4.

Example 4. *A Ship ſails N. E. by N. half Eaſt,* 7968 *Miles; to find the Difference of Latitude and Departure-*

To perform this, you muſt account 1 at the beginning of the Table to be 100; 2, to be 200; 3, 300; 4, 400· And ſo 10 to be 1000, 11 to be 1100; 12, 1200, 13, 1300; 14, 1400· So 20 to be 2000, 30, 3000; 40, 4000; 50, 5000, 60, 6000; 70, 7000, 80, 8000, 90, 9000, and 100, 10000.

According to this Direction, againſt 79 (taken for 7900) and under 3 ¼ Points ſtands 6107. for the Difference of Latitude, and 5012. Miles for the Departure, according to the third Rule. Then take out the Differences of Latitude and Departure for the Remainder 68, according to the firſt Rule, which you ſhall find to be 52 6, and 43 1; ſo the whole Difference of Latitude is 6159.6 Miles. and the Departure 5055.1 Miles

Problem II. *The Courſe and Difference of Latitude being given; to find the Diſtance and Departure.*

Example. *A Ship ſails W N.W. half Weſt, until her Difference of Latitude be* 14.5 *Leagues; to find the Diſtance, and Departure.*

Look over 6 ½ Points the Courſe, in the Column of Latitude. until you find 14.5 and right againſt it you will find the Diſtance 50 Leagues. and the Departure 47 8 Leagues.

Problem III *The Courſe and Departure given, to find the Difference of Latitude and the Diſtance.*

Example

Example *A Ship fails S. W. by S. ¾ W. until her Departure be 47.7 Leagues; to find the Difference of Latitude and Distance.*

Look in the Column of Departure, under 3 ¾ Points, until you find 47 7, and right against it you see 52.6 Leagues, for the Difference of Latitude, and 71 Leagues for the Distance

PROB. IV *The Diff. of Lat. and Distance given, to find the Course and Departure*
    Example *A Ship fails 50 Leagues between the South and the West, until her Difference of Latitude be 14.5 Leagues, to find the Course and Departure*

Look over your several Columns in the Table, until right against 50, the Distance, you find 14 5 in the Column of Latitude, over the Course, which will be 6 ½ Points, and in the Column of Departure you will find your Departure to be 47.8

PROB. V *The Distance and Depart given; to find the Course and Diff of Latitude.*
    Example. *A Ship fails 80 Leag North Westerly, until her Departure be 53.7 Leagues, to find the Course and Difference of Latitude.*

Look over the several Columns in the Table, until right against 80 the Distance, you find 53.7 in the Column of Departure, over it you will see 3 ¾ Points, or N W. by N ¼ W. and the Difference of Latitude (in the Column of Latitude, right against 80) to be 59.3 Leagues.

PROB. VI. *The Difference of Latitude and Departure being given, to find the Course and Distance.*

    Example. *A Ship fails between the North and the East, until her Difference of Latitude be 56.3 Leagues, and her Departure 51.0; to find the Course and Distance.*

Look over your several Columns of Latitude and Departure, until you find 56.3 to stand against 51.0, or the nearest thereto, which will be under 3 ¾ Points, which makes the Course N. E by N. ¾ E. and it stands right against 76 Leag. which is the Distance required.

PROB VII *How to work a Traverse by the Tables of Latitude and Departure.*

These Tables in the working of a Traverse, are both readier and far more exact, than any Instrument commonly used for that purpose.

    Example. *A Ship fails S. W. by S. 37 min. then S. by E. 39 min. then S. E. by S. half E 47 min. then W by N. 59 min. then W N W 62 min. then S W. ½ W 27 min. to find the Difference of Latitude and Departure, and the direct Course and Distance from the first Place.*

Set down the several Courses and Distances, as in the following Table

Course.	Dist.	North	South	East	West.
South West by South.	37		30 8		20.6
South by East	39		38 2	07.6	
S E by S half E	47		36 3	29.8	
West by North.	59	11.5			57.9
West North West	62	23 7			57 3
South West half West.	27		17.1		20.9
		35.2	122.4	37.4	156 7
			35.2		37.4
		Diff Lat	87.2	Dep.	119.2

Then

Then by *Problem* 1. Find the Difference of Latitude and Departure for those Courfes and Diftances feverally, which place in their proper Columns, *viz.* If the Courfe be North-Eafterly, place the Difference of Latitude in the North Column (under *North*) the Departure in the Eaft Column, (under *Eaft* ·) If the Courfe be South-Eafterly, place the Difference of Latitude in the South Column, (under *South*) and the Departure in the Eaft Column. If the Courfe be North-Wefterly, place the Difference of Latitude in the North Column, and Departure in the Weft Column. If the Courfe be South-Wefterly place the Difference of Latitude in the South Column, and the Departure in the Weft Column.

As for Inftance in the foregoing Table, the firft Courfe is South Weft by South the Diftance 37 Becaufe the Courfe is South Wefterly, you muft place the difference of Latitude 30.8 in the South Column, and the Departure 20. 6 in the *Weft* Column, as you fee in the Table.

The like is to be underftood of the reft. Having found the Difference of Latitude and Departure for all your feveral Courfes, and inferted them in their proper Columns, you muft then add up your *North*, *South*, *Eaft* and *Weft* Columns feverally and fubtract the North and South Columns the leffer from the greater; and likewife the Eaft and Weft Columns. So in the Table, the Sum of the North Column is 35. 2, of the South Column 122. 4, of the Eaft Column 37. 4, and of the Weft Column, 156. 7, fubtracting the NorthColumn from the South, the Remainder is 87 2, the Difference of Latitude Southerly; and fubtracting the Eaft Column from the Weft, the Remainder 119. 3, is the Departure *Wefterly.*

Having the Difference of Latitude and Departure, you may find the Courfe and Diftance by *Prob.* 6 But in this Example, becaufe your Difference of Latitude 87 2, and your Departure, 119. 3, out-run the Table, that is to fay, you can find no fuch Numbers in the Table, therefore take the half of your Difference of Latitude, which is 43 6, and the half of your Departure which is 59. 6, According to the Direction in the fixth *Problem*, over 4¾ Points againft 44. 1, in the Column of Latitude, you will find 59 4, in the Column of Departure, (which are the two neareft Numbers in the Table) and in the Column of the Diftance 74, which being doubled, is 148, the Diftance fought. The Courfe is between the South and the *Weft*, becaufe the Difference of Latitude is Southerly, and Departure *Wefterly*, therefore the Courfe is South-weft ¼ *Weft*, which was required.

But one of the Principal Ufes of this Table is *to determine* the Difference of Longitude inDailyReckonings, by having the two Latitudes and Departure given; which it performs with all defirable facility, And is alfo very ufeful for the eafy forming of a Sea Reckoning or Journal, as fhall be inftanced in this following Table, being a Journal from the *Lizard* to the *Barbadoes.*

A Journal of our Voyage, intended by Gods Permiffion from the Lizard in Lat. 49 deg. 55 min. North, Longitude Weft from London 5 deg. 14 min. *To the Ifland of* Barbadoes, *in Lat.* 13 deg. 10 min. *North, and Longitude from* London, 58 deg. 3 min. *Weft The Difference of Longitude* 52 deg. 49 min. *The Courfe South* 49 deg. 53 min. *Weft or S.W.½W. fere. The Diftance* 3422 *Miles. The* Lizard *bears North Diftant* 25 *Miles,* March 22 1716.

Days

Days	Month and Lat. by Obf	The Course Corrected	Dif. in min.	Z North	Sou-thing min.	East-ing min.	West-ing min.	Lat. by reckon D. M.	East Lon. min.	West Long. min.
22	*March*	Lizard South	25		25.0			49. 30		
23		South-West	112		79.2		79.2	48. 11		120. 0
24	47° 00	S.W. by S.½ W.	72		55 6		45.7	47. 15		68. 1
		Correction by Obf			15.0		11.0	47. 00		16. 0
25		S W. by South	96		79 8		53.3	45. 40		75. 2
26		S.W. by South	79		65.7		43.9	44. 34		62. 8
27	42 37	S W by South	138		114.6		76.7	42. 39		106. 2
28		S. S. W. ¼ W.	129		110.7		66 3	40. 48		88. 8
29		S. S. W.	72		66 5		27.6	39. 41		36. 4
30	37 44	S.S. W. ½ W.	102		90.0		48 0	38. 11		62. 0
		Correction by Obf			27.0		16.0	37. 44		20. 0
1	*April*	South West	85		60.1		60.1	36. 44		75. 0
2		W S.W.	20		7.6		18.5	36. 36		24. 1
3		S. by W ½ W.	32		30.6		9.3	36. 05		11. 9
4	34 10	South by W.	120		117.7		23.4	34. 07		27. 9
		Correct. by Obf.	13.			1.0		34. 10	1.0	
5		S. by W. ½ W	164		156.9		47.6	31. 33		56 7
6	29 37	S. S. W.	125		115.5		47.9	29. 37		55. 9
7		S.W. by South	110		91.4		61.2	28. 06		69. 5
8		S.W. by South	122		101.4		67.8	26. 25		76. 2
9	24 43	South West	116		82.0		82.0	25. 03		91. 0
		Correction by Obf.			20 0		11.0	24. 43		12. 0
10		South West	97		68.6		68.6	23. 34		75. 0
11		South West	96		67.9		67.9	22. 26		74. 0
12		South West	114		80.6		80.6	21. 35		87. 0
13		South West	118		83.5		83.5	19. 41		89. 0
14		S. W. by W.	110		61.2		91.4	18. 40		96. 2
15		W. S. W.	91		34.8		84.1	18. 05		89. 4

Days.	Month and Lat. by Obf.		The Courfe Corrected.	Dif. in min	Z North.	Sou-thing. min.	Eaft-ing min.	Weft-ing min.	Lat.by reckon D. M.	Eaft-Lon. min.	Weft-Long. min
	1716		*Brought from the other fide.*						18 05	1·.0	1666.3
16	*April.*		W. S. W.	91		34.8		84.1	17 30		88. 0
17			W. S. W.	84		32.1		77.6	16 58		81. 0
18			W. S. W.	107		41.0		98.9	16 17		103. 7
19			W. S. W.	103		39.5		95.2	15 37		99. 0
20	14	43	W. S. W.	116		44.4		107.2	14 53		111. 0
			Correction by Obf.			10.0		15.9	14 43		16. 0
21			W. by S.	111		21.5		108.9	14 21		112. 6
22			W. by S.	120		23.4		117.7	13 58		121. 2
23			W. by S.	106		20.7		104.0	13 37		107. 0
24			W. by S.	100		19.5		98.1	13 17		100. 8
25			W. by S.	120		23.4		117.7	12 54		120. 7
26			W. by N.	100				98.1	13 13		100. 7
27			Weft.	130				130.0	13 13		133. 5
28			Weft.	136				136.0	13 13		139. 6
29			Weft ¼ South	67		3.3		67.0	13 10		68. 9

The whole difference of Longitude is 3169.0 min. which is
52 deg. 49 min. Wefterly.

The Explanation of this Journal.

In this Journal there are Eleven Columns; The firft contains the Days of the Month; the fecond the Month of the Year, and Latitude by Obfervation; the Third the Courfe Corrected, by the allowance for *Let-way,* or for the *Variation of the Compafs,* if there be any; the fourth the *Diftance failed*; the fifth, fixth, feventh, and eighth, the *Northing, Southing, Eafting, and Wefting,* being the Difference of Latitude and Departure of the feveral *Courfes* and *Diftances*; the ninth, the Latitude by *Dead-Reckoning*; the tenth the *Eaft Diff. Longitude*; the eleventh, the *Weft Diff. Longitude.*

Here I would advife all that are defirous to give a good account of their Reckoning, to any that have Reafon or Authority to demand it, That they keep a particular account of that which they take off the Log-Board every Day at Noon, either in the fame Book where they keep there Reckoning, or elfe in a Book diftinctly for that purpofe, commonly called a *Log-Book.*

K k   Now

Now the manner of proceeeding in this Journal, by the help of the Table of Latitude and Departure is very facile, as follows, the 22d of *March* at Noon, I find the *Lizard* to bear North, and to be distant about 25 Miles or Minutes, therefore I am to the Southward of the *Lizard* 25′, which 25′ I place in the South Column, and that makes my Latitude 49° 30′.

The 22d Day my Courſe is S W and the Diſtance 112′, to find the Difference of Latitude and Departure by the Table of Latitude and Departure, according to *Prob.* 1 The Difference of Latitude is 79.2, and the Departure 79.2 Becauſe the Courſe is South Weſterly, I place the Diff Lat in the South Column, and my Departure in the Weſt Column, 79′, or 1° 19′, ſubtracted from 49° 30′ gives the Latitude 48° 11′.

How to find the Difference of Longitude.

To find the Difference of Longitude, in the two laſt Columns you have both Latitudes 48° 11′, and 49° 30′ (the preſent Latitude, and the Latitude of the Day before) and the Courſe S W. by which you may find the Diff Longitude. according to the Proportion in *Chap.* 6. *Prob* 3. of *Mercator's Sailing*, ſaying, as *Radius* to the *Meridional Diff Lat.* So is the Tang of the Courſe, to the Diff Long. This Proportion being wrought by the Logarithms, or *Gunter's Scale* (which may ſerve in this Caſe) you will find the Diff Longitude 120′ which place in the Weſt Column, becauſe your Courſe is Weſterly.

The 24th Day is wrought after the ſame manner of the 23d. having the Courſe and Diſtance given to find the Diff Latitude, Departure, and Diff. Longitude as was ſhewed before.

And here we thought to have entertained the Reader with Directions for finding the Difference of Longitude by Inſpection, in the Traverſe Table, but our Tables in this Book being only to every Quarter Point of the Compaſs, it is not ſo fit for that purpoſe, and therefore ſhall rather recommend the Learner to the laſt Edition of the *Mariners New Kalendar*, where there is a Traverſe Table to every Degree, and Directions at large, for finding the Longitude thereby.

How to correct your Reckoning by Obſervation of the Latitude.

On the 24th of *March*, by a good Obſervation, I find my Latitude to be 47°, whereas by the Reckoning I ſhould be in the Latit 47° 15′, ſo that the Difference is 15′ more Southerly Therefore to correct my Latitude, I place 15′ in the South Column, which ſubtracted from 47° 15′, makes my Latitude by Reckoning to agree with the Obſervation. To Correct your Departure, you muſt conſider, whether the Fault may be imputed to your Courſe, or to your Diſtance. If your Courſe be well ſteered, and you find no Current, nor any Variation of the Compaſs, then your Diſtance is faulty, but if you cannot truſt to the Courſe ſteered, then your beſt way is to correct your Latitude only, not medling with your Departure. If there be a Current and you know which way the Current ſets, and how faſt, then allow for it, as you are taught in Page 58, of this *Book* But if you only by ſome probable Reaſon conjecture there is a Current, then give what allowance you think meet in Diff Latit. and Departure, and ſee if that will reform your Reckoning in

your

your Latitude. If fo, you have gueffed we'll; but if it will not, it is to be fuppo-
ied that you are miftaken in your conjecture, or that there is fome other caufe of
this Error in your Reckoning

If the Compafs varies (as moft commonly it doth) then finding what the Variation is, and which way it is, you muft allow it in the Ship's Courfe: But if you
cannot impute the Error to any of thefe, then (as I faid before) the Diftance is
faulty; and this is that which ufually makes the Difference between the Latitude obferved, and the Latitude by your Reckoning   And this I take to be the
caufe of the Error this 24th Day of *March*, and generally in this Reckoning

Now to correct your Departure and Diff Longitude, when the Error is in the
Diftance. you muft add up the *North, South, Eaft,* and *Weft Columns,* from the Day
that you correct, to the beginning of your *Journal Tables,* if it be the firft Correc-
tion you have made, or from the Day of Correction to the laft Correction, if it be
the fecond, third, fourth, Correction, &c. then fubtract the Sums of the North and
South Columns from each other, and likewife of the Eaft and Weft, and fay by the
Rule of Proportion   As the Diff of the North and South Columns, to the
Diff of the Eaft and Weft Columns; fo is the Difference between the Latitudes by
Obfervation and Reckoning, to the Diff in the Departure, and for the Diff. Long.
As the Diff. between the Latitudes by Obfervation and Reckoning, to the Meri-
dional Difference of thofe Latitudes, fo is the Diff. in the Departure, to the Diff
in the Longitude.

Example. The 24th Day you will find the Sum of the North Column oo, the
Sum of the South Column (leaving out 15 minutes, the Error) 164 8 minutes,
and therefore their Difference is 164.8. The Sum of the Eaft Column is oo min.
of the Weft Column 124.9 and their Difference 124.9   Then the Operation by
the *Logarithms* will be,

		Co. Ar.
As the Diff. of the North and South Columns, ———	164 8.	7 78304
To the Diff. of the *Eaft* and *Weft* Columns ———	124 9	2 09656
So is the Diff. between the two Latitudes, ——— ———	15 0	1.17609
To the Difference in the Departure ———	11	11.05569

Place this 11 Minutes in the *Weft* Column, becaufe the Sum of the *Weft* Column exceeds the Sum of the *Eaft* Column.

In this Operation we neglect the Tenths of the Departure, as not to be re
garded.

The Operation for the Difference in the Longitude.

The two Latitudes are 47 deg. 15 min and 47 deg. oo min. by which in the
Table of *Meridional Parts* you will find the Meridional Diff Lat. 22 min   Therefore,

		Co. Ar.
As the Diff. between the two Latitudes, —— 15' ———		8.82391
To the Merid. Diff. of thofe Lat. —— 22 ———		1.34242
So is the Diff. in the Departure, ——— 11 ———		1 04139
To the Diff. in the Longitude, ——— 16 ———		11.20772

       This

This 16' is placed in the *West* Column, because the Departure is *Westerly*.

After the same Manner are the Corrections made in this Journal on the 30th of *March*, the 4th, the 9th, and the 20th Days of *April*, the Error being supposed to be in the Computation of the Distance.

If your Ship fail several Courses in 24 Hours, you must find your Diff Latitude and Departure, by working a Traverse, according to *Prob.* 7 in the Use of the Table of Latitude and Departure, your Diff. Lat. will give you what Latitude the Ship is in, then have you two Latitudes, *viz.* the Lat. the Ship was in the Day before at Noon, and the Lat. the Ship is now in, by which you may find the Meridional Diff Lat. by the Table of Merid Parts according to *Chap.* 6. *Prob.* 1. of *Mercator's* Sailing. Then for your Diff. Longitude, say,

> *As the Diff. Latitude found by the Traverse,*
> *To the Diff. Latitude in Meridional Parts*
> *So is the Departure found by the Traverse,*
> *To the Diff. Longitude for the Traverse.*

To find the whole Diff. Longitude of the two Ports between which you make your Voyage

Add up the Columns of the East and West Diff. of Longitude, and subtract the one from the other, the Remainder reduc'd into degrees and minutes, is the Difference of Longitude sought.

In this Journal the Sum of the West Column of Longitude is 3170 0. the Sum of the East Column is 1.0 therefore the Diff of the East and West Columns of Longitude is 3169.0, which reduced into Degrees and Minutes, makes 52° 49', the Diff. Long. between the *Lizard* and the *Barbadoes*.

The Use of the Table of Ten Chiliads, or Ten Thousand Logarithms.

THE first Page of this Table is divided into 6 Columns, of which, the first, third, and fifth are *Natural Numbers*, and against them in the second, fourth, or sixth Columns, you have their *Correspondent Logarithms* ; as for Instance, I desire to know what is the Logarithm of 57 ? I look in the Columns under [*Num.*] and find 57 in the third Column, and against it in the fourth Column, (under *Logar.*) I find 1.755875. the Logarithm of 57 required. This Page contains only all Numbers under 100.

The first Column of the following Pages, contain Numbers, increasing in their Natural Order from 100 to 999, and with the Figures at the top they extend to 9999; for the Use of which,

If your Number consist of 3 Places, as suppose 469, find your Number always in the first Column of the Left-hand Page, and against it, in the second Column under 0) you have 2 6711728, the Logarithm of 469 required

But if your Number contain 4 Places, (as 5678) find the first three Figures (567) in the Left hand Column, and the last Figure (8) at the top, and in the *Common Angle* you have 2 7541954, the Logarithm required, only observe this general Rule, that the first Figure of the Logarithm towards the Left-hand, must always be less by one, then the Number of Places contained in the proposed Absolute Number.

Thus

$$\text{Thus the Logarithm of,} \left\{\begin{array}{l} 5.678 \\ 56\,78 \\ 567.8 \\ 5678 \\ 55780 \end{array}\right\} \text{is} \left\{\begin{array}{l} 0.7541954 \\ 1.7541954 \\ 2.7541954 \\ 3.7541954 \\ 4.7541954 \end{array}\right\} \&c.$$

2 *A Log. being given, to find the correspondent Number.*

Note. If the first Figure of the given Log. be (0) then by the foregoing Rule, the Number sought consists of one Place; if it be (1) it consists of two Places; if it be (2) of three Places; if it be (3) of four Places, &c.

Let the Log. be 0 9030900; this Log will be found in the first Page of the Table against (8), which shews that (8) is the Number sought.

Let the Log. be 1 9190781; the Index or first Figure being 1. the Number contains but two Places, *viz.* under 100. therefore look in the first Page for the given Log. and against it you have 83, the Number required.

Let the Log. be 2.8318698; look down the second Column of the Left-hand Pages, until you find the Logarithm proposed, and against it in the first Column, you have 679, the Number sought.

Let 3.9802761 be the *Log* given; look down the second Column as before, and you will find the nearest less to be 3 9800034, and the Number against it is 955; and crossing the Pages, as before directed, under (6) you will have the given *Log.* Therefore the Number sought is 9556

Let the given *Log.* be 3.9664379; if you look in the Table, according to the former Directions, you cannot find any *Log.* the same with this here given; and this is commonly the Case in the Use of these Tables; but then you must find the nearest, being in this Case less than the *Log.* given, *viz.* 3.9664233 and the Number answering thereto is 9256, which is the nearest in whole Numbers.

Let the given *Log.* be 1.9205407; look down the Left-hand Column as before, for the next less, which is 2.9101233, the Number against which it stands is 832; then looking through the Pages against 832, you find under 8 at the Top 2.9205407, the four figures answering thereto is 8328; but because the Index or first figure of the given *Log.* is 1, the Number must contain but two places, and the rest is a Decimal Fraction, so that 83.28, *viz.* 83 28/100 is the Number required.

The Use of the Table of Artificial, or Logarithmetical Sines, Tangents, and Secants.

THIS Table contains the *Logarithmetical Sines, Tangents,* and *Secants,* of every Degree and Minute of the Quadrant.

1. *To find the Sine, Tangent, or Secant of any Degree and Minute.*

If the Degrees be less than 45, your Sine, Tangent, or Secant, is found in those Columns which are distinguished by the Words (*Sine*) (*Tang*) (*Secant*) at the head of the Table, and their Complements in the Column Titled at the foot.

But if the Degrees exceeds 45, then your Sine, Tangent, or Secant, is found in those Columns which are distinguished by the Words (*Sine*) (*Tang*) (*Secant*) at the foot of the Table, and their Complements in those Titled at the head

Suppo'e

Suppose you were to find the *Log. Sine Tangent or Secant of* 32° 12'. Look for 32° at the head of the Table, and upon the left-hand Page in the Column of Minutes, under the Letter (M) you will find 12', and against 12', and under *Sine* at the head of the Table, you will find 9 7266264, which is the *Log. Sine* of 32° 12', and against 12', and under (*Tang*) you have 9.7991569, the *Log. Tang.* of 32° 12'. and against 12', and under (*Secant*) you have 10.0725305 the *Log. Secant of* 32° 12'

Suppose you were to find the *Log Sine Tangent or Secant* of 37° 47'. Look for 37 deg at the head of the Table, and upon the right-hand Page (because the Minutes exceed 50) in the Column of Min. under (M) you must look for 47 min. and against 47 min. and under (*Sine*) at the head of the Table, you will find 9 7872211, the *Sine* of 37 deg. 47 min. And against 47, and under (*Tang*) you will find 9.8894214, the *Tang.* of 37 deg 47 min And against 47, and under (*Secant*) you will find 10.1021897, the *Secant* of 37 deg 47 min.

Suppose you were to find the *Log Sine, Tangent, or Secant* of 64° 15 · Turn to 64° at the foot of the Table, and upon the right-hand Page, in the Column of Minutes, over the Letter (M) look upwards for 15', against 15', and over (*Sine*) at the foot of the Table, you will find 9 9545793 the *Sine* of 64° 15'; and against 15', and over (*Tang*) you will find 10 3166443 the *Tangent* of 64° 15' And against 15', and over (*Secant*) you will find 10 3620649, the *Secant* of 64° 15'.

Suppose you were to find the *Log. Sine, Tangent, or Secant,* of 78° 45' Turn to 78° at the foot of the Table, and upon the Left-hand Page (because the Minutes exceed 50) in the Column of Minutes, over (M) look for 45, against 45, and over (*Sine*) you find the *Sine* of 78° 45' to be 9 9915739, and the *Tangent* in the same Line over (*Tang*) to be 10 7013382, and the *Secant* over (*Secant*) to be 10.7097643.

2. *A Log. Sine, Tangent, or Secant, being given ; to find the Degree and Minute answering thereto.*

This is but the Converse of the former , but that you may the more readily turn to the deg. and min required, take this brief Direction.

If it be a Sine, and the five first Figures be less than 9.8494, or a Tangent less than *Radius*, or 10.0000000 , or a Secant, and the six first Figures less than 10.15053; then it is a Sine, Tangent, or Secant of less than 45°, and is to be sought in those Columns distinguished with (*Sine*) (*Tangent*) (*Secant*) at the head of the Table ; but if the *Sine, Tangent, or Secant,* exceed these respective Numbers, then the Degrees answering thereto are more than 45, and they are to be found in those Columns distinguished by (*Sine*) (*Tangent*) (*Secant*) at the foot of the Table.

Suppose you were to find the Degree and Minute corresponding to this *Sine* 9 7035329 This being less than 45, I run over the Columns of Sines distinguished by (*Sine*) at the top, and under 30°, and against 21', I find the given Sine.

Suppose I were to find the *Degrees and Minutes corresponding to this Tang.* 10.3862931 : This being greater than 45°, I run over the Columns of Tangents, distinguished by (*Tang.*) at the foot of the Table, and over 67°, and against 39' I find the nearest being greater, viz. 10 3863595, and therefore the deg. and min. corresponding is 67° 40'

1. *Note*, If you are to find the *Sine-Complement, Tangent-Complement, or Secant-Complement* of any Degree and Minute, as suppose you were to find the Sine Complement

plement of 39° 17′, subtract 39° 17′ from 90° 00′, and look the Sine of the Remainder, or Complement to 90°, *viz.* the Sine of 50° 43′, or you may find it as before directed, to save the trouble of Subtraction.

2 *Note*, If you are to find the Sine, Tangent, or Secant, of any Number of Degrees and Minutes exceeding 90°; as suppose you were to find the Tangent of 127° 39′ subtract 127° 39′ from 180° 00′ and find the Tangent of the Remainder, *viz.* the Tangent 52° 21′, which is also the Tangent 127° 39′, as was required.

To find the Complement Arithmetical of any given Logarithm.

The *Co. Ar.* of any Logarithm is what it wants of Radius, *viz.* 10.0000000, or if it be more then Radius, it is what it wants of twice Radius, or 20.0000000; to find which, begin at the Left-hand of your given Logarithm, subtracting every Figure from 9, till you come at the last Figure towards the Right-hand, which subtract from 10, setting down the Remainder, which is the *Co. Ar.* required

Example I desire to know the *Co. Ar.* of Log 2 7581436; you need not set them down as in common Subtraction, but do it by Sight, setting down for every Figure its Complement to 9, thus, for 2, set down 7, for 7, 2, for 5, 4; for 8, 1; for 1, 8; for 4, 5, for 3, 6, for 6 (the last Figure) set its Complement to 10, *viz.* 4; and thus the *Co. Ar* of 2.7581436, is 7.2418564, &c. This Method is to be used in finding the *Co. Ar* of any Sine, Tangent or Logarithm, less then 10 0000000, but for any above 10 0000000 you only reject the first Figure of the Index or Characteristick, and proceed with the rest as before directed, thus the *Co Ar* of 10.8193472, is 9.1806528, &c.

But for more Expedition, and to avoid the trouble of Subtraction, it may be found more readily thus,

$$\text{For } Co. \text{ } Ar. \text{ of} \begin{cases} \text{Sine,} \\ \text{Sine Comp.} \\ \text{Tangent,} \end{cases} \text{Set down} \begin{cases} \text{Secant Comp} \\ \text{Secant,} \\ \text{Tang. Comp.} \end{cases} \begin{matrix} \text{Rejecting the 1} \\ \text{in the Characte-} \\ \text{risttck, which is} \end{matrix}$$

the *Co Ar.* of the Sine, Sine Comp or Tangent (if under 45 Degrees) required.

But for Logarithms which exceed 10.0000000, *viz.* Tangents above 45 Degrees, and all Secants, observe,

$$\text{For } Co. \text{ } Ar. \text{ of} \begin{cases} \text{Tang Comp} \\ \text{Secant,} \\ \text{Secant Comp.} \end{cases} \text{Set down} \begin{cases} \text{Tang.} \\ \text{Sine Comp} \\ \text{Sine.} \end{cases}$$

From hence this General Rule may be deduced.

In any Trigonometrical Proportion, where the *Co. Ar.* is required (which is always when Radius is not one of the three first Terms) if the first Term be a Sine found in the first Column of the Table, set down for its *Co. Ar.* the Secant found in the last Column If it is a Sine found in the second Column, its *Co. Ar.* is the Secant found in the fifth Column, if it is a Tangent found in the third Column, its *Co. Ar.* is the Tangent found in the fourth Column right against it (always rejecting the 1 in the Characteristick) and if the first Term be a Tang. or Secant found in the fourth, fifth or sixth Column, the *Co Ar.* is the Tangent or Sine found in the third, second or first Columns; and having thus taken the *Co. Ar.* of of the firſt Term, and the Sine, Tang *&c* of the ſecond and third Terms, add them all together, and the Sum (rejecting Radius) is the Sine Tang. *&c.* ſought.

Example. As Sine 29° 30', to Sine 56° 15'; So Sine 22 57, to a fourth Sine required. The Sine of 29° 30' is found in the firſt Column, therefore for its *Co. Ar.* ſet down the Secant found againſt it in the laſt Column, rejecting Radius (which is the ſame as if you found *Co Ar.* by Subtraction) and it will ſtand thus.

		Co. Ar.
As Sine	29° 30'	0 3076612
To Sine	56 15	9.9198464
So Sine	22 57	9.5909841
To Sine	41 11	19.8184917

The Reaſon of thus changing Secants for *Co. Ar.* of Sines, *&c.* is evident to thoſe that underſtand the Natural Proportion of the Sines, Tangents and Secants amongſt themſelves, which Proportion may be eaſily Demonſtrated by the Principles, and Natural Conſequences of Geometry.

ADVERTISEMENT.

A

A Table of Logarithms

For Numbers increasing in their Natural Order, from an Unit to 10,000.

With a Table of Artificial *Sines*, *Tangents*, and *Secants*, the *Radius* 10.000000; and to every Degree and Minute of the *Quadrant*.

Num.	Logar.	Num.	Logar.	Num.	Logar.
1	0.0000000	34	1.5314789	67	1.8260748
2	0.3010300	35	1.5440680	68	1.8325089
3	0.4771213	36	1.5563025	69	1.8388491
4	0.6020600	37	1.5682017	70	1.8450980
5	0.6989700	38	1.5797836	71	1.8512583
6	0.7781513	39	1.5910646	72	1.8573325
7	0.8450980	40	1.6020600	73	1.8633229
8	0.9030900	41	1.6127839	74	1.8692317
9	0.9542426	42	1.6232493	75	1.8750613
10	1.0000000	43	1.6334685	76	1.8808136
11	1.0413927	44	1.6434527	77	1.8864907
12	1.0791812	45	1.6532125	78	1.8920946
13	1.1139434	46	1.6627578	79	1.8976271
14	1.1461280	47	1.6720979	80	1.9030900
15	1.1760913	48	1.6812412	81	1.9084850
16	1.2041200	49	1.6901961	82	1.9138139
17	1.2304489	50	1.6989700	83	1.9190781
18	1.2552725	51	1.7075702	84	1.9242793
19	1.2787536	52	1.7160033	85	1.9294189
20	1.3010300	53	1.7242759	86	1.9344985
21	1.3222193	54	1.7323938	87	1.9395193
22	1.3424227	55	1.7403627	88	1.9444827
23	1.3617278	56	1.7481880	89	1.9493900
24	1.3802112	57	1.7558749	90	1.9542425
25	1.3979400	58	1.7634280	91	1.9590414
26	1.4149733	59	1.7708520	92	1.9637878
27	1.4313638	60	1.7781513	93	1.9684829
28	1.4471580	61	1.7853298	94	1.9731279
29	1.4623980	62	1.7923917	95	1.9777236
30	1.4771213	63	1.7993405	96	1.9822712
31	1.4913617	64	1.8061800	97	1.9867717
32	1.5051500	65	1.8129134	98	1.9912261
33	1.5185139	66	1.8195439	99	1.9956352

A TABLE of Logarithms.

Num	0	1	2	3	4
100	2.0000000	2.0004341	2.0008677	2.0013009	2.0017337
101	2.0043214	2.0047511	2.0051805	2.0056094	2.0060379
102	2.0086002	2.0090257	2.0094509	2.0098756	2.0102999
103	2.0128372	2.0132587	2.0136797	2.0141003	2.0145205
104	2.0170333	2.0174507	2.0178677	2.0182843	2.0187005
105	2.0211893	2.0216027	2.0220157	2.0224284	2.0228406
106	2.0253059	2.0257154	2.0261245	2.0265333	2.0269416
107	2.0293838	2.0297895	2.0301948	2.0305997	2.0310043
108	2.0334238	2.0338257	2.0342273	2.0346284	2.0350293
109	2.0374265	2.0378247	2.0382226	2.0386202	2.0390173
110	2.0413927	2.0417873	2.0421816	2.0425755	2.0429691
111	2.0453230	2.0457140	2.0461048	2.0464952	2.0468852
112	2.0492180	2.0496056	2.0499928	2.0503797	2.0507663
113	2.0530784	2.0534626	2.0538464	2.0542299	2.0546130
114	2.0569049	2.0572856	2.0576661	2.0580462	2.0584260
115	2.0606978	2.0610753	2.0614525	2.0618293	2.0622058
116	2.0644580	2.0648322	2.0652061	2.0655797	2.0659530
117	2.0681859	2.0685569	2.0689276	2.0692980	2.0696681
118	2.0718820	2.0722499	2.0726175	2.0729847	2.0733517
119	2.0755470	2.0759118	2.0762762	2.0766404	2.0770043
120	2.0791812	2.0795430	2.0799045	2.0802656	2.0806265
121	2.0827854	2.0831441	2.0835026	2.0838608	2.0842187
122	2.0863598	2.0867157	2.0870712	2.0874264	2.0877814
123	2.0899051	2.0902580	2.0906107	2.0909631	2.0913151
124	2.0934217	2.0937718	2.0941216	2.0944711	2.0948204
125	2.0969100	2.0972573	2.0976043	2.0979511	2.0982975
126	2.1003705	2.1007151	2.1010593	2.1014033	2.1017471
127	2.1038037	2.1041455	2.1044871	2.1048284	2.1051694
128	2.1072100	2.1075491	2.1078880	2.1082266	2.1085650
129	2.1105897	2.1109262	2.1112625	2.1115985	2.1119343
130	2.1139433	2.1142773	2.1146110	2.1149444	2.1152776
131	2.1172713	2.1176027	2.1179338	2.1182647	2.1185954
132	2.1205739	2.1209028	2.1212315	2.1215598	2.1218880
133	2.1238516	2.1241780	2.1245042	2.1248301	2.1251558
134	2.1271048	2.1274288	2.1277525	2.1280760	2.1283993
135	2.1303338	2.1306553	2.1309767	2.1312978	2.1316187
136	2.1335389	2.1338581	2.1341771	2.1344958	2.1348144
137	2.1367206	2.1370374	2.1373541	2.1376705	2.1379867
138	2.1398791	2.1401937	2.1405080	2.1408222	2.1411361
139	2.1430148	2.1433271	2.1436392	2.1439511	2.1442628
140	2.1461280	2.1464381	2.1467480	2.1470577	2.1473671
141	2.1492191	2.1495272	2.1498347	2.1501422	2.1504494
142	2.1522883	2.1525941	2.1528996	2.1532049	2.1535100
143	2.1553360	2.1556396	2.1559430	2.1562462	2.1565491
144	2.1583625	2.1586640	2.1589653	2.1592663	2.1595672
145	2.1613680	2.1616674	2.1619666	2.1622656	2.1625644
146	2.1643528	2.1646502	2.1649474	2.1652443	2.1655411
147	2.1673173	2.1676127	2.1679078	2.1682027	2.1684975
148	2.1702617	2.1705550	2.1708482	2.1711411	2.1714339
149	2.1731863	2.1734776	2.1737688	2.1740598	2.1743506

Num	5	6	7	8	9
100	2.0021661	2.0025980	2.0030295	2.0034605	2.0038912
101	2.0064660	2.0068937	2.0073209	2.0077478	2.0081742
102	2.0107239	2.0111473	2.0115704	2.0119931	2.0124154
103	2.0149403	2.0153597	2.0157787	2.0161973	2.0166155
104	2.0191163	2.0195317	2.0199467	2.0203613	2.0207755
105	2.0232524	2.0236639	2.0240750	2.0244857	2.0248960
106	2.0273496	2.0277572	2.0281644	2.0285712	2.0289777
107	2.0314084	2.0318123	2.0322157	2.0326188	2.0330214
108	2.0354297	2.0358298	2.0362295	2.0366289	2.0370279
109	2.0394141	2.0398105	2.0402066	2.0406023	2.0409977
110	2.0433623	2.0437551	2.0441476	2.0445398	2.0449315
111	2.0472749	2.0476642	2.0480532	2.0484418	
112	2.0511525	2.0515384	2.0519239	2.0523091	2.0526939
113	2.0549958	2.0553783	2.0557625	2.0561423	2.0565237
114	2.0588055	2.0591846	2.0595634	2.0599419	2.0603200
115	2.0625820	2.0629578	2.0633333	2.0637085	2.0640834
116	2.0663259	2.0666985	2.0670708	2.0674428	2.0678145
117	2.0700379	2.0704073	2.0707765	2.0711453	2.0715138
118	2.0737183	2.0740847	2.0744507	2.0748164	2.0751818
119	2.0773679	2.0777312	2.0780941	2.0784568	2.0788192
120	2.0809870	2.0813473	2.0817073	2.0820669	2.0824263
121	2.0845763	2.0849336	2.0852906	2.0856473	2.0860037
122	2.0881361	2.0884905	2.0888446	2.0891984	2.0895519
123	2.0916669	2.0920185	2.0923697	2.0927206	2.0930712
124	2.0951693	2.0955180	2.0958664	2.0962146	2.0965624
125	2.0986437	2.0989896	2.0993353	2.0996806	2.1000257
126	2.1020905	2.1024337	2.1027766	2.1031192	2.1034616
127	2.1055102	2.1058506	2.1061909	2.1065308	2.1068705
128	2.1089031	2.1092410	2.1095785	2.1099159	2.1102529
129	2.1122698	2.1126050	2.1129400	2.1132746	2.1136091
130	2.1156105	2.1159432	2.1162756	2.1166077	2.1169396
131	2.1189257	2.1192559	2.1195858	2.1199154	2.1202448
132	2.1222159	2.1225435	2.1228709	2.1231981	2.1235250
133	2.1254813	2.1258064	2.1261314	2.1264561	2.1267806
134	2.1287223	2.1290450	2.1293676	2.1296899	2.1300119
135	2.1319393	2.1322597	2.1325798	2.1328998	2.1332194
136	2.1351326	2.1354507	2.1357685	2.1360861	2.1364034
137	2.1383027	2.1386184	2.1389339	2.1392492	2.1395643
138	2.1414498	2.1417632	2.1420765	2.1423895	2.1427022
139	2.1445742	2.1448854	2.1451964	2.1455072	2.1458177
140	2.1476763	2.1479853	2.1482941	2.1486026	2.1489110
141	2.1507564	2.1510632	2.1513698	2.1516762	2.1519824
142	2.1538149	2.1541195	2.1544240	2.1547282	2.1550322
143	2.1568519	2.1571544	2.1574568	2.1577589	2.1580608
144	2.1598678	2.1601682	2.1604685	2.1607686	2.1610684
145	2.1628630	2.1631614	2.1634595	2.1637575	2.1640553
146	2.1658376	2.1661340	2.1664301	2.1667260	2.1670218
147	2.1687920	2.1690863	2.1693805	2.1696744	2.1699682
148	2.1717264	2.1720188	2.1723110	2.1726029	2.1728947
149	2.1746412	2.1749316	2.1752218	2.1755118	2.1758016

Num	0	1	2	3	4
150	2.1760913	2.1763807	2.1766699	2.1769590	2.1772478
151	2.1789769	2.1792645	2.1795518	2.1798389	2.1801259
152	2.1818436	2.1821292	2.1824146	2.1826999	2.1829850
153	2.1846914	2.1849752	2.1852588	2.1855421	2.1858253
154	2.1875207	2.1878026	2.1880844	2.1883659	2.1886473
155	2.1903317	2.1906118	2.1908917	2.1911714	2.1914510
156	2.1931246	2.1934029	2.1936810	2.1939590	2.1942367
157	2.1958996	2.1961762	2.1964525	2.1967287	2.1970047
158	2.1986571	2.1989319	2.1992065	2.1994809	2.1997552
159	2.2013971	2.2016702	2.2019431	2.2022158	2.2024883
160	2.2041200	2.2043913	2.2046625	2.2049335	2.2052044
161	2.2068259	2.2070955	2.2073650	2.2076344	2.2079035
162	2.2095150	2.2097830	2.2100508	2.2103185	2.2105860
163	2.2121876	2.2124540	2.2127201	2.2129862	2.2132521
164	2.2148438	2.2151086	2.2153732	2.2156376	2.2159018
165	2.2174839	2.2177471	2.2180100	2.2182728	2.2185355
166	2.2201081	2.2203696	2.2206310	2.2208922	2.2211533
167	2.2227165	2.2229764	2.2232363	2.2234959	2.2237554
168	2.2253093	2.2255677	2.2258260	2.2260841	2.2263421
169	2.2278867	2.2281436	2.2284003	2.2286570	2.2289134
170	2.2304489	2.2307043	2.2309596	2.2312146	2.2314696
171	2.2329961	2.2332500	2.2335038	2.2337574	2.2340108
172	2.2355284	2.2357809	2.2360331	2.2362853	2.2365373
173	2.2380461	2.2382971	2.2385479	2.2387986	2.2390491
174	2.2405492	2.2407988	2.2410481	2.2412974	2.2415465
175	2.2430380	2.2432861	2.2435341	2.2437819	2.2440296
176	2.2455127	2.2457593	2.2460059	2.2462523	2.2464986
177	2.2479733	2.2482186	2.2484637	2.2487087	2.2489536
178	2.2504200	2.2506639	2.2509077	2.2511513	2.2513948
179	2.2528530	2.2530956	2.2533380	2.2535803	2.2538224
180	2.2552725	2.2555137	2.2557548	2.2559957	2.2562365
181	2.2576786	2.2579184	2.2581582	2.2583978	2.2586373
182	2.2600714	2.2603099	2.2605484	2.2607867	2.2610248
183	2.2624511	2.2626883	2.2629255	2.2631625	2.2633993
184	2.2648178	2.2650538	2.2652896	2.2655253	2.2657609
185	2.2671717	2.2674064	2.2676410	2.2678754	2.2681097
186	2.2695129	2.2697464	2.2699797	2.2702128	2.2704459
187	2.2718416	2.2720738	2.2723058	2.2725378	2.2727696
188	2.2741578	2.2743888	2.2746196	2.2748503	2.2750809
189	2.2764618	2.2766915	2.2769211	2.2771506	2.2773800
190	2.2787536	2.2789821	2.2792105	2.2794388	2.2796669
191	2.2810334	2.2812607	2.2814879	2.2817150	2.2819419
192	2.2833012	2.2835274	2.2837534	2.2839793	2.2842051
193	2.2855573	2.2857823	2.2860071	2.2862318	2.2864565
194	2.2878017	2.2880255	2.2882492	2.2884728	2.2886963
195	2.2900346	2.2902573	2.2904798	2.2907022	2.2909246
196	2.2922561	2.2924775	2.2926990	2.2929203	2.2931415
197	2.2944662	2.2946866	2.2949069	2.2951271	2.2953471
198	2.2966652	2.2968845	2.2971036	2.2973227	2.2975417
199	2.2988531	2.2990713	2.2992893	2.2995073	2.2997251

Num	5	6	7	8	9
150	2.1775365	2.1778250	2.1781132	2.1784013	2.1786892
151	2.1804126	2.1806992	2.1809856	2.1812718	2.1815578
152	2.1832698	2.1835545	2.1838390	2.1841233	2.1844075
153	2.1861084	2.1863912	2.1866739	2.1869563	2.1872386
154	2.1889285	2.1892095	2.1894903	2.1897709	2.1900514
155	2.1917304	2.1920096	2.1922886	2.1925674	2.1928461
156	2.1945143	2.1947917	2.1950690	2.1953460	2.1956229
157	2.1972806	2.1975562	2.1978317	2.1981070	2.1983821
158	2.2000293	2.2003032	2.2005769	2.2008505	2.2011239
159	2.2027607	2.2030329	2.2033049	2.2035768	2.2038485
160	2.2054750	2.2057455	2.2060159	2.2062860	2.2065560
161	2.2081725	2.2084413	2.2087100	2.2089785	2.2092468
162	2.2108534	2.2111205	2.2113876	2.2116544	2.2119211
163	2.2135178	2.2137833	2.2140487	2.2143139	2.2145789
164	2.2161659	2.2164298	2.2166936	2.2169572	2.2172206
165	2.2187980	2.2190603	2.2193225	2.2195845	2.2198464
166	2.2214142	2.2216750	2.2219356	2.2221960	2.2224563
167	2.2240148	2.2242740	2.2245331	2.2247921	2.2250507
168	2.2265999	2.2268576	2.2271151	2.2273724	2.2276296
169	2.2291697	2.2294258	2.2296818	2.2299377	2.2301934
170	2.2317244	2.2319790	2.2322335	2.2324879	2.2327421
171	2.2342641	2.2345173	2.2347703	2.2350232	2.2352759
172	2.2367891	2.2370408	2.2372923	2.2375437	2.2377950
173	2.2392995	2.2395497	2.2397998	2.2400498	2.2402996
174	2.2417954	2.2420442	2.1422929	2.2425414	2.2427898
175	2.2442771	2.2445245	2.2447718	2.2450189	2.2452658
176	2.2467447	2.2469907	2.2472365	2.2474823	2.2477278
177	2.2491984	2.2494430	2.2496874	2.2499317	2.2501759
178	2.2516382	2.2518814	2.2521246	2.2523675	2.2526103
179	2.2540645	2.2543063	2.2545481	2.2547897	2.2550312
180	2.2564772	2.2567177	2.2569581	2.2571984	2.2574386
181	2.2588766	2.2591158	2.2593549	2.2595939	2.2598327
182	2.2612629	2.2615008	2.2617385	2.2619762	2.2622137
183	2.2636361	2.2638727	2.2641092	2.2643455	2.2645817
184	2.2659964	2.2662317	2.2664669	2.2667020	2.2669369
185	2.2683439	2.2685780	2.2688119	2.2690457	2.2692794
186	2.2706788	2.2709116	2.2711443	2.2713769	2.2716093
187	2.2730013	2.2732328	2.2734643	2.2736956	2.2739268
188	2.2753113	2.2755417	2.2757719	2.2760020	2.2762320
189	2.2776092	2.2778383	2.2780673	2.2782962	2.2785250
190	2.2798950	2.2801229	2.2803507	2.2805784	2.2808059
191	2.2821688	2.2823955	2.2826221	2.2828486	2.2830750
192	2.2844307	2.2846563	2.2848817	2.2851070	2.2853322
193	2.2866810	2.2869054	2.2871296	2.2873538	2.2875778
194	2.2889196	2.2891428	2.2893659	2.2895889	2.2898118
195	2.2911468	2.2913688	2.2915908	2.2918127	2.2920344
196	2.2933626	2.2935835	2.2938044	2.2940251	2.2942457
197	2.2955671	2.2957869	2.2960067	2.2962263	2.2964458
198	2.2977605	2.2979792	2.2981979	2.2984164	2.2986348
199	2.2999429	2.2001605	2.3003781	2.2005955	2.2008128

Num	0	1	2	3	4
200	2.3010300	2.3012471	2.3014641	2.3016809	2.3018977
201	2.3031951	2.3034121	2.3036280	2.3038438 .	2.3040595
202	2.3053514	2.3055663	2.3057811	2.3059959	2.3062105
203	2.3074960	2.3077099	2.3079237	2.3081374	2.3083509
204	2.3096302	2.3098430	2.3100557	2.3102684	2.3104809
205	2.3117539	2.3119657	2.3121774	2.3123889	2.3126004
206	2.3138672	2.3140780	2.3142887	2.3144992	2.3147097
207	2.3159703	2.3161801	2.3163897	2.3165993	2.3168087
208	2.3180633	2.3182721	2.3184807	2.3186893	2.3188977
209	2.3201463	2.3203540	2.3205617	2.3207692	2.3209767
210	2.3222193	2.3224260	2.3226327	2.3228393	2.3230457
211	2.3242825	2.3244882	2.3246939	2.3248995	2.3251050
212	2.3263359	2.3265407	2.3267454	2.3269500	2.3271545
213	2.3283796	2.3285834	2.3287872	2.3289909	2.3291944
214	2.3304138	2.3306167	2.3308195	2.3310222	2.3312248
215	2.3324385	2.3326404	2.3328423	2.3330440	2.3332457
216	2.3344537	2.3346548	2.3348557	2.3350565	2.3352572
217	2.3364597	2.3366598	2.3368598	2.3370597	2.3372595
218	2.3384565	2.3386557	2.3388547	2.3390537	2.3392526
219	2.3404441	2.3406424	2.3408405	2.3410386	2.3412366
220	2.3424227	2.3426200	2.3428173	2.3430145	2.3432116
221	2.3443923	2.3445887	2.3447851	2.3449814	2.3451776
222	2.3463530	2.3465496	2.3467441	2.3469395	2.3471348
223	2.3483049	2.3484995	2.3486942	2.3488887	2.3490832
224	2.3502480	2.3504419	2.3506356	2.3508293	2.3510228
225	2.3521825	2.3523755	2.3525684	2.3527612	2.3529539
226	2.3541084	2.3543006	2.3544926	2.3546845	2.3548764
227	2.3560259	2.3562171	2.3564083	2.3565994	2.3567905
228	2.3579348	2.3581253	2.3583156	2.3585059	2.3586951
229	2.3598355	2.3600251	2.3602146	2.3604040	2.3605934
230	2.3617278	2.3619166	2.3621053	2.3622939	2.3624825
231	2.3636120	2.3638000	2.3639878	2.3641756	2.3643633
232	2.3654880	2.3656751	2.3658622	2.3660492	2.3662361
233	2.3673559	2.3675423	2.3677285	2.3679147	2.3681008
234	2.3692159	2.3694014	2.3695869	2.3697723	2.3699576
235	2.3710679	2.3712526	2.3714373	2.3716219	2.3718065
236	2.3729120	2.3730960	2.3732799	2.3734637	2.3736475
237	2.3747483	2.3749316	2.3751147	2.3752977	2.3754807
238	2.3765763	2.3767594	2.3769418	2.3771240	2.3773062
239	2.3783979	2.3785796	2.3787612	2.3789427	2.3791241
240	2.3802112	2.3803922	2.3805730	2.3807538	2.3809345
241	2.3820170	2.3821972	2.3823773	2.3825573	2.3827373
242	2.3838154	2.3839948	2.3841741	2.3843534	2.3845326
243	2.3856063	2.3857850	2.3859636	2.3861421	2.3863206
244	2.3873898	2.3875678	2.3877457	2.3879235	2.3881012
245	2.3891661	2.3893433	2.3895205	2.3896975	2.3898746
246	2.3909351	2.3911116	2.3912880	2.3914644	2.3916407
247	2.3926969	2.3928727	2.3930485	2.3932241	2.3933997
248	2.3944517	2.3946268	2.3948018	2.3949767	2.3951516
249	2.3961993	2.3963737	2.3965480	2.3967223	2.3968964

Num	5	6	7	8	9
200	2.3021144	2.3023309	2.3025474	2.3027637	2.3029799
201	2.3042751	2.3044905	2.3047059	2.3049212	2.3051363
202	2.3064250	2.3066394	2.3068537	2.3070679	2.3072820
203	2.3085644	2.3087778	2.3089910	2.3092042	2.3094171
204	2.3106933	2.3109056	2.3111178	2.3113299	2.3115420
205	2.3128118	2.3130231	2.3132343	2.3134454	2.3136563
206	2.3149200	2.3151303	2.3153405	2.3155505	2.3157605
207	2.3170181	2.3172273	2.3174365	2.3176455	2.3178545
208	2.3191061	2.3193143	2.3195225	2.3197305	2.3199384
209	2.3211840	2.3213913	2.3215984	2.3218055	2.3220124
210	2.3232521	2.3234584	2.3236645	2.3238706	2.3240766
211	2.3253104	2.3255157	2.3257209	2.3259260	2.3261310
212	2.3273589	2.3275633	2.3277675	2.3279716	2.3281757
213	2.3293979	2.3296012	2.3298045	2.3300077	2.3302108
214	2.3314273	2.3316297	2.3318320	2.3320343	2.3322364
215	2.3334473	2.3336488	2.3338501	2.3340514	2.3342526
216	2.3354579	2.3356585	2.3358589	2.3360593	2.3362596
217	2.3374593	2.3376589	2.3378584	2.3380579	2.3382572
218	2.3394514	2.3396501	2.3398488	2.3400473	2.3402458
219	2.3414345	2.3416323	2.3418301	2.3420277	2.3422252
220	2.3434086	2.3436055	2.3438023	2.3439991	2.3441957
221	2.3453737	2.3455698	2.3457657	2.3459615	2.3461573
222	2.3473300	2.3475252	2.3477202	2.3479152	2.3481101
223	2.3492775	2.3494718	2.3496660	2.3498601	2.3500541
224	2.3512163	2.3514097	2.3516031	2.3517963	2.3519895
225	2.3531465	2.3533391	2.3535316	2.3537239	2.3539162
226	2.3550682	2.3552599	2.3554515	2.3556430	2.3558345
227	2.3569812	2.3571723	2.3573630	2.3575537	2.3577443
228	2.3588862	2.3590762	2.3592662	2.3594560	2.3596458
229	2.3607827	2.3609719	2.3611610	2.3613500	2.3615399
230	2.3626709	2.3628593	2.3630476	2.3632358	2.3634239
231	2.3645510	2.3647386	2.3649260	2.3651134	2.3653007
232	2.3664230	2.3666097	2.3667954	2.3669830	2.3671695
233	2.3682869	2.3684728	2.3686587	2.3688445	2.3690302
234	2.3701428	2.3703280	2.3705131	2.3706981	2.3708830
235	2.3719909	2.3721753	2.3723596	2.3725438	2.3727279
236	2.3738311	2.3740147	2.3741983	2.3743817	2.3745651
237	2.3756636	2.3758464	2.3760292	2.3762118	2.3763944
238	2.3774884	2.3776704	2.3778524	2.3780343	2.3782161
239	2.3793055	2.3794868	2.3796680	2.3798492	2.3800302
240	2.3811151	2.3812956	2.3814761	2.3816565	2.3818368
241	2.3829171	2.3830969	2.3832766	2.3834563	2.3836359
242	2.3847117	2.3848908	2.3850698	2.3852487	2.3854275
243	2.3864990	2.3866773	2.3868555	2.3870337	2.3872118
244	2.3882789	2.3884565	2.3886340	2.3888114	2.3889888
245	2.3900515	2.3902284	2.3904052	2.3905819	2.3907585
246	2.3918169	2.3919931	2.3921691	2.3923452	2.3925211
247	2.3935752	2.3937506	2.3939260	2.3941013	2.3942765
248	2.3953264	2.3955011	2.3956758	2.3958504	2.3960249
249	2.3970705	2.3972446	2.3974185	2.3975924	2.3977662

Num	0	1	2	3	4
250	2.3979400	2.3981137	2.3982873	2.3984608	2.3986343
251	2.3996737	2.3998467	2.4000196	2.4001925	2.4003653
252	2.4014005	2.4015728	2.4017451	2.4019172	2.4020893
253	2.4031205	2.4032921	2.4034637	2.4036352	2.4038066
254	2.4048337	2.4050047	2.4051755	2.4053464	2.4055171
255	2.4065402	2.4067105	2.4058807	2.4070508	2.4072209
256	2.4082400	2.4084096	2.4085791	2.4087486	2.4089180
257	2.4099331	2.4101021	2.4102710	2.4104398	2.4106085
258	2.4116197	2.4117880	2.4119562	2.4121244	2.4122925
259	2.4132998	2.4134674	2.4136350	2.4138025	2.4139700
260	2.4149733	2.4151404	2.4153073	2.4154742	2.4156410
261	2.4166405	2.4168069	2.4169732	2.4171394	2.4173056
262	2.4183013	2.4184670	2.4186327	2.4187983	2.4189638
263	2.4199557	2.4201208	2.4202859	2.4204509	2.4206158
264	2.4216039	2.4217684	2.4219328	2.4220972	2.4222614
265	2.4232459	2.4234097	2.4235735	2.4237372	2.4239009
266	2.4248816	2.4250449	2.4252080	2.4253712	2.4255342
267	2.4265113	2.4256739	2.4268365	2.4269990	2.4271614
268	2.4281348	2.4282968	2.4284588	2.4286207	2.4287825
269	2.4297523	2.4299137	2.4300751	2.4302364	2.4303976
270	2.4313638	2.4315246	2.4316853	2.4318460	2.4320067
271	2.4329693	2.4331295	2.4332897	2.4334498	2.4336098
272	2.4345689	2.4347285	2.4348881	2.4350476	2.4352071
273	2.4361626	2.4363217	2.4364807	2.4366396	2.4367985
274	2.4377506	2.4379090	2.4380674	2.4382258	2.4383841
275	2.4393327	2.4394906	2.4396484	2.4398062	2.4399639
276	2.4409091	2.4410664	2.4412237	2.4413809	2.4415380
277	2.4424798	2.4426365	2.4427932	2.4429499	2.4431065
278	2.4440448	2.4442010	2.4443571	2.4445132	2.4446692
279	2.4456042	2.4457598	2.4459154	2.4460709	2.4462264
280	2.4471580	2.4473131	2.4474681	2.4476231	2.4477780
281	2.4487063	2.4488608	2.4490153	2.4491697	2.4493241
282	2.4502491	2.4504031	2.4505570	2.4507109	2.4508647
283	2.4517864	2.4519399	2.4520932	2.4522466	2.4523998
284	2.4533183	2.4534712	2.4536241	2.4537769	2.4539296
285	2.4548449	2.4549972	2.4551495	2.4553018	2.4554540
286	2.4563660	2.4565179	2.4566696	2.4568213	2.4569731
287	2.4578819	2.4580332	2.4581844	2.4583356	2.4584868
288	2.4593925	2.4595433	2.4596940	2.4598446	2.4599953
289	2.4608978	2.4610481	2.4611983	2.4613484	2.4614985
290	2.4623980	2.4625477	2.4626974	2.4628470	2.4629966
291	2.4638930	2.4640422	2.4641914	2.4643405	2.4644895
292	2.4653828	2.4655316	2.4656802	2.4658288	2.4659774
293	2.4668676	2.4670158	2.4671640	2.4673120	2.4674601
294	2.4683473	2.4684950	2.4686427	2.4687903	2.4689378
295	2.4698220	2.4699692	2.4701163	2.4702634	2.4704105
296	2.4712917	2.4714384	2.4715850	2.4717317	2.4718782
297	2.4727564	2.4729027	2.4730488	2.4731949	2.4733410
298	2.4742163	2.4743620	2.4745076	2.4746533	2.4747988
299	2.4756712	2.4758164	2.4759616	2.4761067	2.4762518

Num	5	6	7	8	9
250	2.3988077	2.3989811	2.3991543	2.3993275	2.3995007
251	2.4005380	2.4007106	2.4008832	2.4010557	2.4012282
252	2.4022614	2.4024333	2.4026052	2.4027771	2.4029488
253	2.4039780	2.4041492	2.4043205	2.4044916	2.4046627
254	2.4056878	2.4058584	2.4060289	2.4061994	2.4063698
255	2.4073909	2.4075608	2.4077307	2.4079005	2.4080703
256	2.4090874	2.4092567	2.4094259	2.4095950	2.4097641
257	2.4107772	2.4109459	2.4111144	2.4112829	2.4114513
258	2.4124605	2.4126285	2.4127964	2.4129643	2.4131320
259	2.4141374	2.4143047	2.4144719	2.4146391	2.4148063
260	2.4158077	2.4159744	2.4161410	2.4163076	2.4164741
261	2.4174717	2.4176377	2.4178037	2.4179696	2.4181355
262	2.4191293	2.4192947	2.4194601	2.4196254	2.4197906
263	2.4207806	2.4209454	2.4211101	2.4212748	2.4214394
264	2.4224257	2.4225898	2.4227539	2.4229180	2.4230820
265	2.4240645	2.4242281	2.4243915	2.4245550	2.4247183
266	2.4256972	2.4258601	2.4260230	2.4261858	2.4263486
267	2.4273238	2.4274861	2.4276484	2.4278106	2.4279727
268	2.4289443	2.4291060	2.4292677	2.4294293	2.4295908
269	2.4305588	2.4307199	2.4308809	2.4310419	2.4312029
270	2.4321673	2.4323278	2.4324883	2.4326487	2.4328090
271	2.4337698	2.4339298	2.4340896	2.4342494	2.4344092
272	2.4353665	2.4355258	2.4356851	2.4358444	2.4360035
273	2.4369573	2.4371161	2.4372748	2.4374334	2.4375920
274	2.4385423	2.4387005	2.4388587	2.4390167	2.4391747
275	2.4401216	2.4402792	2.4404368	2.4405943	2.4407517
276	2.4416951	2.4418522	2.4420092	2.4421661	2.4423229
277	2.4432630	2.4434195	2.4435759	2.4437322	2.4438885
278	2.4448252	2.4449811	2.4451370	2.4452928	2.4454485
279	2.4463818	2.4465372	2.4466925	2.4468477	2.4470029
280	2.4479329	2.4480877	2.4482424	2.4483971	2.4485517
281	2.4494784	2.4496326	2.4497868	2.4499410	2.4500951
282	2.4510184	2.4511721	2.4513258	2.4514794	2.4516329
283	2.4525531	2.4527062	2.4528593	2.4530124	2.4531654
284	2.4540823	2.4542349	2.4543875	2.4545400	2.4546924
285	2.4556061	2.4557582	2.4559102	2.4560622	2.4562142
286	2.4571246	2.4572762	2.4574277	2.4575791	2.4577305
287	2.4586378	2.4587889	2.4589399	2.4590908	2.4592417
288	2.4601458	2.4602963	2.4604468	2.4605972	2.4607475
289	2.4616486	2.4617986	2.4619485	2.4620984	2.4622482
290	2.4631461	2.4632956	2.4634450	2.4635944	2.4637437
291	2.4646386	2.4647875	2.4649364	2.4650853	2.4652341
292	2.4661259	2.4662743	2.4664227	2.4665711	2.4667194
293	2.4676081	2.4677560	2.4679039	2.4680518	2.4681996
294	2.4690853	2.4692327	2.4693801	2.4695275	2.4696748
295	2.4705575	2.4707044	2.4708513	2.4709982	2.4711450
296	2.4720247	2.4721711	2.4723175	2.4724639	2.4726102
297	2.4734870	2.4736329	2.4737788	2.4739247	2.4740705
298	2.4749443	2.4750898	2.4752352	2.4753806	2.4755259
299	2.4763968	2.4765418	2.4766867	2.4768316	2.4769765

Num	0	1	2	3	4
300	2.4771212	2.4772660	2.4774017	2.4775553	2.4776999
301	2.4785655	2.4787108	2.4788550	2.4789991	2.4791432
302	2.4800069	2.4801507	2.4802945	2.4804381	2.4805818
303	2.4814425	2.4815859	2.4817292	2.4818724	2.4820156
304	2.4828736	2.4830164	2.4831592	2.4833019	2.4834446
305	2.4842998	2.4844422	2.4845845	2.4847268	2.4848690
306	2.4857214	2.4858633	2.4860052	2.4861470	2.4862888
307	2.4871381	2.4872798	2.4874212	2.4875626	2.4877039
308	2.4885507	2.4886917	2.4888326	2.4889735	2.4891144
309	2.4899585	2.4900990	2.4902395	2.4903799	2.4905203
310	2.4913617	2.4915018	2.4916418	2.4917818	2.4919217
311	2.4927602	2.4929000	2.4930396	2.4931791	2.4933186
312	2.4941546	2.4942938	2.4944329	2.4945720	2.4947110
313	2.4955443	2.4956831	2.4958218	2.4959604	2.4960990
314	2.4969296	2.4970679	2.4972062	2.4973444	2.4974825
315	2.4983105	2.4984484	2.4985462	2.4987240	2.4988617
316	2.4996871	2.4998245	2.4999619	2.5000992	2.5002365
317	2.5010593	2.5011962	2.5013332	2.5014701	2.5016069
318	2.5024271	2.5025637	2.5027002	2.5028366	2.5029731
319	2.5037907	2.5039268	2.5040629	2.5041989	2.5043349
320	2.5051500	2.5052857	2.5054213	2.5055569	2.5056925
321	2.5065050	2.5066403	2.5067755	2.5069107	2.5070459
322	2.5078559	2.5079907	2.5081255	2.5082603	2.5083950
323	2.5092025	2.5093370	2.5094713	2.5096057	2.5097400
324	2.5105450	2.5106790	2.5108130	2.5109469	2.5110808
325	2.5118834	2.5120170	2.5121505	2.5122841	2.5124175
326	2.5132176	2.5133508	2.5134840	2.5136171	2.5137501
327	2.5145478	2.5146805	2.5148133	2.5149460	2.5150787
328	2.5158738	2.5160062	2.5161386	2.5162709	2.5164031
329	2.5171959	2.5173279	2.5174598	2.5175917	2.5177236
330	2.5185139	2.5186455	2.5187771	2.5189086	2.5190400
331	2.5198280	2.5199592	2.5200903	2.5202214	2.5203525
332	2.5211381	2.5212689	2.5213996	2.5215303	2.5216610
333	2.5224442	2.5225746	2.5227050	2.5228353	2.5229656
334	2.5237465	2.5238765	2.5240064	2.5241364	2.5242663
335	2.5250448	2.5251744	2.5253040	2.5254335	2.5255631
336	2.5263393	2.5264685	2.5255977	2.5267269	2.5268560
337	2.5276299	2.5277588	2.5278876	2.5280163	2.5281451
338	2.5289167	2.5290452	2.5291736	2.5293020	2.5294303
339	2.5301997	2.5303278	2.5304558	2.5305839	2.5307118
340	2.5314789	2.5316066	2.5317343	2.5318619	2.5319859
341	2.5327544	2.5328817	2.5330090	2.5331363	2.5332635
342	2.5340261	2.5341531	2.5342800	2.5344069	2.5345338
343	2.5352941	2.5354207	2.5355473	2.5356738	2.5358003
344	2.5365584	2.5366847	2.5368109	2.5369370	2.5370631
345	2.5378191	2.5379450	2.5380708	2.5381966	2.5383223
346	2.5390761	2.5392016	2.5393271	2.5394525	2.5395779
347	2.5403295	2.5404546	2.5405797	2.5407048	2.5408298
348	2.5415792	2.5417040	2.5418288	2.5419535	2.5420781
349	2.5428254	2.5429498	2.5430742	2.5431986	2.5433229

Num	5	6	7	8	9
300	2.4778445	2.4779890	2.4781334	2.4782778	2.4784222
301	2.4792873	2.4794313	2.4795753	2.4797192	2.4798631
302	2.4807254	2.4808689	2.4810124	2.4811559	2.4812993
303	2.4821587	2.4823018	2.4824448	2.4825878	2.4827307
304	2.4835873	2.4837299	2.4838725	2.4840150	2.4841574
305	2.4850112	2.4851533	2.4852954	2.4854375	2.4855795
306	2.4864305	2.4865721	2.4867138	2.4868554	2.4869969
307	2.4878451	2.4879863	2.4881275	2.4882686	2.4884097
308	2.4892552	2.4893959	2.4895366	2.4896773	2.4898179
309	2.4906607	2.4908009	2.4909412	2.4910814	2.4912216
310	2.4920616	2.4922014	2.4923413	2.4924810	2.4926207
311	2.4934580	2.4935974	2.4937368	2.4938761	2.4940154
312	2.4948500	2.4949890	2.4951279	2.4952667	2.4954056
313	2.4962375	2.4963761	2.4965145	2.4966529	2.4967913
314	2.4976206	2.4977587	2.4978967	2.4980347	2.5981727
315	2.4989994	2.4991370	2.4992746	2.4994121	2.4995496
316	2.5003737	2.5005109	2.5006481	2.5007852	2.5009222
317	2.5017437	2.5018805	2.5020172	2.5021539	2.5022905
318	2.5031094	2.5032458	2.5033821	2.5035183	2.5036545
319	2.5044709	2.5046068	2.5047426	2.5048785	2.5050142
320	2.5058280	2.5059635	2.5060990	2.5062344	2.5063697
321	2.5071810	2.5073160	2.5074511	2.5075860	2.5077210
322	2.5085297	2.5086644	2.5087990	2.5089335	2.5090680
323	2.5098743	2.5100085	2.5101427	2.5102768	2.5104109
324	2.5112147	2.5113485	2.5114823	2.5116150	2.5117497
325	2.5125510	2.5126844	2.5128178	2.5129511	2.5130844
326	2.5138832	2.5140162	2.5141491	2.5142820	2.5144149
327	2.5152113	2.5153439	2.5154764	2.5156089	2.5157414
328	2.5165354	2.5166676	2.5167997	2.5169318	2.5170639
329	2.5178554	2.5179872	2.5181189	2.5182506	2.5183822
330	2.5191715	2.5193028	2.5194342	2.5195655	2.5196968
331	2.5204835	2.5206145	2.5207455	2.5208764	2.5210073
332	2.5217916	2.5219222	2.5220528	2.5221833	2.5223138
333	2.5230958	2.5232260	2.5233562	2.5234863	2.5236164
334	2.5243961	2.5245259	2.5246557	2.5247854	2.5249151
335	2.5256925	2.5258219	2.5259513	2.5260807	2.5262100
336	2.5269851	2.5271141	2.5272431	2.5273721	2.5275010
337	2.5282738	2.5284024	2.5285311	2.5286596	2.5287882
338	2.5295587	2.5296869	2.5298152	2.5299434	2.5300716
339	2.5308398	2.5309677	2.5310955	2.5312234	2.5313512
340	2.5321171	2.5322446	2.5323721	2.5324996	2.5326270
341	2.5333907	2.5335179	2.5336450	2.5337721	2.5338991
342	2.5346606	2.5347874	2.5349141	2.5350408	2.5351675
343	2.5359267	2.5360532	2.5361795	2.5363059	2.5364322
344	2.5371892	2.5373153	2.5374413	2.5375672	2.5376932
345	2.5384481	2.5385737	2.5386994	2.5388250	2.5389506
346	2.5397032	2.5398286	2.5399538	2.5400791	2.5402043
347	2.5409548	2.5410798	2.5412047	2.5413296	2.5414544
348	2.5422028	2.5423274	2.5424519	2.5425765	2.5427010
349	2.5434472	2.5435714	2.5436956	2.5438198	2.5439439

Num	0	1	2	3	4
350	2.5440680	2.5441921	2.5443161	2.5444401	2.5445641
351	2.5453071	2.5454308	2.5455545	2.5456781	2.5458017
352	2.5455427	2.5466660	2.5467894	2.5469126	2.5470359
353	2.5477747	2.5478977	2.5480207	2.5481436	2.5482665
354	2.5490033	2.5491259	2.5492486	2.5493712	2.5494937
355	2.5502283	2.5503597	2.5504730	2.5505952	2.5507174
356	2.5514500	2.5515720	2.5516939	2.5518158	2.5519377
357	2.5526682	2.5527898	2.5529114	2.5530330	2.5531545
358	2.5538830	2.5540043	2.5541256	2.5542468	2.5543680
359	2.5550944	2.5552154	2.5553362	2.5554572	2.5555781
360	2.5563025	2.5564231	2.5565437	2.5566643	2.5567848
361	2.5575072	2.5576275	2.5577477	2.5578680	2.5579881
362	2.5587086	2.5588285	2.5589484	2.5590683	2.5591882
363	2.5599066	2.5600262	2.5601458	2.5602654	2.5603849
364	2.5611014	2.5612207	2.5613399	2.5614592	2.5615784
365	2.5622929	2.5624118	2.5625308	2.5626497	2.5627685
366	2.5634811	2.5635997	2.5637183	2.5638369	2.5639555
367	2.5646661	2.5647844	2.5649027	2.5650209	2.5651392
368	2.5658478	2.5659658	2.5660838	2.5662017	2.5663196
369	2.5670264	2.5671440	2.5672617	2.5673793	2.5674969
370	2.5682017	2.5683191	2.5684364	2.5685537	2.5686710
371	2.5693739	2.5694910	2.5696080	2.5697249	2.5698419
372	2.5705429	2.5706597	2.5707764	2.5708930	2.5710097
373	2.5717088	2.5718252	2.5719416	2.5720580	2.5721743
374	2.5728716	2.5729877	2.5731038	2.5732198	2.5733358
375	2.5740313	2.5741471	2.5742628	2.5743786	2.5744943
376	2.5751878	2.5753033	2.5754188	2.5755342	2.5756496
377	2.5763413	2.5764565	2.5765717	2.5766868	2.5768016
378	2.5774917	2.5776067	2.5777215	2.5778363	2.5779511
379	2.5786392	2.5787538	2.5788683	2.5789628	2.5790973
380	2.5797836	2.5798979	2.5800121	2.5801263	2.5802405
381	2.5809250	2.5810389	2.5811529	2.5812668	2.5813807
382	2.5820634	2.5821770	2.5822907	2.5824043	2.5825179
383	2.5831988	2.5833122	2.5834255	2.5835388	2.5836521
384	2.5843312	2.5844443	2.5845574	2.5846704	2.5847834
385	2.5854607	2.5855735	2.5856863	2.5857990	2.5859117
386	2.5865873	2.5866998	2.5868123	2.5869247	2.5870371
387	2.5877110	2.5878232	2.5879353	2.5880475	2.5881596
388	2.5888317	2.5889436	2.5890555	2.5891674	2.5892792
389	2.5899496	2.5900612	2.5901728	2.5902844	2.5903959
390	2.5910646	2.5911759	2.5912873	2.5913985	2.5915098
391	2.5921768	2.5922878	2.5923988	2.5925098	2.5926208
392	2.5932861	2.5933968	2.5935076	2.5936183	2.5937290
393	2.5943925	2.5945030	2.5946135	2.5947239	2.5948344
394	2.5954962	2.5956064	2.5957165	2.5958268	2.5959369
395	2.5965971	2.5967070	2.5968169	2.5969268	2.5970367
396	2.5976952	2.5978048	2.5979145	2.5980241	2.5981336
397	2.5987905	2.5988999	2.5990092	2.5991186	2.5992279
398	2.5998831	2.5999922	2.6001013	2.6002103	2.6003193
399	2.6009729	2.6010817	2.6011905	2.6012993	2.6014081

Num	5	6	7	8	9
350	2.5446880	2.5448119	2.5449358	2.5450595	2.5451834
351	2.5459253	2.5460489	2.5461724	2.5462958	2.5464193
352	2.5471591	2.5472823	2.5474055	2.5475286	2.5476517
353	2.5483894	2.5485123	2.5486351	2.5487578	2.5488806
354	2.5496162	2.5497387	2.5498612	2.5499836	2.5501060
355	2.5508396	2.5509618	2.5510839	2.5512059	2.5513280
356	2.5520595	2.5521813	2.5523031	2.5524248	2.5525465
357	2.5532760	2.5533975	2.5535189	2.5536403	2.5537617
358	2.5544892	2.5546103	2.5547314	2.5548524	2.5049735
359	2.5556989	2.5558197	2.5559404	2.5560612	2.5561818
360	2.5569053	2.5570257	2.5571461	2.5572665	2.5573869
361	2.5581083	2.5582284	2.5583485	2.5584686	2.5585886
362	2.5593080	2.5594278	2.5595476	2.5596673	2.5597870
363	2.5605044	2.5606239	2.5607433	2.5608627	2.5609820
364	2.5616975	2.5618167	2.5619358	2.5620548	2.5621739
365	2.5628874	2.5630062	2.5631250	2.5632437	2.5633624
366	2.5640740	2.5641925	2.5643109	2.5644293	2.5645477
367	2.5652573	2.5653755	2.5654936	2.5656117	2.5657298
368	2.5664375	2.5665553	2.5666731	2.5667909	2.5669087
369	2.5676144	2.5677320	2.5678494	2.5679669	2.5680843
370	2.5687882	2.5689054	2.5690226	2.5691397	2.5692568
371	2.5699588	2.5700757	2.5701926	2.5703094	2.5704262
372	2.5711263	2.5712428	2.5713544	2.5714759	2.5715924
373	2.5722906	2.5724069	2.5725231	2.5726393	2.5727555
374	2.5734518	2.5735678	2.5736837	2.5737996	2.5739154
375	2.5746099	2.5747256	2.5748412	2.5749568	2.5750724
376	2.5757650	2.5758803	2.5759956	2.5761109	2.5762261
377	2.5769169	2.5770320	2.5771470	2.5772620	2.5773769
378	2.5780659	2.5781806	2.5782953	2.5784100	2.5785246
379	2.5792118	2.5893262	2.5794406	2.5795550	2.5796693
380	2.5803547	2.5804688	2.5805829	2.5806969	2.5808110
381	2.5814945	2.5816084	2.5817222	2.5818359	2.5819497
382	2.5826314	2.5827450	2.5828584	2.5829719	2.5830854
383	2.5837654	2.5838786	2.5839918	2.5841050	2.5842181
384	2.5848963	2.5850093	2.5851222	2.5852351	2.5853479
385	2.5860244	2.5861370	2.5862496	2.5863622	2.5864748
386	2.5871495	2.5872618	2.5873742	2.5874865	2.5875987
387	2.5882717	2.5883838	2.5884558	2.5886078	2.5887198
388	2.5893910	2.5895028	2.5896145	2.5897262	2.5898379
389	2.5905075	2.5906183	2.5907304	2.5908418	2.5909532
390	2.5916210	2.5917322	2.5918434	2.5919546	2.5920657
391	2.5927318	2.5928427	2.5929536	2.5930644	2.5931753
392	2.5938397	2.5939503	2.5940609	2.5941715	2.5942820
393	2.5949447	2.5950551	2.5951654	2.5952757	2.5953860
394	2.5960470	2.5961571	2.5962671	2.5963771	2.5964871
395	2.5971465	2.5972563	2.5973660	2.5974758	2.5975855
396	2.5982432	2.5983527	2.5984622	2.5985717	2.5986811
397	2.5993371	2.5994464	2.5995556	2.5996648	2.5997739
398	2.6004283	2.6005373	2.6006462	2.6007551	2.6008640
399	2.6015168	2.6016255	2.6017341	2.6018428	2.6019514

Num	0	1	2	3	4
400	2.6020600	2.6021685	2.6022771	2.6023856	2.6024941
401	2.6031444	2.6032527	2.6033609	2.6034692	2.6035774
402	2.6042261	2.6043341	2.6044421	2.6045500	2.6046580
403	2.6053050	2.6054128	2.6055205	2.6056282	2.6057359
404	2.6063814	2.6064888	2.6065963	2.6067037	2.6068111
405	2.6074550	2.6075622	2.6076694	2.6077766	2.6078837
406	2.6085250	2.6086330	2.6087399	2.6088468	2.6089537
407	2.6095944	2.6097011	2.6098078	2.6099144	2.6100210
408	2.6106602	2.6107666	2.6108730	2.6109794	2.6110857
409	2.6117233	2.6118295	2.6119356	2.6120417	2.6121478
410	2.6127859	2.6128898	2.6129957	2.6131015	2.6132073
411	2.6138418	2.6139475	2.6140531	2.6141587	2.6142643
412	2.6148972	2.6150025	2.6151080	2.6152133	2.6153187
413	2.6159501	2.6160552	2.6161603	2.6162654	2.6163705
414	2.6170003	2.6171052	2.6172101	2.6173149	2.6174197
415	2.6180481	2.6181527	2.6182573	2.6183619	2.6184665
416	2.6190933	2.6191977	2.6193021	2.6194064	2.6195107
417	2.6201360	2.6202402	2.6203443	2.6204484	2.6205524
418	2.6211763	2.6212802	2.6213840	2.6214879	2.6215917
419	2.6222140	2.6223177	2.6224213	2.6225249	2.6226284
420	2.6232493	2.6233527	2.6234560	2.6235594	2.6236627
421	2.6242821	2.6243852	2.6244884	2.6245915	2.6246945
422	2.6253124	2.6254153	2.6255182	2.6256211	2.6257239
423	2.6263404	2.6264430	2.6265457	2.6266483	2.6267509
424	2.6273659	2.6274683	2.6275707	2.6276730	2.6277754
425	2.6283889	2.6284911	2.6285933	2.6286954	2.6287975
426	2.6294095	2.6295115	2.6296134	2.6297153	2.6298172
427	2.6304279	2.6305296	2.6306312	2.6307329	2.6308345
428	2.6314438	2.6315452	2.6316467	2.6317481	2.6318495
429	2.6324573	2.6325585	2.6326597	2.6327609	2.6328620
430	2.6334685	2.6335694	2.6336704	2.6337713	2.6338723
431	2.6344773	2.6345780	2.6346788	2.6347795	2.6348801
432	2.6354837	2.6355843	2.6356848	2.6357852	2.6358857
433	2.6364879	2.6365882	2.6366884	2.6367887	2.6368889
434	2.6374897	2.6375898	2.6376898	2.6377898	2.6378898
435	2.6384893	2.6385891	2.6386889	2.6387887	2.6388884
436	2.6394865	2.6395861	2.6396857	2.6397852	2.6398847
437	2.6404814	2.6405808	2.6406802	2.6407795	2.6408788
438	2.6414741	2.6415733	2.6416724	2.6417715	2.6418705
439	2.6424645	2.6425634	2.6426623	2.6427612	2.6428601
440	2.6434527	2.6435514	2.6436500	2.6437487	2.6438473
441	2.6444386	2.6445371	2.6446355	2.6447339	2.6448323
442	2.6454223	2.6455205	2.6456187	2.6457169	2.6458151
443	2.6464037	2.6465017	2.6465997	2.6466977	2.6467957
444	2.6473830	2.6474808	2.6475785	2.6476763	2.6477740
445	2.6483600	2.6484576	2.6485552	2.6486527	2.6487502
446	2.6493349	2.6494322	2.6495295	2.6496269	2.6497242
447	2.6503075	2.6504047	2.6505018	2.6505989	2.6506960
448	2.6512780	2.6513749	2.6514719	2.6515687	2.6516656
449	2.6522463	2.6523430	2.6524397	2.6525364	2.6526331

Num	5	6	7	8	9
400	2.6026025	2.5027109	2.6028193	2.6029277	2.6030361
401	2.6036855	2.6037937	2.6039018	2.6040099	2.6041180
402	2.6047659	2.0048738	2.6049816	2.6050895	2.6051973
403	2.6058435	2.6059512	2.6060587	2.6061663	2.6062738
404	2.6069185	2.6070259	2.6071332	2.6072405	2.6073478
405	2.6079909	2.6080979	2.6082050	2.6083120	2.6084190
406	2.6090605	2.6091674	2.6092742	2.6093809	2.6094877
407	2.6101276	2.6102342	2.6103407	2.6104472	2.6105537
408	2.6111921	2.6112984	2.6114046	2.6115109	2.6116171
409	2.6122539	2.6123599	2.6124660	2.6125720	2.6126779
410	2.6133132	2.6134189	2.6135247	2.6136304	2.6137361
411	2.6143698	2.6144754	2.6145809	2.6146863	2.6147918
412	2.6154240	2.6155292	2.6156345	2.6157397	2.6158449
413	2.6164755	2.6165805	2.6166855	2.6167935	2.6168954
414	2.6175245	2.6176293	2.6177340	2.6178387	2.6179434
415	2.6185710	2.6186755	2.6187800	2.6188845	2.6189889
416	2.6196150	2.6197193	2.6198235	2.6199277	2.6200319
417	2.6206565	2.6207605	2.6208645	2.6209684	2.6210724
418	2.6216955	2.6217992	2.6219030	2.6220067	2.6221104
419	2.6227320	2.6228355	2.6229390	2.6230424	2.6231459
420	2.6237660	2.6238693	2.6239725	2.6240757	2.6241789
421	2.6247976	2.6249006	2.6250036	2.6251066	2.6252095
422	2.6258267	2.6259295	2.6260322	2.6261350	2.6262377
423	2.6268534	2.6269559	2.6270585	2.6271610	2.6272634
424	2.6278777	2.6279800	2.6280823	2.6281845	2.6282867
425	2.6288996	2.6290016	2.6291036	2.6292057	2.6293076
426	2.6299190	2.6300208	2.6301226	2.6302244	2.6303262
427	2.6309361	2.6310377	2.6311392	2.6312408	2.6313423
428	2.6319508	2.6320522	7.6321535	2.6322548	2.6323560
429	2.6329632	2.6330643	2.6331653	2.6332664	2.6333674
430	2.6339732	2.6340740	2.6341749	2.6342757	2.6343765
431	2.6349808	2.6350814	2.6351820	2.6352826	2.6353832
432	2.6359861	2.6360865	2.6361869	2.6362872	2.6363876
433	2.6369891	2.6370893	2.6371894	2.6372895	2.6373896
434	2.6379898	2.6380897	2.6381896	2.6382895	2.6383894
435	2.6389882	2.6390879	2.6391876	2.6392872	2.6393894
436	2.6399842	2.6400837	2.6401832	2.6402826	2.6403820
437	2.6409781	2.6410773	2.6411765	2.6412758	2.6413749
438	2.6419696	2.6420686	2.6421676	2.6422666	2.6423656
439	2.6429589	2.6430577	2.6431565	2.6432552	2.6433540
440	2.6439459	2.6440445	2.6441430	2.6442416	2.6443401
441	2.6449307	2.6450291	2.6451274	2.6452257	2.6453240
442	2.6459133	2.6460114	2.6461095	2.6462076	2.6463057
443	2.6468936	2.6469915	2.6470894	2.6471873	2.6472851
444	2.6478718	2.6479695	2.6480671	2.6481648	2.6482624
445	2.6488477	2.6489452	2.6490426	2.6491401	2.6492375
446	2.6498215	2.6499187	2.6500160	2.6501132	2.6502104
447	2.6507930	2.6508901	2.6509871	2.6510841	2.6511811
448	2.6517624	2.6518593	2.6519561	2.6520528	2.6521496
449	2.6527297	2.6528263	2.6529229	2.6530195	2.6531160

Num	0	1	2	3	4
450	2.6532125	2.6533090	2.6534055	2.6535019	2.6535984
451	2.6541765	2.6542728	2.6543691	2.6544653	2.6545616
452	2.6551384	2.6552345	2.6553306	2.6554266	2.6555226
453	2.6560982	2.6561941	2.6562899	2.6563857	2.6564815
454	2.6570559	2.6571515	2.6572471	2.6573427	2.6574383
455	2.6580114	2.6581068	2.6582023	2.6582976	2.6583930
456	2.6589648	2.6590601	2.6591553	2.6592505	2.6593456
457	2.6599162	2.6600112	2.6601062	2 6602012	2.6602962
458	2.6608655	2.6609603	2.6610551	2.6611499	2.6612446
459	2.6618127	2.6619073	2.6620019	2.6620964	2.6621910
460	2.6627578	2.6628522	2.6629466	2.6630412	2.6631353
461	2.6637009	2.6637951	2.6638893	2·6639835	2.6640776
462	2.6646420	2.6647360	2.6648299	2.6649239	2.6650178
463	2.6655810	2.6656748	2.6657685	2.6658623	2.6659560
464	2.6665180	2.6666116	2.6667051	2.6667987	2.6668922
465	2.6674530	2.6675463	2.6676397	2.6677331	2.6678264
466	2.6683859	2.6684791	2.6685723	2.6686654	2.6687585
467	2.6693169	2.6694099	2.6695028	2.6695958	2.6696887
468	2.6702459	2.6703386	2.6704314	2.6705242	2.6706169
469	2.6711728	2.6712654	2.6713580	2 6714506	2.6715431
470	2.6720979	2.6721903	2.6722826	2.6723750	2.6724673
471	2.6730209	2.6731131	2.6732053	2.6732974	2.6733896
472	2.6739420	2.6740340	2.6741260	2.6742179	2.6743099
473	2.6748611	2.6749529	2.6750447	2.6751365	2.6752283
474	2.6757783	2.6758700	2.6759615	2.6760531	2.6761447
475	2.6766936	2.6767850	2.6768764	2.6769678	2.6770592
476	2.6776069	2.6776982	2.6777894	2.6778806	2.6779718
477	2.6785184	2.6786094	2.6787004	2.6787914	2.6788824
478	2.6794279	2.6795187	2.6796096	2.6797004	2.6797912
479	2.6803355	2.6804262	2.6805168	2.6806074	2.6806980
480	2.6812412	2.6813317	2.6814222	2.6815126	2.6816030
481	2.6821451	2.6822354	2.6823256	2.6824159	2.6825061
482	2.6830470	2.6831371	2.6832272	2.6833173	2.6834073
483	2.6839471	2.6840370	2.6841269	2.6842168	2.6843066
484	2.6848454	2.6849351	2.6850248	2.6851145	2.6852041
485	2.6857417	2.6858313	2.6859208	2.6860103	2.6860998
486	2.6866363	2.6867256	2.6868149	2.6869043	2 6869936
487	2.6875290	2.6876181	2.6877073	2.6877964	2.6878855
488	2.6884198	2.6885088	2.6885978	2.6886867	2.6887757
489	2.6893089	2.6893977	2.6894864	2.6895752	2.6896640
490	2.6901961	2.6902847	2.6903733	2.6904619	2.6905505
491	2.6910815	2.6911699	2.6912584	2.6913468	2.6914352
492	2.6919651	2.6920534	2.6921416	2.6922298	2.6923180
493	2.6928469	2.6929350	2.6930231	2.6931111	2.6931991
494	2.6937269	2.6938148	2.6939027	2.6939906	2.6940785
495	2.6946052	2.6946929	2.6947806	2.6948683	2.6949560
496	2.6954817	2.6955692	2.6956568	2.6957443	2.6958318
497	2.6963564	2.6964438	2.6965311	2.6966185	2.6967058
498	2.6972293	2.6973165	2.6974037	2.6974909	2.6975780
499	2.6981005	2.6981876	2.6982746	2.6983616	2.6984485

Num	5	6	7	8	9
450	2.6536948	2.6537912	2.6538876	2.6539839	2.6540802
451	2.6546578	2.6547539	2.6548501	2.6549462	2.6550423
452	2.6556186	2.6557145	2.6558105	2.6559064	2.6560023
453	2.6565773	2.6566730	2.6567688	2.6568645	2.6569602
454	2.6575339	2.6576294	2.6577250	2.6578205	2.6579159
455	2.6584884	2.6585837	2.6586790	2.6587743	2.6588696
456	2.6594408	2.6595359	2.6596310	2.6597261	2.6598212
457	2.6603911	2.6604860	2.6605809	2.6606758	2.6607706
458	2.6613393	2.6614340	2.6615287	2.6616234	2.6617181
459	2.6622855	2.6623800	2.6624745	2.6625690	2.6626634
460	2.6532296	2.6633239	2.6634182	2.6635125	2.6636067
461	2.6641717	2.6642658	2.6643599	2.6644539	2.6645480
462	2.6651117	2.6652056	2.6652995	2.6653933	2.6654872
463	2.6660497	2.6661434	2.6662371	2.6663307	2.6664244
464	2.6669857	2.6670792	2.6671727	2.6672661	2.6673595
465	2.6679197	2.6680130	2.6681062	2.6681995	2.6682927
466	2.6688516	2.6689447	2.6690378	2.6691308	2.6692239
467	2.6697816	2.6698745	2.6699674	2.6700602	2.6701530
468	2.6707096	2.6708023	2.6708950	2.6709876	2.6710802
469	2.6716356	2.6717281	2.6718206	2.6719130	2.6720054
470	2.6725596	2.6726519	2.6727442	2.6728365	2.6729287
471	2.6734817	2.6735738	2.6736659	2.6737579	2.6738500
472	2.6744018	2.6744937	2.6745856	2.6746775	2.6747693
473	2.6753200	2.6754117	2.6755034	2.6755951	2.6756867
474	2.6762362	2.6763277	2.6764192	2.6765107	2.6766022
475	2.6771505	2.6772418	2.6773332	2.6774244	2.6775157
476	2.6780629	2.6781540	2.6782452	2.6783362	2.6784273
477	2.6789734	2.6790643	2.6791552	2.6792461	2.6793370
478	2.6798819	2.6799727	2.6800634	2.6801541	2.6802448
479	2.6807886	2.6808792	2.6809697	2.6810602	2.6811507
480	2.6816934	2.6817838	2.6818741	2.6819645	2.6820548
481	2.6825963	2.6826865	2.6827766	2.6828668	2.6829569
482	2.6834973	2.6835873	2.6836773	2.6837673	2.6838572
483	2.6843965	2.6844863	2.6845761	2.6846659	2.6847556
484	2.6852938	2.6853834	2.6854730	2.6855626	2.6856522
485	2.6861892	2.6862787	2.6863681	2.6864575	2.6865469
486	2.6870828	2.6871721	2.6872613	2.6873506	2.6874398
487	2.6879746	2.6880537	2.6881528	2.6882418	2.6883308
488	2.6888646	2.6889535	2.6890423	2.6891312	2.6892200
489	2.6897527	2.6898414	2.6899301	2.6900188	2.6901074
490	2.6906390	2.6907275	2.6908161	2.6909046	2.6909930
491	2.6915235	2.6916119	2.6917002	2.6917885	2.6918768
492	2.6924062	2.6924944	2.6925826	2.6926707	2.6927588
493	2.6932872	2.6933752	2.6934631	2.6935511	2.6936390
494	2.6941663	2.6942541	2.6943419	2.6944297	2.6945174
495	2.6950437	2.6951313	2.6952189	2.6953065	2.6953941
496	2.6959193	2.6960067	2.6960942	2.6961816	2.6962690
497	2.6967931	2.6968804	2.6969676	2.6970549	2.6971421
498	2.6976652	2.6977523	2.6978394	2.6979264	2.6980135
499	2.6985355	2.6986224	2.6987093	2.6987963	2.6988831

Num.	0	1	2	3	4
500	2.6989700	2.6990569	2.6991437	2.6992305	2.6993173
501	2.6998377	2.6999244	2.7000111	2.7000977	2.7001843
502	2.7007037	2.7007902	2.7008767	2.7009632	2.7010496
503	2.7015680	2.7016543	2.7017406	2.7018269	2.7019132
504	2.7024305	2.7025167	2.7026028	2.7026890	2.7027751
505	2.7032914	2.7033774	2.7034633	2.7035493	2.7036352
506	2.7041505	2.7042363	2.7043221	2.7044079	2.7044937
507	2.7050080	2.7050936	2.7051792	2.7052649	2.7053505
508	2.7058637	2.7059492	2.7060347	2.7061201	2.7062055
509	2.7067178	2.7068031	2.7068884	2.7069737	2.7070589
510	2.7075702	2.7076553	2.7077405	2.7078256	2.7079107
511	2.7084209	2.7085059	2.7085908	2.7086753	2.7087607
512	2.7092700	2.7093548	2.7094396	2.7095244	2.7096091
513	2.7101174	2.7102020	2.7102865	2.7103713	2.7104559
514	2.7109631	2.7110476	2.7111321	2.7112165	2.7113010
515	2.7118072	2.7118915	2.7119759	2.7120601	2.7121444
516	2.7126497	2.7127339	2.7128180	2.7129021	2.7129862
517	2.7134905	2.7135745	2.7136585	2.7137425	2.7138264
518	2.7143298	2.7144136	2.7144974	2.7145812	2.7146650
519	2.7151674	2.7152510	2.7153347	2.7154183	2.7155019
520	2.7160033	2.7160869	2.7161703	2.7162538	2.7163373
521	2.7168377	2.7169211	2.7170044	2.7170877	2.7171710
522	2.7176705	2.7177537	2.7178369	2.7179200	2.7180032
523	2.7185017	2.7185847	2.7186577	2.7187507	2.7188337
524	2.7193313	2.7194142	2.7194970	2.7195799	2.7196627
525	2.7201593	2.7202420	2.7203247	2.7204074	2.7204901
526	2.7209857	2.7210683	2.7211508	2.7212334	2.7213159
527	2.7218106	2.7218930	2.7219754	2.7220578	2.7221401
528	2.7226339	2.7227162	2.7227984	2.7228806	2.7229628
529	2.7234557	2.7235378	2.7236198	2.7237019	2.7237839
530	2.7242759	2.7243578	2.7244397	2.7245216	2.7246035
531	2.7250945	2.7251763	2.7252581	2.7253398	2.7254216
532	2.7259116	2.7259933	2.7260749	2.7261565	2.7262380
533	2.7267272	2.7268087	2.7268901	2.7269716	2.7270530
534	2.7275413	2.7276226	2.7277039	2.7277852	2.7278664
535	2.7283538	2.7284350	2.7285161	2.7285972	2.7286784
536	2.7291648	2.7292458	2.7293268	2.7294078	2.7294888
537	2.7299743	2.7300552	2.7301360	2.7302168	2.7302977
538	2.7307823	2.7308630	2.7309437	2.7310244	2.7311051
539	2.7315883	2.7316693	2.7317499	2.7318304	2.7319109
540	2.7323938	2.7324742	2.7325546	2.7326350	2.7327153
541	2.7331973	2.7332775	2.7333578	2.7334380	2.7335183
542	2.7339993	2.7340794	2.7341595	2.7342396	2.7343197
443	2.7347998	2.7348798	2.7349598	2.7350397	2.7351196
544	2.7355989	2.7356787	2.7357585	2.7358383	2.7359181
545	2.7363965	2.7364762	2.7365558	2.7366355	2.7367151
546	2.7371926	2.7372722	2.7373517	2.7374312	2.7375107
547	2.7379873	2.7380667	2.7381461	2.7382254	2.7383048
548	2.7387806	2.7388598	2.7389390	2.7390182	2.7390974
549	2.7395723	2.7396514	2.7397305	2.7398096	2.7398887

Num	5	6	7	8	9
500	2.6994041	2.6994908	2.6995776	2.6996643	2.6997510
501	2.7002709	2.7003575	2.7004441	2.7005307	2.7006172
502	2.7011361	2.7012225	2.7013089	2.7013953	2.7014816
503	2.7019995	2.7020857	2.7021719	2.7022582	2.7023444
504	2.7028612	2.7029472	2.7030333	2.7031193	2.7032054
505	2.7037212	2.7038071	2.7038929	2.7039788	2.7040647
506	2.7045794	2.7046652	2.7047509	2.7048366	2.7049223
507	2.7054360	2.7055216	2.7056072	2.7056927	2.7057782
508	2.7062910	2.7063764	2.7064617	2.7065471	2.7066325
509	2.7071442	2.7072294	2.7073146	2.7073998	2.7074850
510	2.7079957	2.7080808	2.7081659	2.7082509	2.7083359
511	2.7088456	2.7089305	2.7090154	2.7091003	2.7091851
512	2.7096939	2.7097786	2.7098633	2.7099480	2.7100327
513	2.7105404	2.7106250	2.7107096	2.7107941	2.7108786
514	2.7113854	2.7114698	2.7115542	2.7116385	2.7117229
515	2.7122287	2.7123129	2.7123971	2.7124813	2.7125655
516	2.7130703	2.7131544	2.7132385	2.7133225	2.7134065
517	2.7139104	2.7139943	2.7140782	2.7141620	2.7142459
518	2.7147488	2.7148325	2.7149162	2.7150000	2.7150837
519	2.7155856	2.7156691	2.7157527	2.7158363	2.7159198
520	2.7164207	2.7165042	2.7165876	2.7166710	2.7167544
521	2.7172543	2.7173376	2.7174209	2.7175041	2.7175873
522	2.7180863	2.7181694	2.7182525	2.7183356	2.7184186
523	2.7189167	2.7189996	2.7190826	2.7191655	2.7192484
524	2.7197455	2.7198283	2.7199111	2.7199938	2.7200766
525	2.7205727	2.7206554	2.7207380	2.7208206	2.7209032
526	2.7213984	2.7214809	2.7215633	2.7216458	2.7217282
527	2.7222225	2.7223048	2.7223871	2.7224694	2.7225517
528	2.7230450	2.7231272	2.7232093	2.7232914	2.7233736
529	2.7238660	2.7239480	2.7240300	2.7241120	2.7241939
530	2.7246854	2.7247672	2.7248491	2.7249309	2.7250127
531	2.7255033	2.7255850	2.7256667	2.7257483	2.7258300
532	2.7263196	2.7264012	2.7264827	2.7265642	2.7266457
533	2.7271344	2.7272158	2.7272972	2.7273786	2.7274599
534	2.7279477	2.7280290	2.7281102	2.7281914	2.7282726
535	2.7287595	2.7288406	2.7289216	2.7290027	2.7290838
536	2.7295697	2.7296507	2.7297316	2.7298125	2.7298934
537	2.7303785	2.7304593	2.7305400	2.7306208	2.7307015
538	2.7311857	2.7312663	2.7313470	2.7314276	2.7315082
539	2.7319914	2.7320719	2.7321524	2.7322329	2.7323133
540	2.7327957	2.7328760	2.7329564	2.7330367	2.7331170
541	2.7335985	2.7336787	2.7337588	2.7338390	2.7339192
542	2.7343997	2.7344798	2.7345598	2.7346398	2.7347198
543	2.7351995	2.7352794	2.7353593	2.7354392	2.7355191
544	2.7359979	2.2360776	2.7361574	2.7362371	2.7363158
545	2.7367948	2.7368744	2.7369540	2.7370335	2.7371131
546	2.7375902	2.7376696	2.7377491	2.7378285	2.7379079
547	2.7383841	2.7384634	2.7385427	2.7386220	2.7387013
548	2.7391766	2.7392558	2.7393350	2.7394141	2.7394932
549	2.7399677	2.7400467	2.7401257	2.7402047	2.7402837

A TABLE of Logarithms.

Num	0	1	2	3	4
550	2.7403627	2.7304416	2.7405206	2.7405995	2.7406784
551	2.7411516	2.7412304	2.7413092	2.7413880	2.7414568
552	2.7419391	2.7420177	2.7420964	2.7421750	2.7422537
553	2.7427251	2.7428037	2.7428822	2.7429607	2.7430392
554	2.7435098	2.7435881	2.7436665	2.7437449	2.7438232
555	2.7442930	2.7443712	2.7444495	2.7445277	2.7446059
556	2.7450748	2.7451529	2.7452310	2.7453091	2.7453871
557	2.7458552	2.7459332	2.7460111	2.7460890	2.7461670
558	2.7466342	2.7467120	2.7467898	2.7468676	2.7469454
559	2.7474118	2.7474895	2.7475672	2.7476448	2.7477225
560	2.7481880	2.7482656	2.7483431	2.7484206	2.7484981
561	2.7489629	2.7490403	2.7491177	2.7491950	2.7492724
562	2.7497363	2.7498136	2.7498908	2.7499681	2.7500453
563	2.7505084	2.7505855	2.7506626	2.7507398	2.7508168
564	2.7512791	2.7513561	2.7514331	2.7515100	2.7515870
565	2.7520484	2.7521253	2.7522022	2.7522790	2.7523558
566	2.7528164	2.7528932	2.7529699	2.7530466	2.7531232
567	2.7535831	2.7536596	2.7537362	2.7538128	2.7538893
568	2.7543443	2.7544248	2.7545012	5.7545777	2.7546541
569	2.7551123	2.7551886	2.7552649	2.7553412	2.7554175
570	2.7558749	2.7559510	2.7560272	2.7561034	2.7561795
571	2.7566351	2.7567122	2.7567882	2.7568642	2.7569402
572	2.7573950	2.7574719	2.7575479	2.7576237	2.7576996
573	2.7581546	2.7582304	2.7583062	2.7583819	2.7584577
574	2.7589119	2.7589875	2.7590632	2.7591388	2.7592144
575	2.7596578	2.7597434	2.7598199	2.7598914	2.7599599
576	2.7604225	2.7604979	2.7605733	2.7606416	2.7607240
577	2.7611758	2.7612511	2.7613263	2.7614016	2.7614768
578	2.7619273	2.7620030	2.7620781	2.7621532	2.7622283
579	2.7626755	2.7627536	2.7628286	2.7629035	2.7629785
580	2.7634230	2.7635029	2.7635777	2.7636525	2.7637274
581	2.7641751	2.7642509	2.7643256	2.7644003	2.7644750
582	2.7649230	2.7649976	2.7650722	2.7651468	2.7652214
583	2.7656686	2.7657430	2.7658175	2.7658920	2.7659664
584	2.7664128	2.7664872	2.7665616	2.7666359	2.7667102
585	2.7671557	2.7672301	2.7673043	2.7673785	2.7674527
586	2.7678976	2.7679717	2.7680453	2.7681199	2.7681940
587	2.7686381	2.7687121	2.7687860	2.7688600	2.7689339
588	2.7693773	2.7694512	2.7695250	2.7695988	2.7696727
589	2.7701153	2.7701890	2.7702627	2.7703364	2.7704101
590	2.7708520	2.7709256	2.7709992	2.7710728	2.7711463
591	2.7715875	2.7716610	2.7717344	2.7718079	2.7718813
592	2.7723217	2.7723951	2.7724684	2.7725417	2.7726150
593	2.7730547	2.7731279	2.7732011	2.7732743	2.7733475
594	2.7737854	2.7738596	2.7739325	2.7740057	2.7740788
595	2.7745170	2.7745899	2.7746529	2.7747359	2.7748088
596	2.7752463	2.7753191	2.7753920	2.7754648	2.7755376
597	2.7759743	2.7760471	2.7761198	2.7761925	2.7762652
598	2.7767012	2.7767733	2.7768464	2.7769190	2.7769916
599	2.7774263	2.7774993	2.7775718	2.7776443	2.7777167

Num	5	6	7	8	9
550	2,7407573	2,7408362	2,7409151	2,7409939	2,7410728
551	2,7415455	2,7416243	2,7417030	2,7417817	2,7418604
552	2,7423323	2,7424109	2,7424895	2,7425680	2,7426466
553	2,7431176	2,7431961	2,7432745	2,7433530	2,7434314
554	2,7439015	2,7439799	2,7440582	2,7441365	2,7442147
555	2,7446841	2,7447622	2,7448404	2,7449185	2,7449967
556	2,7454652	2,7455432	2,7456212	2,7456992	2,7457772
557	2,7462449	2,7463228	2,7464006	2,7464785	2,7465564
558	2,7470232	2,7471009	2,7471787	2,7472564	2,7473341
559	2,7478001	2,7478777	2,7479553	2,7480329	2,7481105
560	2,7485756	2,7486531	2,7487306	2,7488080	2,7488854
561	2,7493498	2,7494271	2,7495044	2,7495817	2,7496590
562	2,7501225	2,7501997	2,7502769	2,7503541	2,7504312
563	2,7508939	2,7509710	2,7510480	2,7511251	2,7512021
564	2,7516639	2,7517409	2,7518178	2,7518947	2,7519716
565	2,7524326	2,7525094	2,7525862	2,7526629	2,7527397
566	2,7531999	2,7532766	2,7533532	2,7534298	2,7535065
567	2,7539659	2,7540424	2,7541189	2,7541954	2,7542719
568	2,7547305	2,7548069	2,7548832	2,7549596	2,7550359
569	2,7554937	2,7555700	2,7556462	2,7557224	2,7557987
570	2,7562556	2,7563318	2,7564079	2,7564840	2,7565600
571	2,7570162	2,7570922	2,7571682	2,7572441	2,7573201
572	2,7577755	2,7578513	2,7579272	2,7580030	2,7580788
573	2,7585334	2,7586091	2,7586848	2,7587605	2,7588362
574	2,7592900	2,7593656	2,7594412	2,7595168	2,7595923
575	2,7600453	2,7601208	2,7601962	2,7602717	2,7603471
576	2,7607993	2,7608746	2,7609500	2,7610253	2,7611005
577	2,7615520	2,7616272	2,7617024	2,7617775	2,7618527
578	2,7623034	2,7623784	2,7624535	2,7625285	2,7626035
579	2,7630534	2,7631284	2,7632033	2,7632782	2,7633531
580	2,7638022	2,7638770	2,7639518	2,7640255	2,7641014
581	2,7645497	2,7646244	2,7646991	2,7647737	2,7648484
582	2,7652959	2,7653705	2,7654450	2,7655195	2,7655941
583	2,7660409	2,7661153	2,7661897	2,7662641	2,7663385
584	2,7667845	2,7668588	2,7669331	2,7670074	2,7670816
585	2,7675269	2,7676011	2,7676752	2,7677494	2,7678235
586	2,7682680	2,7683421	2,7684161	2,7684901	2,7685641
587	2,7690079	2,7690818	2,7691557	2,7692295	2,7693035
588	2,7697465	2,7698203	2,7698940	2,7699678	2,7700416
589	2,7704838	2,7705575	2,7706311	2,7707048	2,7707784
590	2,7712199	2,7712934	2,7713670	2,7714405	2,7715140
591	2,7719547	2,7720282	2,7721016	2,7721750	2,7722483
592	2,7726884	2,7727616	2,7728319	2,7729082	2,7729814
593	2,7734207	2,7734939	2,7735670	2,7736402	2,7737133
594	2,7741519	2,7742249	2,7742979	2,7743710	2,7744440
595	2,7748818	2,7749547	2,7750276	2,7751005	2,7751734
596	2,7756104	2,7756832	2,7757560	2,7758288	2,7759015
597	2,7763379	2,7764106	2,7764833	2,7765559	2,7766286
598	2,7770642	2,7771367	2,7772093	2,7772818	2,7773543
599	2,7777892	2,7778616	2,7779340	2,7780065	2,7780789

Num	0	1	2	3	4
600	2.7781512	2.7782236	2.7782960	2.7783683	2.7784407
601	2.7785745	2.7789467	2.7790190	2.7790912	2.7791634
602	2.7795965	2.7796686	2.7797408	2.7798129	2.7798850
603	2.7803173	2.7803893	2.7804613	2.7805333	2.7806053
604	2.7810359	2.7811088	2.7811807	2.7812525	2.7813245
605	2.7817554	2.7818272	2.7818989	2.7819707	2.7820424
606	2.7824726	2.7825443	2.7826159	2.7826876	2.7827592
607	2.7831887	2.7832602	2.7833318	2.7834033	2.7834748
608	2.7839036	2.7839750	2.7840464	2.7841178	2.7841892
609	2.7846173	2.7846886	2.7847599	2.7848312	2.7849024
610	2.7853298	2.7854010	2.7854722	2.7855434	2.7856145
611	2.7860412	2.7861123	2.7861833	2.7862544	2.7863254
612	2.7867514	2.7868224	2.7868933	2.7869643	2.7870352
613	2.7874605	2.7875313	2.7876021	2.7876730	2.7877438
614	2.7881684	2.7882391	2.7883098	2.7883805	2.7884512
615	2.7888751	2.7889457	2.7890163	2.7890869	2.7891575
616	2.7895807	2.7896512	2.7897217	2.7897922	2.7898626
617	2.7902852	2.7903555	2.7904259	2.7904963	2.7905666
618	2.7909885	2.7910587	2.7911290	2.7911992	2.7912695
619	2.7916906	2.7917608	2.7918309	2.7919011	2.7919712
620	2.7923917	2.7924617	2.7925318	2.7926018	2.7926718
621	2.7930915	2.7931615	2.7932314	2.7933014	2.7933712
622	2.7937904	2.7938602	2.7939300	2.7939998	2.7940696
623	2.7944880	2.7945578	2.7946274	2.7946971	2.7947668
624	2.7951846	2.7952542	2.7953238	2.7953933	2.7954629
625	2.7958800	2.7959495	2.7960191	2.7960884	2.7961578
626	2.7965743	2.7966437	2.7967131	2.7967824	2.7968517
627	2.7972675	2.7973368	2.7974060	2.7974753	2.7975445
628	2.7979596	2.7980288	2.7980979	2.7981671	2.7982362
629	2.7986506	2.7987197	2.7987887	2.7988577	2.7989267
630	2.7993405	2.7994095	2.7994784	2.7995473	2.7996162
631	2.8000294	2.8000982	2.8001670	2.8002358	2.8003046
632	2.8007171	2.8007858	2.8008545	2.8009232	2.8009919
633	2.8014037	2.8014723	2.8015409	2.8016095	2.8016781
634	2.8020893	2.8021578	2.8022262	2.8022947	2.8023632
635	2.8027737	2.8028421	2.8029105	2.8029789	2.8030472
636	2.8034571	2.8035254	2.8035937	2.8036619	2.8037302
637	2.8041394	2.8042076	2.8042758	2.8043439	2.8044121
638	2.8048207	2.8048887	2.8049568	2.8050248	2.8050929
639	2.8055009	2.8055688	2.8056368	2.8057047	2.8057726
640	2.8061800	2.8062478	2.8063157	2.8063835	2.8064513
641	2.8068580	2.8069258	2.8069935	2.8070612	2.8071290
642	2.8075350	2.8076027	2.8076703	2.8077379	2.8078055
643	2.8082110	2.8082785	2.8083460	2.8084136	2.8084811
644	2.8088849	2.8089533	2.8090207	2.8090881	2.8091555
645	2.8095597	2.8096271	2.8096944	2.8097617	2.8098290
646	2.8102325	2.8102997	2.8103670	2.8104342	2.8105013
647	2.8109043	2.8109714	2.8110385	2.8111056	2.8111727
648	2.8115750	2.8116420	2.8117090	2.8117760	2.8118430
649	2.8122447	2.8123116	2.8123785	2.8124454	2.8125123

Num	5	6	7	8	9
600	2.7785130	2.7785853	2.7786576	2.7787299	2.7788022
601	2.7792356	2.7793078	2.7793800	2.7794522	2.7795243
602	2.7799571	2.7800291	2.7801012	2.7801732	2.7802453
603	2.7806773	2.7807492	2.7808212	2.7808931	2.7809650
604	2.7813963	2.7814681	2.7815400	2.7816118	2.7816836
605	2.7821141	2.7821859	2.7822576	2.7823293	2.7824010
606	2.7828308	2.7829024	2.7829740	2.7830456	2.7831171
607	2.7835463	2.7836178	2.7836892	2.7837607	2.7838321
608	2.7842606	2.7843319	2.7844033	2.7844746	2.7845460
609	2.7849737	2.7850450	2.7851162	2.7851874	2.7852586
610	2.7856857	2.7857558	2.7858279	2.7858990	2.7859701
611	2.7863965	2.7864675	2.7865385	2.7866094	2.7866805
612	2.7871061	2.7871770	2.7872479	2.7873188	2.7873896
613	2.7878146	2.7878853	2.7879561	2.7880269	2.7880976
614	2.7885219	2.7885926	2.7886632	2.7887339	2.7888045
615	2.7892281	2.7892986	2.7893691	2.7894397	2.7895102
616	2.7899331	2.7900035	2.7900739	2.7901444	2.7902148
617	2.7906370	2.7907073	2.7907776	2.7908479	2.7909182
618	2.7913397	2.7914099	2.7914801	2.7915503	2.7916205
619	2.7920413	2.7921114	2.7921815	2.7922516	2.7923216
620	2.7927418	2.7928118	2.7928817	2.7929517	2.7930217
621	2.7934411	2.7935110	2.7935809	2.7936507	2.7937206
622	2.7941394	2.7942091	2.7942789	2.7943486	2.7944183
623	2.7948365	2.7949061	2.7949757	2.7950454	2.7951150
624	2.7955324	2.7956020	2.7956715	2.7957410	2.7958105
625	2.7962273	2.7962967	2.7963662	2.7964356	2.7965050
626	2.7969211	2.7969904	2.7970597	2.7971290	2.7971983
627	2.7976137	2.7976829	2.7977521	2.7978213	2.7978905
628	2.7983053	2.7983744	2.7984435	2.7985125	2.7985816
629	2.7989957	2.7990647	2.7991337	2.7992027	2.7992716
630	2.7996851	2.7997540	2.7998228	2.7998917	2.7999605
631	2.8003734	2.8004421	2.8005109	2.8005796	2.8006484
632	2.8010605	2.8011292	2.8011978	2.8012665	2.8013351
633	2.8017466	2.8018152	2.8018837	2.8019522	2.8020208
634	2.8024316	2.8025001	2.8025685	2.8026369	2.8027053
635	2.8031156	2.8031839	2.8032522	2.8033205	2.8033888
636	2.8037984	2.8038666	2.8039348	2.8040031	2.8040712
637	2.8044802	2.8045483	2.8045164	2.8046845	2.8047526
638	2.8051609	2.8052289	2.8052969	2.8053649	2.8054329
639	2.8058405	2.8059085	2.8059763	2.8060442	2.8061121
640	2.8065191	2.8065869	2.8066547	2.8067225	2.8067903
641	2.8071967	2.8072643	2.8073320	2.8073997	2.8074574
642	2.8078731	2.8079407	2.8080083	2.8080759	2.8081434
643	2.8085485	2.8086160	2.8086835	2.8087510	2.8088184
644	2.8092229	2.8092903	2.8093577	2.8094250	2.8094924
645	2.8098962	2.8099635	2.8100308	2.8100980	2.8101653
646	2.8105685	2.8106357	2.8107029	2.8107700	2.8108371
647	2.8112398	2.8113068	2.8113739	2.8114409	2.8115080
648	2.8119100	2.8119769	2.8120439	2.8121108	2.8121778
649	2.8125792	2.8126460	2.8127129	2.8127797	2.8128465

Num	0	1	2	3	4
650	2.8129134	2.8129802	2.8130470	2.8131138	2.8131805
651	2.8135810	2.8136477	2.8137144	2.8137811	2.8138478
652	2.8142476	2.8143142	2.8143808	2.8144474	2.8145140
653	2.8149132	2.8149797	2.8150452	2.8151127	2.8151791
654	2.8155777	2.8156441	2.8157105	2.8157769	2.8158433
655	2.8162413	2.8163076	2.8163739	2.8164402	2.8165064
656	2.8169038	2.8169700	2.8170362	2.8171024	2.8171686
657	2.8175654	2.8176315	2.8176975	2.8177636	2.8178297
658	2.8182259	2.8182919	2.8183579	2.8184239	2.8184898
659	2.8188854	2.8189513	2.8190172	2.8190831	2.8191489
660	2.8195439	2.8196097	2.8196755	2.8197413	2.8198071
661	2.8202015	2.8202672	2.8203328	2.8203985	2.8204642
662	2.8208580	2.8209236	2.8209892	2.8210548	2.8211203
663	2.8215135	2.8215790	2.8216445	2.8217100	2.8217755
664	2.8221681	2.8222335	2.8222989	2.8223643	2.8224296
665	2.8228216	2.8228869	2.8229521	2.8230175	2.8230828
656	2.8234742	2.8235394	2.8236046	2.8236698	2.8237350
657	2.8241258	2.8241909	2.8242560	2.8243211	2.8243862
658	2.8247765	2.8248415	2.8249065	2.8249715	2.8250364
669	2.8254261	2.8254910	2.8255559	2.8256208	2.8256857
670	2.8260748	2.8261396	2.8262044	2.8262692	2.8263340
671	2.8267225	2.8267872	2.8268519	2.8269166	2.8269813
672	2.8273693	2.8274339	2.8274985	2.8275631	2.8276277
673	2.8280151	2.8280796	2.8281441	2.8282086	2.8282731
674	2.8286599	2.8287243	2.8287887	2.8288532	2.8289176
675	2.8293038	2.8293681	2.8294324	2.8294967	2.8295611
676	2.8299467	2.8300109	2.8300752	2.8301394	2.8302036
677	2.8305887	2.8306528	2.8307169	2.8307811	2.8308452
678	2.8312297	2.8312937	2.8313578	2.8314218	2.8314858
679	2.8318698	2.8319337	2.8319977	2.8320616	2.8321255
680	2.8325089	2.8325728	2.8326365	2.8327005	2.8327643
681	2.8331471	2.8332109	2.8332746	2.8333384	2.8334021
682	2.8337844	2.8338480	2.8339117	2.8339754	2.8340390
683	2.8344207	2.8344843	2.8345479	2.8346114	2.8346750
684	2.8350561	2.8351195	2.8351831	2.8352465	2.8353100
685	2.8356906	2.8357540	2.8358174	2.8358807	2.8359441
686	2.8363241	2.8363874	2.8364507	2.8365140	2.8365773
687	2.8369567	2.8370199	2.8370832	2.8371463	2.8372095
688	2.8375884	2.8376516	2.8377147	2.8377778	2.8378409
689	2.8382192	2.8382822	2.8383453	2.8384083	2.8384713
690	2.8388491	2.8389120	2.8389750	2.8390379	2.8391008
691	2.8394780	2.8395409	2.8396037	2.8396666	2.8397294
692	2.8401061	2.8401688	2.8402316	2.8402944	2.8403571
693	2.8407332	2.8407959	2.8408586	2.8409212	2.8409838
694	2.8413595	2.8414220	2.8414846	2.8415472	2.8416097
695	2.8419848	2.8420473	2.8421098	2.8421722	2.8422347
696	2.8426092	2.8426716	2.8427340	2.8427964	2.8428588
697	2.8432328	2.8432951	2.8433574	2.8434197	2.8434819
698	2.8438554	2.8439176	2.8439798	2.8440420	2.8441042
699	2.8444772	2.8445393	2.8446014	2.8446635	2.8447256

Num	5	6	7	8	9
650	2.8132473	2.8133141	2.8133808	2.8134475	2.8135143
651	2.8139144	2.8139811	2.8140477	2.8141144	2.8141810
652	2.8145805	2.8146471	2.8147136	2.8147801	2.8148467
653	2.8152456	2.8153120	2.8153785	2.8154449	2.8155113
654	2.8159096	2.8159760	2.8160423	2.8161087	2.8161750
655	2.8165727	2.8166389	2.8167052	2.8167714	2.8168376
656	2.8172347	2.8173009	2.8173670	2.8174331	2.8174993
657	2.8178958	2.8179618	2.8180278	2.8180939	2.8181599
658	2.8185558	2.8186217	2.8186877	2.8187536	2.8188195
659	2.8192148	2.8192806	2.8193465	2.8194123	2.8194781
660	2.8198728	2.8199386	2.8200043	2.8200700	2.8201358
661	2.8205298	2.8205955	2.8206511	2.8207268	2.8207924
662	2.8211859	2.8212514	2.8213170	2.8213825	2.8214480
663	2.8218409	2.8219064	2.8219718	2.8220372	2.8221027
664	2.8224950	2.8225603	2.8226257	2.8226910	2.8227563
665	2.8231481	2.8232133	2.8232786	2.8233438	2.8234090
666	2.8238002	2.8238653	2.8239305	2.8239956	2.8240607
667	2.8244513	2.8245163	2.8245814	2.8246464	2.8247114
668	2.8251014	2.8251664	2.8252313	2.8252963	2.8253612
669	2.8257506	2.8258154	2.8258803	2.8259451	2.8260100
670	2.8263988	2.8264635	2.8265283	2.8265931	2.8266578
671	2.8270460	2.8271107	2.8271753	2.8272400	2.8273046
672	2.8276923	2.8277569	2.8278214	2.8278860	2.8279505
673	2.8283376	2.8284021	2.8284665	2.8285310	2.8285955
674	2.8289820	2.8290463	2.8291107	2.8291751	2.8292394
675	2.8296254	2.8296896	2.8297539	2.8298182	2.8298824
676	2.8302678	2.8303320	2.8303962	2.8304603	2.8305245
677	2.8309093	2.8309734	2.8310375	2.8311016	2.8311656
678	2.8315499	2.8316139	2.8316778	2.8317418	2.8318058
679	2.8321895	2.8322534	2.8323173	2.8323812	2.8324450
680	2.8328281	2.8328919	2.8329558	2.8330195	2.8330833
681	2.8334659	2.8335296	2.8335933	2.8336570	2.8337207
682	2.8341027	2.8341663	2.8342299	2.8342935	2.8343571
683	2.8347385	2.8348021	2.8348656	2.8349291	2.8349926
684	2.8353735	2.8354369	2.8355003	2.8355638	2.8356272
685	2.8360075	2.8360708	2.8361341	2.8361975	2.8362608
686	2.8366405	2.8367038	2.8367670	2.8368303	2.8368935
687	2.8372727	2.8373359	2.8373990	2.8374622	2.8375253
688	2.8379039	2.8379670	2.8380301	2.8380931	2.8381562
689	2.8385343	2.8385973	2.8386602	2.8387232	2.8387861
690	2.8391637	2.8392266	2.8392895	2.8393523	2.8394152
691	2.8397922	2.8398550	2.8399178	2.8399806	2.8400433
692	2.8404198	2.8404825	2.8405452	2.8406079	2.8406706
693	2.8410465	2.8411091	2.8411717	2.8412343	2.8412969
694	2.8416722	2.8417348	2.8417973	2.8418598	2.8419223
695	2.8422971	2.8423596	2.8424220	2.8424844	2.8425468
696	2.8429211	2.8429835	2.8430458	2.8431081	2.8431705
697	2.8435442	2.8436065	2.8436687	2.8437310	2.8437932
698	2.8441664	2.8442286	2.8442907	2.8443529	2.8444150
699	2.8447877	2.8448498	2.8449119	2.8449739	2.8450360

Ddd

A TABLE of Logarithms.

Num	0	1	2	3	4
700	2.8450980	2.8451601	2.8452221	2.8452841	2.8453461
701	2.8457130	2.8457800	2.8458419	2.8459038	2.8459658
702	2.8463371	2.8463990	2.8464608	2.8465227	2.8465845
703	2.8469553	2.8470171	2.8470789	2.8471406	2.8472024
704	2.8475727	2.8476343	2.8476960	2.8477577	2.8478193
705	2.8481891	2.8482507	2.8483123	2.8483739	2.8484355
706	2.8488047	2.8488662	2.8489277	2.8489892	2.8490507
707	2.8494194	2.8494808	2.8495423	2.8496037	2.8496651
708	2.8500333	2.8500946	2.8501559	2.8502172	2.8502786
709	2.8506462	2.8507075	2.8507687	2.8508300	2.8508912
710	2.8512583	2.8513195	2.8513807	2.8514418	2.8515030
711	2.8518696	2.8519307	2.8519917	2.8520528	2.8521139
712	2.8524800	2.8525410	2.8526020	2.8526629	2.8527239
713	2.8530895	2.8531504	2.8532113	2.8532722	2.8533331
714	2.8536982	2.8537590	2.8538198	2.8538806	2.8539414
715	2.8543060	2.8543668	2.8544275	2.8544882	2.8545489
716	2.8549130	2.8549737	2.8550343	2.8550949	2.8551556
717	2.8555192	2.8555797	2.8556403	2.8557008	2.8557614
718	2.8561244	2.8561849	2.8562454	2.8563059	2.8563663
719	2.8567289	2.8567893	2.8568497	2.8569101	2.8569704
720	2.8573325	2.8573928	2.8574531	2.8575134	2.8575737
721	2.8579353	2.8579955	2.8580557	2.8581159	2.8581761
722	2.8585372	2.8585973	2.8586575	2.8587176	2.8587777
723	2.8591383	2.8591984	2.8592584	2.8593185	2.8593785
724	2.8597386	2.8597985	2.8598585	2.8599185	2.8599784
725	2.8603380	2.8603979	2.8604578	2.8605177	2.8605776
726	2.8609365	2.8609964	2.8610562	2.8611160	2.8611758
727	2.8615344	2.8615941	2.8616539	2.8617136	2.8617733
728	2.8621314	2.8621910	2.8622507	2.8623103	2.8623699
729	2.8627275	2.8627871	2.8628457	2.8629062	2.8629658
730	2.8633229	2.8633823	2.8634418	2.8635013	2.8635608
731	2.8639174	2.8639768	2.8640362	2.8640956	2.8641550
732	2.8645111	2.8645704	2.8646297	2.8646890	2.8647483
733	2.8651040	2.8651632	2.8652225	2.8652817	2.8653409
734	2.8656961	2.8657552	2.8658144	2.8658735	2.8659327
735	2.8662873	2.8663464	2.8664055	2.8664646	2.8665236
736	2.8668778	2.8669368	2.8669958	2.8670548	2.8671138
737	2.8674675	2.8675264	2.8675853	2.8676442	2.8677031
738	2.8680564	2.8681152	2.8681740	2.8682329	2.8682917
739	2.8686444	2.8687032	2.8687620	2.8688207	2.8688794
740	2.8692317	2.8692904	2.8693491	2.8694077	2.8694664
741	2.8698182	2.8698768	2.8699354	2.8699940	2.8700526
742	2.8704039	2.8704624	2.8705209	2.8705795	2.8706380
743	2.8709888	2.8710473	2.8711057	2.8711641	2.8712226
744	2.8715729	2.8716313	2.8716897	2.8717480	2.8718064
745	2.8721563	2.8722146	2.8722728	2.8723311	2.8723894
746	2.8727388	2.8727970	2.8728552	2.8729134	2.8729716
747	2.8733206	2.8733788	2.8734369	2.8734950	2.8735531
748	2.8739016	2.8739597	2.8740177	2.8740757	2.8741338
749	2.8744818	2.8745398	2.8745978	2.8746557	2.8747137

Num	5	6	7	8	9
700	2.8454081	2.8454701	2.8455321	2.8455941	2.8455561
701	2.8460277	2.8460896	2.8461515	2.8452134	2.8462752
702	2.8466463	2.8467081	2.8457700	2.8453313	2.8453935
703	2.8472641	2.8473258	2.8473875	2.8474493	2.8475110
704	2.8478810	2.8479426	2.8480043	2.8480659	2.8481275
705	2.8484970	2.8485586	2.8486201	2.8486817	2.8487432
706	2.8491122	2.8491736	2.8492351	2.8492965	2.8493580
707	2.8497264	2.8497878	2.8498492	2.8499106	2.8499719
708	2.8503399	2.8504011	2.8504624	2.8505237	2.8505850
709	2.8509524	2.8510136	2.8510748	2.8511360	2.8511972
710	2.8515641	2.8516252	2.8516863	2.8517474	2.8518085
711	2.8521749	2.8522359	2.8522970	2.8523580	2.8524190
712	2.8527849	2.8528458	2.8529068	2.8529677	2.8530286
713	2.8533940	2.8534548	2.8535157	2.8535765	2.8536374
714	2.8540022	2.8540630	2.8541238	2.8541845	2.8542453
715	2.8546096	2.8546703	2.8547310	2.8547917	2.8548524
716	2.8552162	2.8552768	2.8553374	2.8553980	2.8554586
717	2.8558219	2.8558824	2.8559429	2.8560035	2.8560640
718	2.8564268	2.8564872	2.8565476	2.8566081	2.8566685
719	2.8570308	2.8570912	2.8571515	2.8572118	2.8572722
720	2.8576340	2.8576943	2.8577545	2.8578148	2.8578750
721	2.8582363	2.8582965	2.8583567	2.8584169	2.8584770
722	2.8588379	2.8588980	2.8589581	2.8590181	2.8590782
723	2.8594385	2.8594986	2.8595586	2.8596186	2.8596786
724	2.8600384	2.8600983	2.8601583	2.8602182	2.8602781
725	2.8606374	2.8606973	2.8607571	2.8608170	2.8608768
726	2.8612356	2.8612954	2.8613552	2.8614149	2.8614747
727	2.8618330	2.8618927	2.8619524	2.8620120	2.8620717
728	2.8624296	2.8624892	2.8625488	2.8626084	2.8626679
729	2.8630253	2.8630848	2.8631443	2.8632039	2.8632634
730	2.8636202	2.8636797	2.8637391	2.8637985	2.8638580
731	2.8642143	2.8642737	2.8643331	2.8643924	2.8644517
732	2.8648076	2.8648669	2.8649262	2.8649855	2.8650447
733	2.8654001	2.8654593	2.8655185	2.8655777	2.8656369
734	2.8659918	2.8660509	2.8661100	2.8661691	2.8662282
735	2.8665827	2.8666417	2.8667008	2.8667598	2.8668188
736	2.8671728	2.8672317	2.8672907	2.8673496	2.8674086
737	2.8677620	2.8678209	2.8678798	2.8679387	2.8679975
738	2.8683505	2.8684033	2.8684681	2.8685269	2.8685857
739	2.8689382	2.8689969	2.8690556	2.8691143	2.8691730
740	2.8695251	2.8695837	2.8696423	2.8697010	2.8697596
741	2.8701112	2.8701677	2.8702283	2.8702868	2.8703454
742	2.8706965	2.8707549	2.8708134	2.8708719	2.8709304
743	2.8712810	2.8713394	2.8713978	2.8714562	2.8715146
744	2.8718547	2.8719230	2.8719814	2.8720397	2.8720980
745	2.8724476	2.8725059	2.8725641	2.8726224	2.8726806
746	2.8730298	2.8730880	2.8731461	2.8732043	2.8732625
747	2.8736112	2.8736693	2.8737274	2.8737855	2.8738435
748	2.8741918	2.8742498	2.8743078	2.8743658	2.8744238
749	2.8747719	2.8748296	2.8748875	2.8749454	2.8750034

Num	0	1	2	3	4
750	2.8750613	2.8751192	2.8751771	2.8752349	2.8752928
751	2.8756399	2.8756978	2.8757556	2.8758134	2.8758712
752	2.8762178	2.8762756	2.8763333	2.8763911	2.8764488
753	2.8767950	2.8768526	2.8769103	2.8769680	2.8770256
754	2.8773713	2.8774289	2.8774865	2.8775441	2.8776017
755	2.8779469	2.8780045	2.8780620	2.8781195	2.8781770
756	2.8785218	2.8785792	2.8786367	2.8786941	2.8787515
757	2.8790959	2.8791532	2.8792106	2.8792650	2.8793253
758	2.8796692	2.8797265	2.8797838	2.5798411	2.8798983
759	2.8802418	2.8802990	2.8803562	2.8804134	2.8804706
760	2.8808136	2.8808707	2.8809279	2.8809850	2.8810421
761	2.8813847	2.8814417	2.8814988	2.8815558	2.8816129
762	2.8819550	2.8820120	2.8820689	2.8821259	2.8821829
763	2.8825245	2.8825815	2.8826384	2.8826953	2.8827522
764	2.8830934	2.8831502	2.8832070	2.8832639	2.8833207
765	2.8836614	2.8837182	2.8837750	2.8838317	2.8838885
766	2.8842288	2.8842855	2.8843421	2.8843988	2.8844555
767	2.8847954	2.8848520	2.8849086	2.8849652	2.8850218
768	2.8853612	2.8854178	2.8854743	2.8855308	2.8855874
769	2.8859263	2.8859828	2.8860393	2.8860957	2.8861522
770	2.8864907	2.8865471	2.8866035	2.8866599	2.8867163
771	2.8870544	2.8871107	2.8871670	2.8872233	2.8872795
772	2.8876173	2.8876736	2.8877298	2.8877860	2.8878423
773	2.8881795	2.8882357	2.8882918	2.8883480	2.8884042
774	2.8887410	2.8887971	2.8888532	2.8889093	2.8889653
775	2.8893017	2.8893577	2.8894138	2.8894598	2.8895258
776	2.8898617	2.8899177	2.8899736	2.8900296	2.8900855
777	2.8904210	2.8904769	2.8905328	2.8905887	2.8906445
778	2.8909796	2.8910354	2.8910912	2.8911470	2.8912028
779	2.8915375	2.8915932	2.8916489	2.8917047	2.8917604
780	2.8920946	2.8921503	2.8922059	2.8922616	2.8923173
781	2.8926510	2.8927066	2.8927622	2.8928178	2.8928734
782	2.8932058	2.8932623	2.8933178	2.8933733	2.8934288
783	2.8937618	2.8938172	2.8938727	2.8939281	2.8939836
784	2.8943161	2.8943715	2.8944268	2.8944822	2.8945376
785	2.8948697	2.8949250	2.8949803	2.8950356	2.8950909
786	2.8954225	2.8954778	2.8955330	2.8955883	2.8956435
787	2.8959747	2.8960299	2.8960851	2.8961403	2.8961954
788	2.8965252	2.8965813	2.8966364	2.8966915	2.8967466
789	2.8970770	2.8971320	2.8971871	2.8972421	2.8972971
790	2.8976271	2.8976821	2.8977370	2.8977920	2.8978469
791	2.8981765	2.8982314	2.8982863	2.8983412	2.8983960
792	2.8987252	2.8987800	2.8988348	2.8988897	2.8989445
793	2.8992732	2.8993279	2.8993827	2.8994375	2.8994922
794	2.8998205	2.8998752	2.8999299	2.8999846	2.9000392
795	2.9003671	2.9004218	2.9004764	2.9005310	2.9005856
796	2.9009131	2.9009676	2.9010222	2.9010767	2.9011313
797	2.9014583	2.9015128	2.9015673	2.9016218	2.9016762
798	2.9020029	2.9020573	2.9021117	2.9021661	2.9022205
799	2.9025468	2.9026011	2.9026555	2.9027098	2.9027641

A TABLE of Logarithms.

z

Num	5	6	7	8	9
750	2.8753507	2.8754086	2.8754664	2.8755243	2.8755821
751	2.8759290	2.8759868	2.8760445	2.8761023	2.8761601
752	2.8765065	2.8765642	2.8766219	2.8766796	2.8767373
753	2.8770833	2.8771409	2.8771985	2.8772561	2.8773137
754	2.8776592	2.8777168	2.8777743	2.8778319	2.8778894
755	2.8782345	2.8782919	2.8783494	2.8784069	2.8784643
756	2.8788089	2.8788663	2.8789237	2.8789811	2.8790385
757	2.8793826	2.8794400	2.8794973	2.8795546	2.8796119
758	2.8799556	2.8800128	2.8800701	2.8801273	2.8801846
759	2.8805278	2.8805850	2.8806421	2.8806993	2.8807564
760	2.8810992	2.8811563	2.8812134	2.8812705	2.8813276
761	2.8816699	2.8817269	2.8817840	2.8818410	2.8818980
762	2.8822398	2.8822968	2.8823537	2.8824107	2.8824676
763	2.8828090	2.8828659	2.8829228	2.8829797	2.8830365
764	2.8833775	2.8834343	2.8834911	2.8835479	2.8836047
765	2.8839452	2.8840019	2.8840586	2.8841154	2.8841721
766	2.8845122	2.8845688	2.8846255	2.8846821	2.8847387
767	2.8850784	2.8851350	2.8851915	2.8852481	2.8853047
768	2.8856439	2.8857004	2.8857569	2.8858134	2.8858699
769	2.8862086	2.8862651	2.8863215	2.8863779	2.8864343
770	2.8867726	2.8868290	2.8868854	2.8869417	2.8869980
771	2.8873359	2.8873922	2.8874485	2.8875048	2.8875610
772	2.8878985	2.8879547	2.8880109	2.8880671	2.8881233
773	2.8884603	2.8885165	2.8885726	2.8886287	2.8886848
774	2.8890214	2.8890775	2.8891336	2.8891896	2.8892457
775	2.8895818	2.8896378	2.8896938	2.8897498	2.8898058
776	2.8901415	2.8901974	2.8902533	2.8903092	2.8903651
777	2.8907004	2.8907562	2.8908121	2.8904679	2.8909238
778	2.8912586	2.8913144	2.8913702	2.8914259	2.8914887
779	2.8918161	2.8918718	2.8919275	2.8919832	2.8920389
780	2.8923729	2.8924285	2.8924842	2.8925398	2.8925954
781	2.8929290	2.8929846	2.8930401	2.8930957	2.8931512
782	2.8934843	2.8935398	2.8935953	2.8936508	2.8937063
783	2.8940390	2.8940944	2.8941498	2.8942053	2.8942607
784	2.8945929	2.8946483	2.8947037	2.8947590	2.8948143
785	2.8951462	2.8952015	2.8952568	2.8953120	2.8953673
786	2.8956987	2.8957539	2.8958091	2.8958643	2.8959195
787	2.8962506	2.8963057	2.8963608	2.8964160	2.8964711
788	2.8968017	2.8968568	2.8969118	2.8969669	2.8970220
789	2.8973521	2.8974071	2.8974621	2.8975171	2.8975721
790	2.8979019	2.8979568	2.8980117	2.8980667	2.8981216
791	2.8984509	2.8985058	2.8985606	2.8986155	2.8986703
792	2.8989993	2.8990541	2.8991089	2.8991636	2.8992184
793	2.8995469	2.8996017	2.8996564	2.8997111	2.8997658
794	2.9000939	2.9001486	2.9002032	2.9002579	2.9003125
795	2.9006402	2.9006948	2.9007494	2.9008039	2.9008585
796	2.9011858	2.9012403	2.9012948	2.9013493	2.9014038
797	2.9017307	2.9017851	2.9018396	2.9018940	2.9019485
798	2.9022749	2.9023293	2.9023837	2.9024381	2.9024924
799	2.9028185	2.9028728	2.9029271	2.9029814	2.9030357

Num	0	1	2	3	4
800	2.9030900	2.9031443	2.9031985	2.9032528	2.9033071
801	2.9036325	2.9036867	2.9037409	2.9037951	2.9038493
802	2.9041744	2.9042285	2.9042827	2.9043369	2.9043909
803	2.9047155	2.9047696	2.9048237	2.9048778	2.9049318
804	2.9052560	2.9053101	2.9053641	2.9054181	2.9054721
805	2.9057960	2.9058498	2.9059038	2.9059577	2.9060116
806	2.9063351	2.9063889	2.9064428	2.9064967	2.9065505
807	2.9068735	2.9069273	2.9069812	2.9070350	2.9070887
808	2.9074114	2.9074651	2.9075188	2.9075726	2.9076263
809	2.9079485	2.9080022	2.9080559	2.9081095	2.9081632
810	2.9084850	2.9085386	2.9085922	2.9086458	2.9086994
811	2.9090209	2.9090744	2.9091279	2.9091815	2.9092350
812	2.9095560	2.9096095	2.9096630	2.9097165	2.9097699
813	2.9100905	2.9101440	2.9101974	2.9102508	2.9103042
814	2.9106244	2.9106778	2.9107311	2.9107845	2.9108378
815	2.9111576	2.9112109	2.9112642	2.9113174	2.9113707
816	2.9116902	2.9117434	2.9117967	2.9118499	2.9119030
817	2.9122220	2.9122752	2.9123284	2.9123815	2.9124346
818	2.9127533	2.9128064	2.9128595	2.9129126	2.9129656
819	2.9132839	2.9133369	2.9133899	2.9134430	2.9134960
820	2.9138139	2.9138668	2.9139198	2.9139727	2.9140257
821	2.9143432	2.9143961	2.9144490	2.9145018	2.9145547
822	2.9148718	2.9149246	2.9149775	2.9150303	2.9150831
823	2.9153998	2.9154526	2.9155054	2.9155581	2.9156109
824	2.9159272	2.9159799	2.9160326	2.9160853	2.9161380
825	2.9164539	2.9165066	2.9165592	2.9166118	2.9166645
826	2.9169800	2.9170326	2.9170852	2.9171378	2.9171903
827	2.9175055	2.9175580	2.9176105	2.9176630	2.9177155
828	2.9180303	2.9180828	2.9181352	2.9181877	2.9182401
829	2.9185545	2.9186069	2.9186593	2.9187117	2.9187640
830	2.9190781	2.9191304	2.9191827	2.9192350	2.9192873
831	2.9196010	2.9196533	2.9197055	2.9197578	2.9198100
832	2.9201233	2.9201755	2.9202277	2.9202799	2.9203321
833	2.9206450	2.9206971	2.9207493	2.9208014	2.9208535
834	2.9211661	2.9212181	2.9212702	2.9213222	2.9213743
835	2.9216865	2.9217385	2.9217905	2.9218425	2.9218945
836	2.9222063	2.9222582	2.9223102	2.9223621	2.9224140
837	2.9227255	2.9227773	2.9228292	2.9228811	2.9229330
838	2.9232440	2.9232958	2.9233477	2.9233995	2.9234513
839	2.9237520	2.9238137	2.9238655	2.9239172	2.9239690
840	2.9242793	2.9243310	2.9243827	2.9244344	2.9244860
841	2.9247960	2.9248476	2.9248993	2.9249509	2.9250025
842	2.9253121	2.9253637	2.9254152	2.9254668	2.9255184
843	2.9258276	2.9258791	2.9259306	2.9259821	2.9260336
844	2.9263424	2.9263939	2.9264453	2.9264968	2.9265482
845	2.9268567	2.9269081	2.9269595	2.9270109	2.9270622
846	2.9273704	2.9274217	2.9274730	2.9275243	2.9275757
847	2.9278834	2.9279347	2.9279859	2.9280372	2.9280885
848	2.9283959	2.9284471	2.9284983	2.9285495	2.9286007
849	2.9289077	2.9289588	2.9290100	2.9290611	2.9291123

Num	5	6	7	8	9
800	2.9033613	2.9034156	2.9034698	2.9035241	2.9035783
801	2.9039035	2.9039577	2.9040119	2.9040661	2.9041202
802	2.9044450	2.9044992	2.9045533	2.9046074	2.9046615
803	2.9049859	2.9050399	2.9050940	2.9051480	2.9052020
804	2.9055261	2.9055800	2.9056340	2.9056880	2.9057420
805	2.9060656	2.9061195	2.9061734	2.9062273	2.9062812
806	2.9066044	2.9066582	2.9067121	2.9067659	2.9068197
807	2.9071425	2.9071963	2.9072501	2.9073038	2.9073576
808	2.9076800	2.9077337	2.9077674	2.9078411	2.9078948
809	2.9082169	2.9082705	2.9083241	2.9083778	2.9084314
810	2.9087530	2.9088066	2.9088602	2.9089137	2.9089673
811	2.9092885	2.9093420	2.9093955	2.9094490	2.9095025
812	2.9098234	2.9098768	2.9099303	2.9099837	2.9100371
813	2.9103576	2.9104109	2.9104643	2.9105177	2.9105710
814	2.9108911	2.9109444	2.9109977	2.9110510	2.9111043
815	2.9114240	2.9114772	2.9115305	2.9115837	2.9116369
816	2.9119562	2.9120094	2.9120626	2.9121157	2.9121689
817	2.9124878	2.9125409	2.9125940	2.9126471	2.9127002
818	2.9130187	2.9130717	2.9131248	2.9131778	2.9132309
819	2.9135490	2.9136019	2.9136549	2.9137079	2.9137609
820	2.9140786	2.9141315	2.9141844	2.9142373	2.9142903
821	2.9146076	2.9146604	2.9147133	2.9147661	2.9148190
822	2.9151359	2.9151887	2.9152415	2.9152943	2.9153471
823	2.9156636	2.9157163	2.9157691	2.9158218	2.9158745
824	2.9161907	2.9162433	2.9162960	2.9163487	2.9164013
825	2.9167171	2.9167697	2.9168223	2.9168749	2.9169275
826	2.9172429	2.9172954	2.9173479	2.9174005	2.9174530
827	2.9177680	2.9178205	2.9178730	2.9179254	2.9179779
828	2.9182925	2.9183449	2.9183973	2.9184497	2.9185021
829	2.9188164	2.9188687	2.9189211	2.9189734	2.9190258
830	2.9193396	2.9193919	2.9194442	2.9194965	2.9195488
831	2.9198623	2.9199145	2.9199667	2.9200189	2.9200711
832	2.9203842	2.9204364	2.9204886	2.9205407	2.9205929
833	2.9209056	2.9209577	2.9210098	2.9210619	2.9211140
834	2.9214263	2.9214784	2.9215304	2.9215824	2.9216345
835	2.9219465	2.9219984	2.9220504	2.9221024	2.9221543
836	2.9224659	2.9225179	2.9225698	2.9226217	2.9226736
837	2.9229848	2.9230367	2.9230885	2.9231404	2.9231922
838	2.9235031	2.9235549	2.9236066	2.9236584	2.9237102
839	2.9240208	2.9240724	2.9241242	2.9241759	2.9242276
840	2.9245377	2.9245894	2.9246410	2.9246927	2.9247444
841	2.9250541	2.9251057	2.9251573	2.9252089	2.9252605
842	2.9255699	2.9256215	2.9256730	2.9257245	2.9257761
843	2.9260851	2.9261366	2.9261880	2.9262395	2.9262910
844	2.9265997	2.9266511	2.9267025	2.9267539	2.9268053
845	2.9271136	2.9271650	2.9272163	2.9272677	2.9273190
846	2.9276270	2.9276783	2.9277296	2.9277808	2.9278321
847	2.9281397	2.9281909	2.9282422	2.9282934	2.9283446
848	2.9286518	2.9287030	2.9287542	2.9288054	2.9288565
849	2.9291634	2.9292145	2.9292656	2.9293167	2.9293678

Num	0	1	2	3	4
850	2.9294189	2.9294700	2.9295211	2.9295722	2.9296233
851	2.9299295	2.9299805	2.9300315	2.9300826	2.9301336
852	2.9304395	2.9304906	2.9305415	2.9305925	2.9306434
853	2.9309490	2.9309999	2.9310508	2.9311017	2.9311526
854	2.9314579	2.9315087	2.9315596	2.9316104	2.9316612
855	2.9319662	2.9320169	2.9320677	2.9321185	2.9321692
856	2.9324738	2.9325245	2.9325752	2.9326259	2.9326767
857	2.9329808	2.9330315	2.9330822	2.9331328	2.9331835
858	2.9334873	2.9335379	2.9335885	2.9336391	2.9336897
859	2.9339932	2.9340437	2.9340943	2.9341448	2.9341953
860	2.9344984	2.9345489	2.9345994	2.9346499	2.9347004
861	2.9350032	2.9350536	2.9351040	2.9351544	2.9352049
862	2.9355073	2.9355576	2.9356080	2.9356584	2.9357087
863	2.9360103	2.9360611	2.9361114	2.9361617	2.9362120
864	2.9365137	2.9365640	2.9366143	2.9366645	2.9367148
865	2.9370161	2.9370653	2.9371155	2.9371657	2.9372169
866	2.9375179	2.9375680	2.9376182	2.9376683	2.9377184
867	2.9380191	2.9380692	2.9381193	2.9381693	2.9382194
868	2.9385197	2.9385698	2.9386198	2.9386698	2.9387198
869	2.9390198	2.9390697	2.9391197	2.9391697	2.9392196
870	2.9395193	2.9395692	2.9396191	2.9396690	2.9397189
871	2.9400182	2.9400680	2.9401179	2.9401677	2.9402176
872	2.9405165	2.9405663	2.9406161	2.9406659	2.9407157
873	2.9410142	2.9410640	2.9411137	2.9411635	2.9412132
874	2.9415114	2.9415611	2.9416108	2.9416605	2.9417101
875	2.9420081	2.9420577	2.9421073	2.9421569	2.9422065
876	2.9425041	2.9425537	2.9426032	2.9426528	2.9427024
877	2.9429996	2.9430491	2.9430986	2.9431481	2.9431976
878	2.9434945	2.9435440	2.9435934	2.9436429	2.9436923
879	2.9439889	2.9440383	2.9440877	2.9441371	2.9441865
880	2.9444827	2.9445320	2.9445814	2.9446307	2.9446800
881	2.9449759	2.9450252	2.9450745	2.9451238	2.9451730
882	2.9454686	2.9455178	2.9455671	2.9456163	2.9456655
883	2.9459607	2.9460099	2.9460591	2.9461082	2.9461574
884	2.9464523	2.9465014	2.9465505	2.9465976	2.9466487
885	2.9469433	2.9469923	2.9470414	2.9470905	2.9471395
886	2.9474337	2.9474827	2.9475317	2.9475807	2.9476297
887	2.9479236	2.9479726	2.9480215	2.9480705	2.9481194
888	2.9484130	2.9484519	2.9485108	2.9485597	2.9486085
889	2.9489018	2.9489506	2.9489994	2.9490483	2.9490971
890	2.9493900	2.9494388	2.9494876	2.9495364	2.9495851
891	2.9498777	2.9499264	2.9499752	2.9500239	2.9500726
892	2.9503649	2.9504135	2.9504622	2.9505109	2.9505596
893	2.9508515	2.9509001	2.9509487	2.9509973	2.9510459
894	2.9513375	2.9513861	2.9514347	2.9514832	2.9515318
895	2.9518230	2.9518716	2.9519201	2.9519686	2.9520171
896	2.9523080	2.9523565	2.9524049	2.9524534	2.9525018
897	2.9527924	2.9528409	2.9528893	2.9529377	2.9529861
898	2.9532763	2.9533247	2.9533730	2.9534214	2.9534697
899	2.9537597	2.9538080	2.9538563	2.9539046	2.9539529

Num	5	6	7	8	9
850	2.9296743	2.9297254	2.9297764	2.9298275	2.9298785
851	2.9301847	2.9302357	2.9302865	2.9303376	2.9303886
852	2.9306944	2.9307453	2.9307963	2.9308472	2.9308981
853	2.9312035	2.9312544	2.9313053	2.9313561	2.9314070
854	2.9317121	2.9317629	2.9318137	2.9318645	2.9319153
855	2.9322200	2.9322708	2.9323215	2.9323723	2.9324230
856	2.9327274	2.9327781	2.9328288	2.9328795	2.9329301
857	2.9332341	2.9332848	2.9333354	2.9333860	2.9334367
858	2.9337403	2.9337909	2.9338415	2.9338920	2.9339426
859	2.9342459	2.9342964	2.9343469	2.9343974	2.9344479
860	2.9347509	2.9348013	2.9348518	2.9349022	2.9349527
861	2.9352553	2.9353057	2.9353561	2.9354065	2.9354569
862	2.9357591	2.9358095	2.9358598	2.9359101	2.9359605
863	2.9362623	2.9363126	2.9363629	2.9364132	2.9364635
864	2.9367650	2.9368152	2.9368655	2.9369157	2.9369659
865	2.9372671	2.9373172	2.9373674	2.9374176	2.9374677
866	2.9377686	2.9378187	2.9378688	2.9379189	2.9379690
867	2.9382695	2.9383195	2.9383696	2.9384196	2.9384697
868	2.9387698	2.9388198	2.9388698	2.9389198	2.9389698
869	2.9392696	2.9393195	2.9393695	2.9394194	2.9394693
870	2.9397688	2.9398187	2.9398685	2.9399184	2.9399683
871	2.9402674	2.9403172	2.9403670	2.9404169	2.9404667
872	2.9407654	2.9408152	2.9408650	2.9409147	2.9409645
873	2.9412629	2.9413126	2.9413623	2.9414120	2.9414617
874	2.9417598	2.9418095	2.9418591	2.9419088	2.9419584
875	2.9422561	2.9423058	2.9423553	2.9424049	2.9424545
876	2.9427519	2.9428015	2.9428510	2.9429005	2.9429501
877	2.9432471	2.9432966	2.9433461	2.9433956	2.9434450
878	2.9437418	2.9437912	2.9438406	2.9438900	2.9439395
879	2.9442358	2.9442852	2.9443346	2.9443840	2.9444333
880	2.9447294	2.9447787	2.9448280	2.9448773	2.9449266
881	2.9452223	2.9452716	2.9453208	2.9453701	2.9454193
882	2.9457147	2.9457639	2.9458131	2.9458623	2.9459115
883	2.9462066	2.9462557	2.9463048	2.9463540	2.9464031
884	2.9466978	2.9467469	2.9467960	2.9468451	2.9468942
885	2.9471886	2.9472376	2.9472866	2.9473357	2.9473847
886	2.9476787	2.9477277	2.9477767	2.9478257	2.9478747
887	2.9481684	2.9482173	2.9482662	2.9483151	2.9483641
888	2.9486574	2.9487063	2.9487552	2.9488040	2.9488529
889	2.9491460	2.9491948	2.9492436	2.9492924	2.9493412
890	2.9496339	2.9496827	2.9497314	2.9497802	2.9498290
891	2.9501213	2.9501701	2.9502188	2.9502675	2.9503162
892	2.9506082	2.9506569	2.9507055	2.9507542	2.9508028
893	2.9510946	2.9511432	2.9511918	2.9512404	2.9512889
894	2.9515803	2.9516289	2.9516774	2.9517260	2.9517745
895	2.9520656	2.9521141	2.9521626	2.9522111	2.9522595
896	2.9525503	2.9525987	2.9526472	2.9526956	2.9527440
897	2.9530345	2.9530828	2.9531312	2.9531796	2.9532280
898	2.9535181	2.9535664	2.9536147	2.9536631	2.9537114
899	2.9540012	2.9540494	2.9540977	2.9541460	2.9541943

Numb	0	1	2	3	4
900	2.9542425	2.9542908	2.9543390	2.9543872	2.9544355
901	2.9547248	2.9547730	2.9548212	2.9548694	2.9549176
902	2.9552065	2.9552547	2.9553028	2.9553510	2.9553991
903	2.9556877	2.9557358	2.9557839	2.9558320	2.9558801
904	2.9561684	2.9562165	2.9562545	2.9563125	2.9563605
905	2.9566486	2.9566966	2.9567445	2.9567925	2.9568405
906	2.9571282	2.9571761	2.9572241	2.9572720	2.9573199
907	2.9576073	2.9576552	2.9577030	2.9577509	2.9577988
908	2.9580858	2.9581337	2.9581815	2.9582293	2.9582771
909	2.9585639	2.9586117	2.9586594	2.9587072	2.9587549
910	2.9590414	2.9590891	2.9591368	2.9591845	2.9592322
911	2.9595184	2.9595660	2.9596137	2.9596614	2.9597090
912	2.9599948	2.9600425	2.9600901	2.9601377	2.9601853
913	2.9604708	2.9605183	2.9605659	2.9606135	2.9606610
914	2.9609462	2.9609937	2.9610412	2.9610887	2.9611362
915	2.9614211	2.9614636	2.9615160	3.9615635	2.9616129
916	2.9618955	2.9619429	2.9619903	2.9620377	2.9620851
917	2.9623693	2.9624167	2.9624640	2.9925114	2.9625587
918	2.9628427	2.9628900	2.9629373	2.9629846	2.9630319
919	2.9633155	2.9633628	2.9634100	2.9634573	2.9635045
920	2.9637878	2.9638350	2.9638822	2.9639294	2.9639766
921	2.9642595	2.9643068	2.9643539	2.9644011	2.96444821
922	2.9647309	2.9647780	2.9648251	2.9648722	2.9649193
923	2.9652017	2.9652488	2.9652958	2.9653428	2.9653599
924	2.9656720	2.9657190	2.9657650	2.9658130	2.9658599
925	2.9661417	2.9661887	2.9662356	2.9662826	2.9663295
926	2.9666110	2.9666579	2.9667048	2.9667517	2.9667985
927	2.9670797	2.9671266	2.9671734	2.9672203	2.9672671
928	2.9675480	2.9675948	2.9676416	2.9676883	2.9677351
929	2.9680157	2.9680625	2.9681092	2.9681559	2.9682027
930	2.9684829	2.9685296	2.9685763	2.9686230	2.9686697
931	2.9689497	2.9689963	2.9690430	2.9690895	2.9691362
932	2.9694159	2.9694625	2.9695091	2.9695557	2.9696023
933	2.9698816	2.9699282	2.9699747	2.9700213	2.9700678
934	2.9703469	2.9703934	2.9704399	2.9704863	2.9705328
935	2.9708116	2.9708581	2.9709045	2.9709509	2.9709974
936	2.9712758	2.9713222	2.9713586	2.9714150	2.9714614
937	2.9717396	2.9717859	2.9718323	2.9718786	2.9719249
938	2.9722028	2.9722491	2.9722954	2.9723417	2.9723880
939	2.9726656	2.9727118	2.9727581	2.9728043	2.9728506
940	2.9731278	2.9731741	2.9732202	2.9732564	2.9733126
941	2.9735896	2.9736358	2.9736819	2.9737281	2.9737742
942	2.9740529	2.9740970	2.9741431	2.9741892	2.9742353
943	2.9745117	2.9745577	2.9746038	2.9746498	2.9746959
944	2.9749720	2.9750180	2.9750640	2.9751100	2.9751560
945	2.9754318	2.9754778	2.9755237	2.9755697	2.9756156
946	2.9758911	2.9759370	2.9759829	2.9760288	2.9760747
947	2.9763500	2.9763958	2.9764417	2.9764875	2.9765334
948	2.9768083	2.9768541	2.9768999	2.9769457	2.9769915
949	2.9772652	2.9773120	2.9773577	2.9774035	2.9774492

Num	5	6	7	8	9
900	2.9544837	2.9545319	2.9545802	2.9546284	2.9546766
901	2.9549657	2.9550139	2.9550621	2.9551102	2.9551584
902	2.9554472	2.9554953	2.9555434	2.9555915	2.9556397
903	2.9559282	2.9559762	2.9560243	2.9560723	2.9561204
904	2.9564086	2.9564566	2.9565046	2.9565526	2.9566006
905	2.9568885	2.9569364	2.9569844	2.9570323	2.9570803
906	2.9573678	2.9574157	2.9574636	2.9575115	2.9575594
907	2.9578466	2.9578945	2.9579423	2.9579902	2.9580380
908	2.9583249	2.9583727	2.9584205	2.9584683	2.9585161
909	2.9588027	2.9588505	2.9588982	2.9589459	2.9589937
910	2.9592799	2.9593276	2.9593753	2.9594230	2.9594707
911	2.9597567	2.9598043	2.9598520	2.9598996	2.9599472
912	2.9602329	2.9602805	2.9603280	2.9603756	2.9604232
913	2.9607086	2.9607561	2.9608036	2.9608512	2.9608987
914	2.9611837	2.9612312	2.9612787	2.9613262	2.9613736
915	2.9616583	2.9617058	2.9617532	2.9618006	2.9618481
916	2.9621325	2.9621799	2.9622272	2.9622746	2.9623220
917	2.9626061	2.9626534	2.9627007	2.9627481	2.9627954
918	2.9630792	2.9631264	2.9631737	2.9632210	2.9632683
919	2.9635517	2.9635990	2.9636462	2.9636934	2.9637406
920	2.9640238	2.9640710	2.9641181	2.9641653	2.9642125
921	2.9644953	2.9645425	2.9645896	2.9646367	2.9646838
922	2.9649664	2.9650134	2.9650605	2.9651076	2.9651546
923	2.9654369	2.9654839	2.9655309	2.9655780	2.9656250
924	2.9659069	2.9659539	2.9660009	2.9660478	2.9660948
925	2.9663764	2.9664233	2.9664703	2.9665172	2.9665641
926	2.9668454	2.9668923	2.9669392	2.9669860	2.9670329
927	2.9673139	2.9673607	2.9674076	2.9674544	2.9675012
928	2.9677819	2.9678287	2.9678754	2.9679222	2.9679690
929	2.9682494	2.9682961	2.9683428	2.9683895	2.9684362
930	2.9687164	2.9687630	2.9688097	2.9688564	2.9689030
931	2.9691829	2.9692295	2.9692761	2.9693227	2.9693693
932	2.9696488	2.9696954	2.9697420	2.9697885	2.9698351
933	2.9701143	2.9701608	2.9702074	2.9702539	2.9703004
934	2.9705793	2.9706258	2.9706722	2.9707187	2.9707652
935	2.9710438	2.9710902	2.9711366	2.9711830	2.9712294
936	2.9715078	2.9715542	2.9716005	2.9716469	2.9716932
937	2.9719713	2.9720176	2.9720639	2.9721102	2.9721565
938	2.9724343	2.9724805	2.9725268	2.9725731	2.9726193
939	2.9728968	2.9729430	2.9729892	2.9730354	2.9730816
940	2.9733588	2.9734050	2.9734511	2.9734973	2.9735435
941	2.9738203	2.9738664	2.9739126	2.9739587	2.9740048
942	2.9742814	2.9743274	2.9743735	2.9744196	2.9744655
943	2.9747419	2.9747879	2.9748340	2.9748800	2.9749260
944	2.9752020	2.9752479	2.9752939	2.9753399	2.9753858
945	2.9756615	2.9757075	2.9757534	2.9757993	2.9758452
946	2.9761206	2.9761665	2.9762124	2.9762582	2.9763041
947	2.9765792	2.9766251	2.9766709	2.9767167	2.9767625
948	2.9770373	2.9770831	2.9771289	2.9771747	2.9772204
949	2.9774950	2.9775407	2.9775864	2.9776322	2.9776779

A TABLE of Logarithms.

Num	0	1	2	3	4
950	2.9777236	2.9777593	2.9778150	2.9778607	2.9779064
951	2.9781805	2.9782262	2.9782718	2.9783175	2.9783631
952	2.9786369	2.9786826	2.9787282	2.9787738	2.9788194
953	2.9790929	2.9791385	2.9791840	2.9792296	2.9792751
954	2.9795484	2.9795939	2.9796394	2.9796849	2.9797304
955	2.9800034	2.9800488	2.9800943	2.9801398	2.9801852
956	2.9804579	2.9805033	2.9805487	2.9805942	2.9806396
957	2.9809119	2.9809573	2.9810027	2.9810481	2.9810934
958	2.9813655	2.9814108	2.9814562	2.9815015	2.9815468
959	2.9818186	2.9818639	2.9819092	2.9819544	2.9819997
960	2.9822712	2.9823165	2.9823617	2.9824069	2.9824522
961	2.9827234	2.9827686	2.9828138	2.9828589	2.9829041
962	2.9831751	2.9832202	2.9832654	2.9833105	2.9833556
963	2.9836263	2.9836714	2.9837165	2.9837616	2.9838066
964	2.9840770	2.9841221	2.9841671	2.9842122	2.9842572
965	2.9845273	2.9845723	2.9846173	2.9846623	2.9847073
966	2.9849771	2.9850221	2.9850670	2.9851120	2.9851569
967	2.9854265	2.9854714	2.9855163	2.9855612	2.9856061
968	2.9858754	2.9859202	2.9859651	2.9860099	2.9860548
969	2.9863238	2.9863686	2.9864134	2.9864582	2.9865030
970	2.9867717	2.9868165	2.9868613	2.9869060	2.9869508
971	2.9872192	2.9872640	2.9873087	2.9873534	2.9873981
972	2.9876663	2.9877109	2.9877556	2.9878003	2.9878449
973	2.9881128	2.9881575	2.9882021	2.9882467	2.9882913
974	2.9885590	2.9886035	2.9886481	2.9886927	2.9887373
975	2.9890046	2.9890492	2.9890937	2.9891382	2.9891828
976	2.9894498	2.9894943	2.9895388	2.9895833	2.9896278
977	2.9898946	2.9899390	2.9899835	2.9900279	2.9900723
978	2.9903389	2.9903833	2.9904277	2.9904721	2.9905164
979	2.9907729	2.9908270	2.9908714	2.9909158	2.9909601
980	2.9912261	2.9912704	2.9913147	2.9913590	2.9914033
981	2.9916690	2.9917133	2.9917575	2.9918018	2.9918461
982	2.9921115	2.9921557	2.9921999	2.9922441	2.9922884
983	2.9925535	2.9925977	2.9926419	2.9926860	2.9927302
984	2.9929951	2.9930392	2.9930834	2.9931275	2.9931716
985	2.9934362	2.9934803	2.9935244	2.9935685	2.9936126
986	2.9938769	2.9939210	2.9939650	2.9940090	2.9940531
987	2.9943172	2.9943612	2.9944051	2.9944491	2.9944931
988	2.9947569	2.9948009	2.9948448	2.9948888	2.9949327
989	2.9951963	2.9952402	2.9952841	2.9953280	2.9953719
990	2.9956352	2.9956791	2.9957229	2.9957668	2.9958106
991	2.9960737	2.9961175	2.9961613	2.9962051	2.9962489
992	2.9965117	2.9965554	2.9965992	2.9966430	2.9966868
993	2.9969492	2.9969930	2.9970367	2.9970804	2.9971242
994	2.9973864	2.9974301	2.9974738	2.9975174	2.9975611
995	2.9978231	2.9978667	2.9979104	2.9979540	2.9979975
996	2.9982593	2.9983029	2.9983465	2.9983901	2.9984337
997	2.9986952	2.9987387	2.9987823	2.9988258	2.9988694
998	2.9991305	2.9991740	2.9992176	2.9992611	2.9993046
999	2.9995655	2.9996090	2.9996524	2.9996959	2.9997393

Num	5	6	7	8	9
950	2.9779521	2.9779978	2.9780435	2.9780892	2.9781348
951	2.9784088	2.9784544	2.9785001	2.9785457	2.9785913
952	2.9788650	2.9789106	2.9789562	2.9790017	2.9790473
953	2.9793207	.29793662	2.9794118	2.9794573	2.9795028
954	2.9797759	2.9798214	2.9798669	2.9799124	2.9799579
955	2.9802307	2.9802761	2.9803216	2.9803670	2.9804125
956	2.9806850	2.9807304	2.9807758	2.9808212	2.9808666
957	2.9811388	2.9811841	2.9812295	2.9812748	2.9813202
958	2.9815921	2.9816374	2.9816827	2.9817280	2.9817733
959	2.9820450	2.9820902	2.9821355	2.9821807	2.9822260
960	2.9824974	2.9825426	2.9825878	2.9826330	2.9826782
961	2.9829493	2.9829945	2.9830396	2.9830848	2.9831299
962	2.9834007	2.9834459	2.9834910	2.9835361	2.9835812
963	2.9838517	2.9838968	2.9839419	2.9839869	2.9840320
964	2.9843022	2.9843743	2.9843923	2.9844373	2.9844823
965	2.9847523	2.9847973	2.9848422	2.9848872	2.9849322
966	2.9852019	2.9852468	2.9852917	2.9853366	2.9853816
967	2.9856510	2.9856959	2.9857407	2.9857856	2.9858305
968	2.9860996	2.9861445	2.9861893	2.9862341	2.9862790
969	2.9865478	2.9865926	2.9866374	2.9866822	2.9867270
970	2.9869955	2.9870403	2.9870850	2.9871298	2.9871745
971	2.9874428	2.9874875	2.9875322	2.9875769	2.9876216
972	2.9878896	2.9879343	2.9879789	2.9880236	2.9880682
973	2.9883360	2.9883806	2.9884252	2.9884698	2.9885144
974	2.9887818	2.9888264	2.9888710	2.9889155	2.9889601
975	2.9892273	2.9892718	2.9893163	2.9893608	2.9894053
976	2.9896722	2.9897167	2.9897612	2.9898056	2.9898501
977	2.9901168	2.9901612	2.9902056	2.9902500	2.9902944
978	2.9905608	2.9906052	2.9906496	2.9906940	2.9907383
979	2.9910044	2.9910488	2.9910931	2.9911374	2.9911818
980	2.9914476	2.9914919	2.9915362	2.9915805	2.9916247
981	2.9918903	2.9919345	2.9919788	2.9920230	2.9920673
982	2.9923326	2.9923768	2.9924210	2.9924651	2.9925093
983	2.9927744	2.9928185	2.9928627	2.9929068	2.9929510
984	2.9932157	2.9932598	2.9933039	2.9933480	2.9933921
985	2.9936566	2.9937007	2.9937448	2.9937888	2.9938329
986	2.9940971	2.9941411	2.9941851	2.9942291	2.9942731
987	2.9945371	2.9945811	2.9946251	2.9946690	2.9947130
988	2.9949767	2.9950206	2.9950645	2.9951085	2.9951524
989	2.9954158	2.9954597	2.9955036	2.9955474	2.9955913
990	2.9958545	2.9958983	2.9959422	2.9959860	2.9960298
991	2.9962927	2.9963365	2.9963803	2.9964241	2.9964679
992	2.9967305	2.9967743	2.9968180	2.9968618	2.9969055
993	2.9971679	2.9972116	2.9972553	2.9972990	2.9973427
994	2.9976048	2.9976485	2.9976921	2.9977358	2.9977794
995	2.9980413	2.9980849	2.9981285	2.9981721	2.9982157
996	2.9984773	2.9985209	2.9985645	2.9986080	2.9986516
997	2.9989129	2.9989564	2.9990000	2.9990435	2.9990870
998	2.9993481	2.9993916	2.9994350	2.9994785	2.9995220
999	2.9997828	2.9998262	2.9998697	2.9999131	2.9999566

0 Degrees.

M	Sine.		Tang.		Secant		
0	0.000000	10.000000	0.000000	Infinite.	10.0000000	Infinite.	60
1	6.463720?	9.9999999	6.4637261	13.5362739	10.0000000	13.5362739	59
2	6.764756	9.9999999	6.7647562	13.2352438	10.0000001	13.2352439	58
3	6.940847?	9.9999998	6.9408475	13.0591525	10.0000002	13.0591527	57
4	7.065786?	9.9999997	7.0657863	12.9342137	10.0000003	12.9342140	56
5	7.162696	9.9999995	7.1626964	12.8373036	10.0000005	12.8373042	55
6	7.241877?	9.9999993	7.2418778	12.7581222	10.0000007	12.7581229	54
7	7.308824?	9.9999991	7.3088248	12.6911752	10.0000009	12.6911761	53
8	7.366516?	9.9999988	7.3668169	12.6331831	10.0000012	12.6331843	52
9	7.417963?	9.9999985	7.4179696	12.5820304	10.0000015	12.5820319	51
10	7.463725?	9.9999982	7.4637273	12.5362727	10.0000018	12.5362745	50
11	7.505113?	9.9999978	7.5051203	12.4948797	10.0000022	12.4948819	49
12	7.542906	9.9999974	7.5429091	12.4570909	10.0000026	12.4570935	48
13	7.577668	9.9999969	7.5776715	12.4223285	10.0000031	12.4223316	47
14	7.609853	9.9999964	7.6098566	12.3901434	10.0000036	12.3901470	46
15	7.639816	9.9999959	7.6398201	12.3601799	10.0000041	12.3601840	45
16	7.667844	9.9999953	7.6678492	12.3321508	50.0000047	12.3321555	44
17	7.694173	9.9999947	7.6941786	12.3058214	10.0000053	12.3058267	43
18	7.718996	9.9999940	7.7190026	12.2809974	10.0000060	12.2810034	42
19	7.742477	9.9999933	7.7424841	12.2575159	10.0000066	12.2575225	41
20	7.764753	9.9999927	7.7647612	12.2352390	10.0000073	12.2352463	40
21	7.785942	9.9999910	7.7859508	12.2140492	10.0000081	12.2140573	39
22	7.806145	9.9999911	7.8061547	12.1938453	10.0000089	12.1938542	38
23	7.825457	9.9999903	7.8254604	12.1745396	10.0000097	12.1745493	37
24	7.843933	9.9999894	7.8439444	12.1560556	10.0000106	12.1560662	36
25	7.861562	9.9999885	7.8616738	12.1383262	10.0000115	12.1383377	35
26	7.878595	9.9999876	7.8787077	12.1212923	10.0000124	12.1213047	34
27	7.895085	9.9999866	7.8950988	12.1049012	10.0000134	12.1049146	33
28	7.910879	9.9999856	7.9108938	12.0891062	10.0000144	12.0891207	32
29	7.926119	9.9999845	7.9261344	12.0738656	10.0000155	12.0738810	31
30	7.940541	9.9999835	7.9405584	12.0591416	10.0000165	12.0591581	30
	Sine.		Tang.		Secant		

89 Degrees.

0 *Degrees.*

M	Sine.		Tang.		Secant.		
30	7.9408419	9.9999835	7.9408584	12.0591416	10.0000165	12.0591581	30
31	7.9558819	9.9999823	7.9550996	12.0449004	10.0000177	12.0449181	29
32	7.9688698	9.9999812	7.9688886	12.0311114	10.0000188	12.0311302	28
33	7.9822334	9.9999800	7.9822534	12.0177466	10.0000200	12.0177666	27
34	7.9951980	9.9999788	7.9952192	12.0047808	10.0000212	12.0048020	26
35	8.0077867	9.9999775	8.0078092	11.9921908	10.0000225	11.9922133	25
36	8.0200207	9.9999762	8.0200445	11.9799555	10.0000238	11.9799793	24
37	8.0319195	9.9999748	8.0319446	11.9680554	10.0000252	11.9680805	23
38	8.0435009	9.9999735	8.0435274	11.9564726	10.0000265	11.9564991	22
39	8.0547814	9.9999721	8.0548094	11.9451906	10.0000279	11.9452186	21
40	8.0657763	9.9999706	8.0658057	11.9341943	10.0000294	11.9342237	20
41	8.0764997	9.9999691	8.0765306	11.9234694	10.0000309	11.9235003	19
42	8.0869646	9.9999676	8.0869970	11.9130030	10.0000324	11.9130354	18
43	8.0971832	9.9999660	8.0972172	11.9027828	10.0000340	11.9028168	17
44	8.1071669	9.9999644	8.1072025	11.8927975	10.0000356	11.8928331	16
45	8.1169262	9.9999628	8.1169634	11.8830366	10.0000372	11.8830738	15
46	8.1264710	9.9999611	8.1265099	11.8734901	10.0000389	11.8735290	14
47	8.1358104	9.9999594	8.1358510	11.8641490	10.0000406	11.8641896	13
48	8.1449532	9.9999577	8.1449956	11.8550044	10.0000423	11.8550468	12
49	8.1539075	9.9999559	8.1539516	11.8460484	10.0000441	11.8460925	11
50	8.1626808	9.9999541	8.1627267	11.8372733	10.0000459	11.8373192	10
51	8.1716804	9.9999522	8.1713282	11.8286718	10.0000478	11.8287196	9
52	8.1797129	9.9999503	8.1797626	11.8202374	10.0000497	11.8202871	8
53	8.1879848	9.9999484	8.1880364	11.8119636	10.0000516	11.8120152	7
54	8.1961020	9.9999464	8.1961556	11.8038444	10.0000536	11.8038980	6
55	8.2040703	9.9999444	8.2041259	11.7958741	10.0000556	11.7959297	5
56	8.2118949	9.9999424	8.2119526	11.7880474	10.0000576	11.7881051	4
57	8.2195811	9.9999403	8.2196408	11.7803592	10.0000597	11.7804189	3
58	8.2271335	9.9999382	8.2271953	11.7728047	10.0000618	11.7728665	2
59	8.2345568	9.9999360	8.2346208	11.7653792	10.0000640	11.7654432	1
60	8.2418553	9.9999338	8.2419215	11.7580785	10.0000662	11.7581447	0
	Sine.		Tang.		Secant.		M

89 *Degrees.*

1 Degree.

M	Sine.		Tang.		Secant.		
	8.24 1553	9.9999953	8.241921	11.7580785	10.0000662	11.7581447	60
1	8.247 332	9.9999516	8.2491015	11.7508985	10.0000684	11.7509668	59
2	8.255094	9.9999294	8.2551645	11.7443635	10.0000706	11.7439057	58
3	8.262642	9.9999271	8.2631153	11.7368847	10.0000729	11.7363576	57
4	8.269831	9.9999247	8.2699563	11.7300437	10.0000753	11.7301190	56
5	8.276613	9.9999224	8.2766912	11.7233088	10.0000775	11.7233864	55
6	8.283243	9.9999200	8.2833234	11.7166756	10.0000800	11.7167566	54
7	8.289773	9.9999176	8.2898559	11.7101441	10.0000825	11.7102266	53
8	8.296200	9.9999150	8.2962917	11.7037083	10.0000850	11.7037933	52
9	8.302544	9.9999125	8.3026335	11.6973665	10.0000875	11.6974540	51
10	8.308794	9.9999100	8.3088842	11.6911158	10.0000900	11.6912059	50
11	8.314953	9.9999074	8.3150462	11.6849538	10.0000926	11.6850464	49
12	8.321029	9.9999047	8.3211221	11.6788779	10.0000953	11.6789731	48
13	8.327016	9.9999021	8.3271143	11.6728857	10.0000979	11.6729837	47
14	8.332923	9.9998994	8.3330249	11.6669751	10.0001006	11.6670757	46
15	8.338752	9.9998966	8.3388563	11.6611437	10.0001034	11.6612471	45
16	8.344504	9.9998939	8.3446105	11.6553895	10.0001061	11.6554957	44
17	8.350180	9.9998911	8.3502895	11.6497105	10.0001089	11.6498195	43
18	8.355783	9.9998882	8.3558953	11.6441047	10.0001118	11.6442165	42
19	8.361315	9.9998853	8.3614297	11.6385703	10.0001147	11.6386850	41
20	8.366776	9.9998824	8.3668945	11.6331055	10.0001176	11.6332231	40
21	8.372171	9.9998794	8.3722915	11.6277085	10.0001206	11.6278290	39
22	8.377498	9.9998764	8.3776223	11.6223777	10.0001236	11.6225012	38
23	8.382762	9.9998734	8.3828886	11.6171114	10.0001266	11.6172380	37
24	8.387962	9.9998703	8.3880918	11.6119082	10.0001297	11.6120379	36
25	8.393100	9.9998672	8.3932336	11.6067664	10.0001328	11.6068992	35
26	8.398179	9.9998641	8.3983152	11.6016848	10.0001359	11.6018207	34
27	8.403199	9.9998609	8.4033381	11.5966619	10.0001391	11.5968010	33
28	8.408161	9.9998577	8.4083037	11.5916963	10.0001423	11.5918386	32
29	8.413067	9.9998544	8.4132132	11.5867868	10.0001456	11.5869324	31
30	8.417919	9.9998512	8.4180679	11.5819321	10.0001488	11.5820810	30

| | Sine. | | Tang. | | Secant. | | M |

88 Degrees.

1 Degree.

M	Sine.		Tang.		Secant.		
30	8.4179190	9.9998512	8.4180679	11.5819321	10.0001488	11.5820810	30
31	8.4227100	9.9998478	8.4228690	11.5771310	10.0001522	11.5772832	29
32	8.4274621	9.9998445	8.4276176	11.5723824	10.0001555	11.5725379	28
33	8.4321561	9.9998411	8.4323150	11.5676850	10.0001589	11.5678430	27
34	8.4357999	9.9998376	8.4369621	11.5630378	10.0001624	11.5632001	26
35	8.4413941	9.9998342	8.4415601	11.5584390	10.0001659	11.5586056	25
36	8.4459400	9.9998306	8.4461103	11.5538897	10.0001694	11.5540591	24
37	8.4504400	9.9998271	8.4506131	11.5493869	10.0001729	11.5495598	23
38	8.4548934	9.9998235	8.4550699	11.5449301	10.0001765	11.5451066	22
39	8.4593015	9.9998199	8.4594814	11.5405186	10.0001801	11.5406985	21
40	8.4636649	9.9998162	8.4638486	11.5361514	10.0001838	11.5363351	20
41	8.4679850	9.9998124	8.4681725	11.5318275	10.0001875	11.5320150	19
42	8.4722620	9.9998088	8.4724533	11.5275467	10.0001912	11.5277379	18
43	8.4764984	9.9998050	8.4766933	11.5233067	10.0001950	11.5235016	17
44	8.4806934	9.9998012	8.4808924	11.5191080	10.0001988	11.5193068	16
45	8.4848474	9.9997974	8.4850505	11.5149495	10.0002026	11.5151521	15
46	8.4889032	9.9997935	8.4891696	11.5108304	10.0002065	11.5110368	14
47	8.4930398	9.9997896	8.4932502	11.5067498	10.0002104	11.5069602	13
48	8.4970764	9.9997856	8.4972928	11.5027072	10.0002144	11.5029216	12
49	8.5010798	9.9997817	8.5012982	11.4987018	10.0002183	11.4989202	11
50	8.5050447	9.9997776	8.5052672	11.4947328	10.0002224	11.4949553	10
51	8.5089736	9.9997736	8.5092001	11.4907999	10.0002264	11.4910264	9
52	8.5128673	9.9997695	8.5130978	11.4869022	10.0002305	11.4871327	8
53	8.5167264	9.9997653	8.5169610	11.4830390	10.0002347	11.4832736	7
54	8.5205514	9.9997612	8.5207902	11.4792098	10.0002388	11.4794486	6
55	8.5243430	9.9997570	8.5245860	11.4754140	10.0002430	11.4756570	5
56	8.5281017	9.9997527	8.5283490	11.4716510	10.0002473	11.4718983	4
57	8.5318281	9.9997484	8.5320797	11.4679203	10.0002516	11.4681719	3
58	8.5355228	9.9997441	8.5357787	11.4642213	10.0002559	11.4644772	2
59	8.5391863	9.9997398	8.5394466	11.4605534	10.0002602	11.4608137	1
60	8.5428192	9.9997354	8.5430838	11.4569162	10.0002646	11.4571808	0

| | Sine. | | Tang. | | Secant. | | M |

88 Degrees.

A Table of Artificial Sines,

2 Degrees.

	Sine.		Tang.		Secant.		
0	8.5428192	9.9997354	8.5430838	11.4569162	10.0002646	11.4571808	60
1	8.5464218	9.9973709	8.5466909	11.4533091	10.000269	11.4535782	59
2	8.5497948	9.9997265	8.5502683	11.4497317	10.000273	11.4500052	58
3	8.5535356	9.9997220	8.5538166	11.4461834	10.000280	11.4464514	57
4	8.5570536	9.9997174	8.5573362	11.4426638	10.0002826	11.4429464	56
5	8.5605404	9.9997128	8.5608276	11.4391724	10.0002872	11.4394596	55
6	8.5639994	9.9997082	8.5642912	11.4357088	10.0002918	11.4360006	54
7	8.5674310	9.9997036	8.5677275	11.4322725	10.0002964	11.4325690	53
8	8.5708357	9.9996989	8.5711368	11.4288632	10.0003011	11.4291643	52
9	8.5742139	9.9996942	8.5745197	11.4254803	10.0003058	11.4257861	51
10	8.5775660	9.9996894	8.5778766	11.4221234	10.0003106	11.4224340	50
11	8.5808923	9.9996846	8.5812077	11.4187923	10.0003154	11.4191077	49
12	8.5841983	9.9996798	8.5845136	11.4154864	10.0003202	11.4158067	48
13	8.5974649	9.9996749	8.5877945	11.4122055	10.0003251	11.4125306	47
14	8.5907209	9.9996700	8.5910509	11.4089491	10.0003300	11.4092791	46
15	8.5939483	9.9996650	8.5942832	11.4057168	10.0003350	11.4060517	45
16	8.5971517	9.9996601	8.5974917	11.4025083	10.0003399	11.4028483	44
17	8.6003317	9.9996550	8.6006767	11.3993233	10.0003450	11.3996683	43
18	8.6034886	9.9996500	8.6038386	11.3961614	10.0003500	11.3965114	42
19	8.6065226	9.9996449	8.6069777	11.3930223	10.0003551	11.3933774	41
20	8.6097341	9.9996398	8.6100943	11.3899057	10.0003602	11.3902659	40
21	8.6128235	9.9996346	8.6131889	11.3868111	10.0003654	11.3871765	39
22	8.6158910	9.9996294	8.6162616	11.3837384	10.0003706	11.3841090	38
23	8.6189369	9.9996242	8.6193127	11.3806873	10.0003758	11.3810631	37
24	8.6219616	9.9996189	8.6223427	11.3776573	10.0003811	11.3780384	36
25	8.6249653	9.9996136	8.6253518	11.3746482	10.0003864	11.3750347	35
26	8.6279484	9.9996082	8.6283402	11.3716598	10.0003918	11.3720516	34
27	8.6309111	9.9996028	8.6313083	11.3686917	10.0003972	11.3690889	33
28	8.6338537	9.9995974	8.6342563	11.3657437	10.0004026	11.3661463	32
29	8.6367764	9.9995919	8.6371845	11.3628155	10.0004081	11.3632236	31
30	8.6396796	9.9995865	8.6400931	11.3599069	10.0004135	11.3603204	30
	Sine.		Tang.		Secant.		M

87 Degrees.

2 Degrees.

M	Sine.		Tang.		Secant.		
30	8.6396796	9.9995865	8.6400931	11.3599069	10.0004135	11.3603204	30
31	8.6425634	9.9995809	8.6429825	11.3570175	10.0004191	11.3574365	29
32	8.6454282	9.9995753	8.6458529	11.3541472	10.0004247	11.3545718	28
33	8.6482742	9.9995697	8.6487044	11.3512956	10.0004303	11.3517258	27
34	8.6511016	9.9995641	8.6515375	11.3484625	10.0004359	11.3488984	26
35	8.6539107	9.9995584	8.6543522	11.3456478	10.0004416	11.3460893	25
36	8.6567017	9.9995527	8.6571490	11.3428510	10.0004473	11.3432983	24
37	8.6594748	9.9995469	8.6599279	11.3400721	10.0004531	11.3405252	23
38	8.6622303	9.9995411	8.6626891	11.3373109	10.0004589	11.3377697	22
39	8.6649684	9.9995353	8.6654331	11.3345669	10.0004647	11.3350316	21
40	8.6676893	9.9995295	8.6681598	11.3318402	10.0004705	11.3323107	20
41	8.6703932	9.9995236	8.6708697	11.3291303	10.0004764	11.3296068	19
42	8.6730804	9.9995176	8.6735628	11.3264372	10.0004824	11.3269196	18
43	8.6757510	9.9995116	8.6762393	11.3237607	10.0004884	11.3242490	17
44	8.6784052	9.9995056	8.6788996	11.3211004	10.0004944	11.3215948	16
45	8.6810433	9.9994996	8.6815437	11.3184563	10.0005004	11.3189567	15
46	8.6836654	9.9994935	8.6841719	11.3158281	10.0005065	11.3163346	14
47	8.6862718	9.9994874	8.6867844	11.3132156	10.0005126	11.3137284	13
48	8.6888625	9.9994812	8.6893813	11.3106187	10.0005188	11.3111375	12
49	8.6914379	9.9994750	8.6919629	11.3080371	10.0005250	11.3085621	11
50	8.6939980	9.9994688	8.6945292	11.3054708	10.0005312	11.3060020	10
51	8.6965431	9.9994625	8.6970806	11.3029194	10.0005375	11.3034569	9
52	8.6990734	9.9994562	8.6996172	11.3003828	10.0005438	11.3009266	8
53	8.7015889	9.9994498	8.7021390	11.2978610	10.0005502	11.2984111	7
54	8.7040899	9.9994435	8.7046465	11.2953535	10.0005565	11.2959101	6
55	8.7065766	9.9994370	8.7071395	11.2928605	10.0005630	11.2934234	5
56	8.7090490	9.9994306	8.7096185	11.2903815	10.0005694	11.2909510	4
57	8.7115075	9.9994241	8.7120834	11.2879166	10.0005759	11.2884925	3
58	8.7139520	9.9994176	8.7145345	11.2854655	10.0005824	11.2860480	2
59	8.7163829	9.9994110	8.7169719	11.2830281	10.0005890	11.2836171	1
60	8.7188002	9.9994044	8.7193958	11.2806042	10.0005956	11.2811998	0
	Sine.		Tang.		Secant.		M

87 Degrees.

3 Degrees.

M	Sine.		Tang.		Secant.		
0	8.7188002	9.9994044	8.7193958	11.2806042	0.0000595	11.2811998	60
1	8.7212040	9.9993978	8.7218063	11.2781937	10.0000602	11.2787960	59
2	8.7235946	9.9993911	8.7242035	11.2757965	0.0000608	11.2764054	58
3	8.7259721	9.9993844	8.7265877	11.2734123	10.0000615	11.2740279	57
4	8.7283366	9.9993778	8.7289589	11.2710411	10.0000622	11.2716634	56
5	8.7306882	9.9993708	8.7313174	11.2686826	10.0000629	11.2693118	55
6	8.7330272	9.9993640	8.7336631	11.2663369	10.0000636	11.2669728	54
7	8.7353535	9.9993572	8.7359964	11.2640036	10.0000642	11.2646465	53
8	8.7376671	9.9993503	8.7383172	11.2616828	10.0000649	11.2623325	52
9	8.7399691	9.9993433	8.7406258	11.2593742	10.0000656	11.2600309	51
10	8.7422586	9.9993364	8.7429222	11.2570778	10.0000663	11.2577414	50
11	8.7445362	9.9993293	8.7452067	11.2547933	10.0000670	11.2554640	49
12	8.7468014	9.9993223	8.7474792	11.2525208	10.0000677	11.2531985	48
13	8.7490555	9.9993150	8.7497400	11.2502600	10.0000684	11.2509447	47
14	8.7512973	9.9993081	8.7519892	11.2480108	10.0000691	11.2487027	46
15	8.7535278	9.9993009	8.7542269	11.2457731	10.0000699	11.2464722	45
16	8.7557460	9.9992938	8.7564531	11.2435469	10.0007062	11.2442531	44
17	8.7579546	9.9992866	8.7586681	11.2413319	10.0007135	11.2420454	43
18	8.7601512	9.9992793	8.7608719	11.2391281	10.0007207	11.2398486	42
19	8.7623366	9.9992720	8.7630647	11.2369353	10.0007280	11.2376624	41
20	8.7645111	9.9992646	8.7652465	11.2347535	10.0007354	11.2354889	40
21	8.7666747	9.9992572	8.7674175	11.2325825	10.0007428	11.2333253	39
22	8.7688275	9.9992498	8.7695777	11.2304223	10.0007502	11.2311725	38
23	8.7709697	9.9992424	8.7717274	11.2282726	10.0007576	11.2290303	37
24	8.7731014	9.9992345	8.7738665	11.2261335	10.0007651	11.2268986	36
25	8.7752226	9.9992274	8.7759952	11.2240048	10.0007726	11.2247774	35
26	8.7773332	9.9992198	8.7781136	11.2218864	10.0007802	11.2226666	34
27	8.7794344	9.9992122	8.7802218	11.2197782	10.0007878	11.2205660	33
28	8.7815244	9.9992046	8.7823199	11.2176801	10.0007954	11.2184756	32
29	8.7836048	9.9991969	8.7844079	11.2155921	10.0008031	11.2163952	31
30	8.7856753	9.9991892	8.7864861	11.2135139	10.0008108	11.2143247	30
	Sine.		Tang.		Secant.		M

86 Degrees.

3 *Degrees.*

′	Sine.		Tang.		Secant.		
3	.7856753	9.9991892	8.7864361	11.2135139	10.0008102	11.2143247	30
31	.7877354	9.9991815	8.7885544	11.2114456	10.0008185	11.2122641	29
2	.7897867	9.9991737	8.7906132	11.2093870	10.0008263	11.2102133	28
33	8.7918278	9.9991659	8.7926620	11.2073380	10.0008341	11.2081722	27
34	8.7928594	9.9991580	8.7947014	11.2052986	10.0008420	11.2061406	26
35	8.7958814	9.9991501	8.7967313	11.2032687	10.0008499	11.2041186	25
36	8.7978941	9.9991422	8.7987519	11.2012481	10.0008578	11.2021059	24
37	8.7998974	9.9991342	8.8007632	11.1992368	10.0008658	11.2001026	23
38	8.8018915	9.9991262	8.8027653	11.1972347	10.0008738	11.1981085	22
39	8.8038764	9.9991182	8.8047583	11.1952417	10.0008818	11.1961236	21
40	8.8058523	9.9991101	8.8067422	11.1932578	10.0008899	11.1941477	20
41	8.8078192	9.9991020	8.8087172	11.1912828	10.0008980	11.1921808	19
42	8.8097772	9.9990938	8.8106834	11.1893166	10.0009062	11.1902228	18
43	8.8117264	9.9990856	8.8126407	11.1873593	10.0009144	11.1882736	17
44	8.8136668	9.9990774	8.8145894	11.1854106	10.0009226	11.1863332	16
45	8.8155985	9.9990691	8.8165294	11.1834706	10.0009309	11.1844015	15
46	8.8175217	9.9990608	8.8184608	11.1815392	10.0009392	11.1824783	14
47	8.8194363	9.9990525	8.8203838	11.1796162	10.0009475	11.1805637	13
48	8.8213425	9.9990441	8.8222984	11.1777016	10.0009559	11.1786575	12
49	8.8232404	9.9990357	8.8242046	11.1757954	10.0009643	11.1767596	11
50	8.8251299	9.9990273	8.8261026	11.1738974	10.0009727	11.1748701	10
51	8.8270112	9.9990188	8.8279924	11.1720076	10.0009812	11.1729888	9
52	8.8288844	9.9990103	8.8298741	11.1701259	10.0009897	11.1711156	8
53	8.8307495	9.9990017	8.8317478	11.1682522	10.0009983	11.1692505	7
54	8.8326066	9.9989931	8.8336134	11.1663866	10.0010069	11.1673934	6
55	8.8344557	9.9989845	8.8354712	11.1645288	10.0010155	11.1655443	5
56	8.8362969	9.9989758	8.8373211	11.1626789	10.0010242	11.1637031	4
57	8.8381304	9.9989671	8.8391633	11.1608367	10.0010329	11.1618696	3
58	8.8399561	9.9989584	8.8409977	11.1590023	10.0010416	11.1600439	2
59	8.8417741	9.9989496	8.8428245	11.1571755	10.0010504	11.1582259	1
60	8.8435845	9.9989408	8.8446437	11.1553563	10.0010592	11.1564155	0
	Sine.		Tang.		Secant		M

86 *Degrees.*

4 Degrees.

M	Sine.		Tang.		Secant.		
	8.8435845	9.9989428	8.8446437	11.1553563	10.0010592	11.1564155	60
1	8.8453587	9.9989319	8.8464554	11.1535446	10.0010681	11.1546126	59
2	8.8471827	9.9989230	8.8482597	11.1517403	10.0010770	11.1528173	58
3	8.8489707	9.9989141	8.8500566	11.1499434	10.0010859	11.1510293	57
4	8.8507512	9.9989052	8.8518461	11.1481539	10.0010948	11.1492488	56
5	8.8525245	9.9988962	8.8536283	11.1463717	10.0011038	11.1474755	55
6	8.8542905	9.9988871	8.8554034	11.1445966	10.0011129	11.1457095	54
7	8.8560494	9.9988780	8.8571713	11.1428287	10.0011220	11.1439507	53
8	8.8578016	9.9988689	8.8589321	11.1410679	10.0011311	11.1421990	52
9	8.8595457	9.9988599	8.8606859	11.1393141	10.0011402	11.1404543	51
10	8.8612933	9.9988506	8.8624327	11.1375673	10.0011494	11.1387167	50
11	8.8630133	9.9988416	8.8641725	11.1358275	10.0011586	11.1369861	49
12	8.8647376	9.9988321	8.8659055	11.1340945	10.0011679	11.1352624	48
13	8.8664545	9.9988228	8.8676317	11.1323683	10.0011772	11.1335455	47
14	8.8681646	9.9988135	8.8693511	11.1306489	10.0011865	11.1318354	46
15	8.8698681	9.9988041	8.8710638	11.1289362	10.0011959	11.1301320	45
16	8.8715646	9.9987947	8.8727699	11.1272301	10.0012053	11.1284354	44
17	8.8732546	9.9987853	8.8744694	11.1255306	10.0012147	11.1267454	43
18	8.8749381	9.9987758	8.8761623	11.1238377	10.0012242	11.1250619	42
19	8.8766150	9.9987663	8.8778487	11.1221513	10.0012337	11.1233850	41
20	8.8782854	9.9987567	8.8795286	11.1204714	10.0012433	11.1217146	40
21	8.8799493	9.9987471	8.8812022	11.1187978	10.0012529	11.1200507	39
22	8.8816069	9.9987375	8.8828694	11.1171306	10.0012625	11.1183931	38
23	8.8832581	9.9987276	8.8845303	11.1154697	10.0012722	11.1167419	37
24	8.8849031	9.9987181	8.8861850	11.1138150	10.0012819	11.1150969	36
25	8.8865418	9.9987084	8.8878334	11.1121666	10.0012916	11.1134582	35
26	8.8881743	9.9986986	8.8894757	11.1105243	10.0013014	11.1118257	34
27	8.8898007	9.9986888	8.8911119	11.1088881	10.0013112	11.1101993	33
28	8.8914209	9.9986790	8.8927420	11.1072580	10.0013210	11.1085791	32
29	8.8930351	9.9986691	8.8943660	11.1056340	10.0013309	11.1069649	31
30	8.8946433	9.9986591	8.8959842	11.1040158	10.0013409	11.1053567	30

	Sine.		Tang.		Secant.	M

85 Degrees.

4 Degrees.

M	Sine.		Tang.		Secant.		
30	8.8946433	9.9986591	8.8959842	11.1040158	10.0013409	11.1053567	30
31	8.8962455	9.9986492	8.8975963	11.1024037	10.0013508	11.1037545	29
32	8.8978418	9.9986392	8.8992026	11.1007974	10.0013608	11.1021582	28
33	8.8994322	9.9986292	8.9008030	11.0991970	10.0013708	11.1005678	27
34	8.9010168	9.9986191	8.9023977	11.0976023	10.0013809	11.0989832	26
35	8.9025955	9.9986090	8.9039866	11.0960134	10.0013910	11.0974045	25
36	8.9041685	9.9985988	8.9055697	11.0944303	10.0014012	11.0958315	24
37	8.9057358	9.9985886	8.9071472	11.0928528	10.0014114	11.0942642	23
38	8.9072975	9.9985784	8.9087190	11.0912810	10.0014216	11.0927025	22
39	8.9088535	9.9985682	8.9102853	11.0897147	10.0014318	11.0911465	21
40	8.9104039	9.9985579	8.9118460	11.0881540	10.0014421	11.0895961	20
41	8.9119487	9.9985475	8.9134012	11.0865988	10.0014525	11.0880513	19
42	8.9134881	9.9985372	8.9149509	11.0850491	10.0014628	11.0865119	18
43	8.9150219	9.9985268	8.9164952	11.0835048	10.0014732	11.0849781	17
44	8.9165504	9.9985163	8.9180340	11.0819660	10.0014837	11.0834496	16
45	8.9180734	9.9985058	8.9195675	11.0804325	10.0014942	11.0819266	15
46	8.9195911	9.9984953	8.9210957	11.0789043	10.0015047	11.0804089	14
47	8.9211034	9.9984848	8.9226186	11.0773814	10.0015152	11.0788966	13
48	8.9226105	9.9984742	8.9241363	11.0758637	10.0015258	11.0773895	12
49	8.9241123	9.9984636	8.9256487	11.0743513	10.0015364	11.0758877	11
50	8.9256089	9.9984529	8.9271560	11.0728440	10.0015471	11.0743911	10
51	8.9271003	9.9984422	8.9286581	11.0713419	10.0015578	11.0728997	9
52	8.9285866	9.9984315	8.9301552	11.0698448	10.0015685	11.0714134	8
53	8.9300678	9.9984207	8.9316471	11.0683529	10.0015793	11.0699322	7
54	8.9315439	9.9984099	8.9331340	11.0668660	10.0015901	11.0684561	6
55	8.9330150	9.9983990	8.9346160	11.0653840	10.0016010	11.0669850	5
56	8.9344811	9.9983881	8.9360929	11.0639071	10.0016119	11.0655189	4
57	8.9359422	9.9983772	8.9375650	11.0624350	10.0016228	11.0640578	3
58	8.9373983	9.9983663	8.9390321	11.0609679	10.0016337	11.0626017	2
59	8.9388496	9.9983553	8.9404944	11.0595056	10.0016447	11.0611504	1
60	8.9402960	9.9983442	8.9419518	11.0580482	10.0016558	11.0597040	0
	Sine.		Tang.		Secant		M

85 Degrees.

5 Degrees.

M	Sine.		Tang.		Secant.		
0	8.9402960	9.9983442	8.9419518	11.0580482	10.0016558	11.0597040	60
1	8.9417376	9.9983332	8.9434044	11.0565956	10.0016668	11.0582624	59
2	8.9431743	9.9983220	8.9448525	11.0551477	10.0016780	11.0568257	58
3	8.9446063	9.9983109	8.9462954	11.0537046	10.0016891	11.0553937	57
4	8.9460335	9.9982997	8.9477338	11.0522652	10.0017003	11.0539665	56
5	8.9474561	9.9982886	8.9491676	11.0508324	10.0017115	11.0525439	55
6	8.9488739	9.9982772	8.9505967	11.0494033	10.0017228	11.0511261	54
7	8.9502871	9.9982660	8.9520211	11.0479789	10.0017340	11.0497129	53
8	8.9516957	9.9982546	8.9534410	11.0465590	10.0017454	11.0483043	52
9	8.9530996	9.9982435	8.9548564	11.0451436	10.0017567	11.0469004	51
10	8.9544991	9.9982315	8.9562672	11.0437328	10.0017682	11.0455009	50
11	8.9558940	9.9982204	8.9576735	11.0423265	10.0017796	11.0441060	49
12	8.9572843	9.9982089	8.9590754	11.0409246	10.0017911	11.0427157	48
13	8.9586703	9.9981974	8.9604728	11.0395272	10.0018026	11.0413297	47
14	8.9600517	9.9981854	8.9618659	11.0381341	10.0018141	11.0399483	46
15	8.9614288	9.9981743	8.9632545	11.0367455	10.0018257	11.0385712	45
16	8.9628014	9.9981626	8.9646388	11.0353612	10.0018374	11.0371986	44
17	8.9641697	9.9981510	8.9660188	11.0339812	10.0018490	11.0358303	43
18	8.9655337	9.9981393	8.9673944	11.0326056	10.0018607	11.0344663	42
19	8.9668934	9.9981275	8.9687658	11.0312342	10.0018725	11.0331066	41
20	8.9682487	9.9981156	8.9701330	11.0298670	10.0018842	11.0317513	40
21	8.9695999	9.9981040	8.9714959	11.0285041	10.0018960	11.0304001	39
22	8.9709468	9.9980921	8.9728547	11.0271453	10.0019079	11.0290532	38
23	8.9722895	9.9980802	8.9742092	11.0257908	10.0019198	11.0277105	37
24	8.9736280	9.9980682	8.9755597	11.0244403	10.0019317	11.0263720	36
25	8.9749624	9.9980563	8.9769060	11.0230940	10.0019437	11.0250376	35
26	8.9762926	9.9980443	8.9782483	11.0217517	10.0019557	11.0237074	34
27	8.9776188	9.9980323	8.9795865	11.0204135	10.0019677	11.0223812	33
28	8.9789408	9.9980202	8.9809206	11.0190794	10.0019798	11.0210592	32
29	8.9802589	9.9980081	8.9822507	11.0177493	10.0019919	11.0197411	31
30	8.9815729	9.9979960	8.9835769	11.0164231	10.0020040	11.0184271	30
	Sine.		Tang.		Secant.		M

84 Degrees.

5 *Degrees.*

M	Sine.		Tang.		Secant.		
30	8.9815729	9.9979960	9.9835769	11.0164231	10.0020040	11.018247	
31	8.9828829	9.9979838	9.9848991	11.0151009	10.0021162	11.0171171	29
32	8.9841889	9.9979714	8.9862173	11.0137827	10.0020284	11.0158111	
33	8.9854910	9.9979593	8.9875317	11.0124683	10.0020407	11.0145090	27
34	8.9867891	9.9979470	8.9888421	11.0111579	10.0020530	11.0132109	26
35	8.9880834	9.9979347	8.9901487	11.0098513	10.0020653	11.0119166	25
36	8.9893737	9.9979223	8.9914514	11.0085486	10.0020777	11.0106263	24
37	8.9906602	9.9979099	8.9927503	11.0072497	10.0020901	11.0093398	23
38	8.9919429	9.9978975	8.9940454	11.0059546	10.0021025	11.0080571	22
39	8.9932217	9.9978850	8.9953367	11.0046633	10.0021150	11.0067783	21
40	8.9944968	9.9978725	8.9966243	11.0033757	10.0021275	11.0055032	20
41	8.9957681	9.9978590	8.9979081	11.0020919	10.0021410	11.0042319	19
42	8.9970356	9.9978473	8.9991883	11.0008117	10.0021527	11.0029644	18
43	8.9982994	9.9978347	9.0004647	10.9995353	10.0021653	11.0017006	17
44	8.9995595	9.9978220	9.0017375	10.9982625	10.0021780	11.0004405	16
45	9.0008160	9.9978093	9.0030066	10.9969934	10.0021907	10.9991840	15
46	9.0020687	9.9977966	9.0042721	10.9957279	10.0022034	10.9979313	14
47	9.0033179	9.9977838	9.0055340	10.9944660	10.0022162	10.9966821	13
48	9.0045634	9.9977710	9.0067924	10.9932076	10.0022290	10.9954366	12
49	9.0058053	9.9977582	9.0080471	10.9919529	10.0022418	10.9941947	11
50	9.0070436	9.9977453	9.0092984	10.9907016	10.0022547	10.9929564	10
51	9.0082784	9.9977323	9.0105461	10.9894539	10.0022677	10.9917216	9
52	9.0095096	9.9977194	9.0117903	10.9882097	10.0022806	10.9904904	8
53	9.0107374	9.9977064	9.0130310	10.9869690	10.0022936	10.9892626	7
54	9.0119616	9.9976933	9.0142682	10.9857318	10.0023067	10.9880384	6
55	9.0131823	9.9976803	9.0155021	10.9844979	10.0023197	10.9868177	5
56	9.0143996	9.9976672	9.0167325	10.9832675	10.0023328	10.9856004	4
57	9.0156135	9.9976540	9.0179594	10.9820406	10.0023460	10.9843865	3
58	9.0168239	9.9976408	9.0191831	10.9808169	10.0023592	10.9831761	2
59	9.0180309	9.9976276	9.0204033	10.9795967	10.0023724	10.9819691	1
60	9.0192346	9.9976143	9.0216202	10.9783798	10.0023857	10.9807654	0
	Sine.		Tang.		Secant.		M

. 84 *Degrees.*

A Table of Artificial Sines,

6 Degrees.

M	Sine.		Tang.		Secant.		
0	9.0192345	9.9976143	9.0216202	10.9783798	10.0023857	10.9807554	60
1	9.0204348	9.9976011	9.0228338	10.9771662	10.0023989	10.9795652	59
2	9.0216318	9.9975877	9.0240441	10.9759559	10.0024123	10.9783682	58
3	9.0228254	9.9975743	9.0252510	10.9747490	10.0024257	10.9771746	57
4	9.0240157	9.9975609	9.0264546	10.9735452	10.0024391	10.9759843	56
5	9.0252027	9.9975475	9.0276552	10.9723448	10.0024525	10.9747973	55
6	9.0263865	9.9975340	9.0288524	10.9711476	10.0024660	10.9736135	54
7	9.0275669	9.9975205	9.0300464	10.9699536	10.0024795	10.9724331	53
8	9.0287442	9.9975069	9.0312373	10.9687627	10.0024931	10.9712558	52
9	9.0299182	9.9974933	9.0324249	10.9675751	10.0025067	10.9700818	51
10	9.0310890	9.9974797	9.0336093	10.9663907	10.0025203	10.9689110	50
11	9.0322567	9.9974660	9.0347906	10.9652094	10.0025340	10.9677433	49
12	9.0334212	9.9974523	9.0359688	10.9640312	10.0025477	10.9665788	48
13	9.0345825	9.9974386	9.0371439	10.9628561	10.0025614	10.9654175	47
14	9.0357407	9.9974245	9.0383159	10.9616841	10.0025752	10.9642593	46
15	9.0368958	9.9974110	9.0394845	10.9605152	10.0025890	10.9631042	45
16	9.0380477	9.9973971	9.0406506	10.9593494	10.0026029	10.9619523	44
17	9.0391966	9.9973833	9.0418134	10.9581866	10.0026167	10.9608034	43
18	9.0403424	9.9973693	9.0429731	10.9570269	10.0026307	10.9596576	42
19	9.0414852	9.9973554	9.0441299	10.9558701	10.0026446	10.9585148	41
20	9.0426247	9.9973414	9.0452836	10.9547164	10.0026586	10.9573751	40
21	9.0437617	9.9973273	9.0464343	10.9535657	10.0026727	10.9562383	39
22	9.0448954	9.9973132	9.0475821	10.9524179	10.0026868	10.9551046	38
23	9.0460261	9.9972991	9.0487270	10.9512730	10.0027009	10.9539739	37
24	9.0471538	9.9972850	9.0498689	10.9501311	10.0027150	10.9528462	36
25	9.0482786	9.9972708	9.0510078	10.9489922	10.0027292	10.9517214	35
26	9.0494005	9.9972566	9.0521439	10.9478561	10.0027434	10.9505995	34
27	9.0505193	9.9972423	9.0532771	10.9467229	10.0027577	10.9494806	33
28	9.0516354	9.9972280	9.0544074	10.9455926	10.0027720	10.9483646	32
29	9.0527485	9.9972137	9.0555349	10.9444651	10.0027863	10.9472515	31
30	9.0538588	9.9971993	9.0566595	10.9433405	10.0028007	10.9461412	30
	Sine.		Tang.		Secant.		M

83 Degrees.

6 Degrees.

M	Sine.		Tang.		Secant.		
30	9.0538588	9.9971993	9.0566595	10.9433405	10.0028007	10.9461412	30
31	9.0549661	9.9971849	9.0577813	10.9422187	10.0028151	10.9450339	29
32	9.0560706	9.9971704	9.0589202	10.9410998	10.0028296	10.9439294	28
33	9.0571723	9.9971559	9.0600164	10.9399836	10.0028441	10.9428377	27
34	9.0582711	9.9971414	9.0611297	10.9388703	10.0028585	10.9417289	26
35	9.0593672	9.9971268	9.0622403	10.9377597	10.0028732	10.9406328	25
36	9.0604604	9.9971122	9.0633482	10.9366518	10.0028878	10.9395396	24
37	9.0615509	9.9970976	9.0644533	10.9355467	10.0029024	10.9384491	23
38	9.0626380	9.9970829	9.0655556	10.9344444	10.0029171	10.9373614	22
39	9.0637235	9.9970682	9.0666553	10.9333447	10.0029318	10.9362765	21
40	9.0648057	9.9970535	9.0677522	10.9322478	10.0029465	10.9351943	20
41	9.0658852	9.9970387	9.0688465	10.9311535	10.0029613	10.9341148	19
42	9.0669619	9.9970239	9.0699381	10.9300619	10.0029761	10.9330381	18
43	9.0680360	9.9970090	9.0710270	10.9289730	10.0029910	10.9319640	17
44	9.0691074	9.9969941	9.0721133	10.9278867	10.0030059	10.9308926	16
45	9.0701761	9.9969792	9.0731969	10.9268031	10.0030208	10.9298239	15
46	9.0712421	9.9969642	9.0742779	10.9257221	10.0030358	10.9287579	14
47	9.0723055	9.9969492	9.0753563	10.9246437	10.0030508	10.9276945	13
48	9.0733663	9.9969342	9.0764321	10.9235679	10.0030658	10.9266337	12
49	9.0744244	9.9969191	9.0775053	10.9224947	10.0030809	10.9255756	11
50	9.0754799	9.9969040	9.0785760	10.9214240	10.0030960	10.9245201	10
51	9.0765329	9.9968888	9.0796441	10.9203559	10.0031112	10.9234671	9
52	9.0775832	9.9968736	9.0807096	10.9192904	10.0031264	10.9224168	8
53	9.0786310	9.9968584	9.0817726	10.9182274	10.0031416	10.9213690	7
54	9.0796762	9.9968431	9.0828331	10.9171669	10.0031569	10.9203238	6
55	9.0807189	9.9968278	9.0838911	10.9161089	10.0031722	10.9192811	5
56	9.0817590	9.9968125	9.0849466	10.9150534	10.0031875	10.9182410	4
57	9.0827966	9.9967971	9.0859996	10.9140004	10.0032029	10.9172034	3
58	9.0838317	9.9967817	9.0870501	10.9129499	10.0032183	10.9161683	2
59	9.0848643	9.9967662	9.0880981	10.9119019	10.0032338	10.9151357	1
60	9.0858945	9.9967507	9.0891438	10.9108562	10.0032493	10.9141055	0
	Sine.		Tang.		Secant.		M

83 Degrees.

7 Degrees.

M	Sine.		Tang.		Secant.		
0	9.0858945	9.9967507	9.0891435	10.9108562	10.0032493	10.9141055	60
1	9.0869221	9.9967352	9.090186,	10.9098131	10.0032648	10.9130779	59
2	9.0879473	9.9967196	9.0912277	10.9087723	10.0032804	10.9120527	58
3	9.0889700	9.9967040	9.0922660	10.9077340	10.0032960	10.9110300	57
4	9.0899903	9.9966884	9.0933020	10.9066980	10.0033115	10.9100097	56
5	9.0910082	9.9966727	9.0943355	10.9056645	10.0033273	10.9089918	55
6	9.0920237	9.9966570	9.0953667	10.9046333	10.0033430	10.9079763	54
7	9.0930367	9.9966412	9.0963955	10.9036045	10.0033588	10.9069633	53
8	9.0940474	9.9966254	9.0974219	10.9025781	10.0033746	10.9059526	52
9	9.0950556	9.9966096	9.0984460	10.9015540	10.0033904	10.9049444	51
10	9.0960615	9.9965937	9.0994678	10.9005322	10.0034063	10.9039385	50
11	9.0970651	9.9965778	9.1004872	10.8995128	10.0034222	10.9029349	49
12	9.0980662	9.9965619	9.1015044	10.8984956	10.0034381	10.9019338	48
13	9.0990651	9.9965459	9.1025172	10.8974808	10.0034541	10.9009349	47
14	9.1000615	9.9965299	9.1035317	10.8964683	10.0034701	10.8999384	46
15	9.1010558	9.9965138	9.1045420	10.8954580	10.0034862	10.8989442	45
16	9.1020477	9.9964977	9.1055500	10.8944500	10.0035023	10.8979523	44
17	9.1030373	9.9964816	9.1065557	10.8934443	10.0035184	10.8969627	43
18	9.1040246	9.9964655	9.1075591	10.8924409	10.0035345	10.8959575	42
19	9.1050096	9.9964493	9.1085604	10.8914396	10.0035507	10.8949904	41
20	9.1059924	9.9964330	9.1095594	10.8904406	10.0035670	10.8940076	40
21	9.1069729	9.9964167	9.1105562	10.8894438	10.0035833	10.8930271	39
22	9.1079512	9.9964004	9.1115528	10.8884492	10.0035996	10.8920488	38
23	9.1089272	9.9963841	9.1125431	10.8874569	10.0036159	10.8910728	37
24	9.1099010	9.9963677	9.1135333	10.8864667	10.0036323	10.8900990	36
25	9.1108726	9.9963513	9.1145213	10.8854787	10.0036487	10.8891274	35
26	9.1118423	9.9963348	9.1155072	10.8844928	10.0036652	10.8881580	34
27	9.1128092	9.9963182	9.1164909	10.8835091	10.0036817	10.8871908	33
28	9.1137742	9.9963018	9.1174724	10.8825276	10.0036982	10.8862258	32
29	9.1147373	9.9962852	9.1184518	10.8815482	10.0037148	10.8852630	31
30	9.1156977	9.9962686	9.1194291	10.8805709	10.0037314	10.8843023	30
	Sine.		Tang.		Secant.		M

82 Degrees.

7 Degrees.

M	Sine.		Tang.		Secant.		M
30	9.1156977	9.9962686	9.1194429	10.8805570	10.0037314	10.8843302	30
31	9.1166562	9.9962519	9.1204044	10.8795956	10.0037481	10.8833443	29
32	9.1176125	9.9962352	9.1213773	10.8786227	10.0037548	10.8823574	28
33	9.1185667	9.9962185	9.1223482	10.8776518	10.0037815	10.8814633	27
34	9.1195188	9.9962017	9.1233171	10.8766829	10.0037983	10.8804451	26
35	9.1204688	9.9961849	9.1242839	10.8757161	10.0038151	10.8795531	25
36	9.1214167	9.9961681	9.1252486	10.8747514	10.0038319	10.8788583	24
37	9.1223624	9.9961512	9.1262112	10.8737888	10.0038488	10.8776376	23
38	9.1233061	9.9961343	9.1271718	10.8728282	10.0038657	10.8766939	22
39	9.1242477	9.9961174	9.1281303	10.8718697	10.0038826	10.8757523	21
40	9.1251872	9.9961004	9.1290868	10.8709132	10.0038996	10.8748128	20
41	9.1261246	9.9960834	9.1300413	10.8699587	10.0039166	10.8738754	19
42	9.1270600	9.9960663	9.1309937	10.8690063	10.0039337	10.8729400	18
43	9.1279934	9.9960492	9.1319442	10.8680558	10.0039508	10.8720066	17
44	9.1289247	9.9960321	9.1328926	10.8671074	10.0039679	10.8710753	16
45	9.1298539	9.9960149	9.1338391	10.8661609	10.0039851	10.8701461	15
46	9.1307812	9.9959977	9.1347835	10.8652165	10.0040023	10.8692188	14
47	9.1317064	9.9959804	9.1357260	10.8642740	10.0040195	10.8682936	13
48	9.1326297	9.9959631	9.1366665	10.8633335	10.0040369	10.8673703	12
49	9.1335509	9.9959458	9.1376051	10.8623949	10.0040542	10.8664491	11
50	9.1344702	9.9959284	9.1385417	10.8614583	10.0040716	10.8655298	10
51	9.1353875	9.9959111	9.1394764	10.8605236	10.0040889	10.8646125	9
52	9.1363028	9.9958936	9.1404092	10.8595908	10.0041064	10.8636972	8
53	9.1372161	9.9958761	9.1413400	10.8586600	10.0041239	10.8627835	7
54	9.1381275	9.9958586	9.1422689	10.8577311	10.0041414	10.8618725	6
55	9.1390370	9.9958411	9.1431959	10.8568041	10.0041589	10.8609630	5
56	9.1399445	9.9958235	9.1441210	10.8558790	10.0041765	10.8600555	4
57	9.1408501	9.9958059	9.1450442	10.8549558	10.0041941	10.8591499	3
58	9.1417537	9.9957882	9.1459655	10.8540345	10.0042118	10.8582463	2
59	9.1426555	9.9957705	9.1468850	10.8531150	10.0042295	10.8573445	1
60	9.1335553	9.9957528	9.1478025	10.8521975	10.0042472	10.8564447	0
	Sine.		Tang.		Secant.		M

82 Degrees.

8 *Degrees*.

M	Sine.		Tang.		Secant.		
0	9.143555	9.9957525	9.1478025	10.852197	10.0042472	10.8564447	60
1	9.144453	9.9957355	9.1487162	10.851281	10.0042650	10.8555468	59
2	9.145349	9.9957174	9.1496321	10.8503675	10.0042828	10.8546507	58
3	9.146219	9.9956999	9.1505441	10.849455	10.0043007	10.8537565	57
4	9.147135	9.9956815	9.1514545	10.8484515	10.0043185	10.8528642	56
5	9.148022	9.9956635	9.1523647	10.8476357	10.0043365	10.8519738	55
6	9.148913	9.9956456	9.152729	10.8467308	10.0043544	10.851085	54
7	9.149801	9.9956276	9.1541735	10.8458261	10.0043724	10.8501985	53
8	9.150685	9.9956095	9.1550767	10.8449231	10.0043905	10.8493136	52
9	9.151569	9.9955915	9.1559785	10.8440228	10.0044085	10.848430C	51
10	9.152452	9.9955734	9.1568773	10.8431227	10.0044266	10.8475493	50
11	9.153330	9.9955552	9.1577748	10.8422252	10.0044448	10.8466699	49
12	9.154207	9.9955370	9.1586726	10.8413294	10.0044630	10.8457924	48
13	9.155083	9.9955158	9.1595646	10.8404354	10.0044812	10.8449166	47
14	9.155957	9.9955005	9.1604569	10.8395431	10.0044995	10.8440426	46
15	9.156829	9.9954822	9.1613473	10.8386527	10.0045178	10.8431704	45
16	9.157700	9.9954639	9.1622361	10.8377639	10.0045361	10.8423000	44
17	9.158565	9.9954455	9.1631231	10.8368769	10.0045545	10.8414314	43
18	9.159435	9.9954271	9.1640083	10.8359917	10.0045729	10.8405646	42
19	9.160300	9.9954087	9.1648919	10.8351081	10.0045913	10.8396995	41
20	9.161163	9.9953902	9.1657737	10.8342263	10.0046098	10.8388361	40
21	9.162025	9.9953717	9.1666538	10.8333462	10.0046283	10.837974C	39
22	9.162885	9.9953531	9.1675322	10.8324678	10.0046469	10.8371147	38
23	9.163743	9.9953345	9.1684089	10.8315911	10.0046655	10.8362566	37
24	9.164599	9.9953159	9.1692839	10.8307161	10.0046841	10.8354002	36
25	9.165454	9.9952972	9.1701572	10.8298428	10.0047029	10.8345456	35
26	9.166307	9.9952785	9.1710289	10.8289711	10.0047215	10.8336926	34
27	9.167158	9.9952597	9.1718989	10.8281011	10.0047403	10.8328414	33
28	9.168000	9.9952409	9.1727672	10.8272328	10.0047591	10.8319919	32
29	9.168855	9.9952221	9.1736338	10.8263664	10.0047779	10.8311441	31
30	9.169702	9.9952033	9.1744988	10.8255012	10.0047967	10.8302979	30

	Sine.		Tang.		Secant.		M

81 *Degrees*.

8 Degrees.

M	Sine.		Tang.		Secant.		
30	9.1697021	9.9952033	9.1744988	10.825501	10.0047967	10.8302975	30
31	9.1705465	9.9951844	9.1753622	10.8246375	10.0048156	10.8294535	29
32	9.1713892	9.9951654	9.1762239	10.8237761	10.0048346	10.8286109	28
33	9.1722305	9.9951464	9.1770840	10.8229160	10.0048536	10.8277695	27
34	9.1730699	9.9951274	9.1779425	10.8220575	10.0048726	10.8269301	26
35	9.1739077	9.9951084	9.1787993	10.8212007	10.0048916	10.8260923	25
36	9.1747439	9.9950893	9.1796546	10.8203454	10.0049107	10.8252561	24
37	9.1755784	9.9950702	9.1805082	10.8194918	10.0049298	10.8244216	23
38	9.1764112	9.9950510	9.1813602	10.8186398	10.0049490	10.8235888	22
39	9.1772425	9.9950318	9.1822106	10.8177894	10.0049682	10.8227575	21
40	9.1780721	9.9950126	9.1830595	10.8169405	10.0049874	10.8219279	20
41	9.1789001	9.9949933	9.1839068	10.8160932	10.0050067	10.8210999	19
42	9.1797265	9.9949740	9.1847525	10.8152475	10.0050260	10.8202735	18
43	9.1805512	9.9949546	9.1855966	10.8144034	10.0050454	10.8194488	17
44	9.1813744	9.9949352	9.1864392	10.8135608	10.0050648	10.8186256	16
45	9.1821960	9.9949158	9.1872802	10.8127198	10.0050842	10.8178040	15
46	9.1830160	9.9948964	9.1881196	10.8118804	10.0051036	10.8169840	14
47	9.1838344	9.9948769	9.1889575	10.8110425	10.0051231	10.8161656	13
48	9.1846512	9.9948573	9.1897939	10.8102061	10.0051427	10.8153488	12
49	9.1854665	9.9948377	9.1906287	10.8093713	10.0051623	10.8145335	11
50	9.1862802	9.9948181	9.1914621	10.8085379	10.0051819	10.8137198	10
51	9.1870923	9.9947985	9.1922939	10.8077061	10.0052015	10.8129077	9
52	9.1879029	9.9947788	9.1931241	10.8068759	10.0052212	10.8120971	8
53	9.1887120	9.9947591	9.1939529	10.8060471	10.0052409	10.8112880	7
54	9.1895195	9.9947393	9.1947802	10.8052198	10.0052607	10.8104805	6
55	9.1903254	9.9947195	9.1956059	10.8043941	10.0052805	10.8096746	5
56	9.1911299	9.9946997	9.1964302	10.8035698	10.0053003	10.8088701	4
57	9.1919328	9.9946798	9.1972530	10.8027470	10.0053202	10.8080672	3
58	9.1927342	9.9946599	9.1980743	10.8019257	10.0053401	10.8072658	2
59	9.1935341	9.9946399	9.1988941	10.8011059	10.0053601	10.8064659	1
60	9.1943324	9.9946199	9.1997125	10.8002875	10.0053801	10.8056676	0
	Sine.		Tang.		Secant.		M

81 Degrees.

9 Degrees.

M.	Sine.		Tang.		Secant.		
0	9.1943324	9.9945199	9.1997125	10.8002875	10.0053801	10.8056676	60
1	9.1951293	9.9945599	9.2005294	10.7994706	10.0054001	10.8048707	59
2	9.1959247	9.9945799	9.2013445	10.7986551	10.0054202	10.8040755	58
3	9.1967186	9.9945599	9.2021588	10.7978412	10.0054403	10.8032814	57
4	9.1975111	9.9945354	9.2029714	10.7970286	10.0054604	10.8024890	56
5	9.1983019	9.9944599	9.2037825	10.7962175	10.0054806	10.8016981	55
6	9.1990913	9.9944399	9.2045922	10.7954078	10.0055008	10.8009087	54
7	9.1998779	9.9944799	9.2054004	10.7945996	10.0055211	10.8001207	53
8	9.2006658	9.9944589	9.2062072	10.7937928	10.0055413	10.7993344	52
9	9.2014509	9.9944383	9.2070126	10.7929874	10.0055617	10.7985491	51
10	9.2022234	9.9944180	9.2078165	10.7921835	10.0055820	10.7977765	50
11	9.2030167	9.9943975	9.2086191	10.7913809	10.0056025	10.7969833	49
12	9.2037974	9.9943771	9.2094203	10.7905797	10.0056229	10.7962026	48
13	9.2045766	9.9943566	9.2102200	10.7897800	10.0056434	10.7954234	47
14	9.2053545	9.9943361	9.2110184	10.7889816	10.0056639	10.7946455	46
15	9.2061309	9.9943156	9.2118153	10.7881847	10.0056844	10.7938691	45
16	9.2069059	9.9942950	9.2126109	10.7873891	10.0057050	10.7930941	44
17	9.2076795	9.9942743	9.2134051	10.7865949	10.0057257	10.7923205	43
18	9.2084516	9.9942537	9.2141980	10.7858020	10.0057463	10.7915484	42
19	9.2092224	9.9942330	9.2149894	10.7850106	10.0057670	10.7907776	41
20	9.2099917	9.9942122	9.2157795	10.7842205	10.0057878	10.7900083	40
21	9.2107597	9.9941914	9.2165683	10.7834317	10.0058086	10.7892403	39
22	9.2115263	9.9941706	9.2173556	10.7826444	10.0058294	10.7884737	38
23	9.2122914	9.9941498	9.2181417	10.7818583	10.0058502	10.7877086	37
24	9.2130552	9.9941289	9.2189264	10.7810736	10.0058711	10.7869448	36
25	9.2138175	9.9941079	9.2197097	10.7802903	10.0058921	10.7861825	35
26	9.2145787	9.9940870	9.2204917	10.7795083	10.0059130	10.7854213	34
27	9.2153384	9.9940659	9.2212724	10.7787276	10.0059341	10.7846616	33
28	9.2160967	9.9940449	9.2220518	10.7779482	10.0059551	10.7839033	32
29	9.2168537	9.9940238	9.2228298	10.7771702	10.0059762	10.7831463	31
30	9.2176092	9.9940027	9.2236066	10.7763934	10.0059973	10.7823908	30
	Sine.		Tang.		Secant		M.

80 Degrees.

9 Degrees.

M	Sine.		Tang.		Secant.		
30	9.2176092	9.9940027	9.2236065	10.7763935	10.0059973	10.7823909	30
31	9.2183638	9.9939815	9.2243819	10.7756181	10.0060185	10.7816365	29
32	9.2191164	9.9939603	9.2251561	10.7748439	10.0060397	10.7808836	28
33	9.2198680	9.9939391	9.2259289	10.7740711	10.0060609	10.7801320	27
34	9.2206184	9.9939178	9.2267004	10.7732996	10.0060822	10.7793816	26
35	9.2213671	9.9938965	9.2274706	10.7725294	10.0061035	10.7786329	25
36	9.2221147	9.9938752	9.2282395	10.7717605	10.0061248	10.7778853	24
37	9.2228609	9.9938538	9.2290071	10.7709929	10.0061462	10.7771391	23
38	9.2236059	9.9938324	9.2297735	10.7702265	10.0061676	10.7763941	22
39	9.2243495	9.9938109	9.2305386	10.7694614	10.0061891	10.7756505	21
40	9.2250918	9.9937894	9.2313024	10.7686976	10.0062106	10.7749082	20
41	9.2258328	9.9937679	9.2320650	10.7679350	10.0062321	10.7741672	19
42	9.2265725	9.9937463	9.2328262	10.7671738	10.0062537	10.7734275	18
43	9.2273110	9.9937247	9.2335863	10.7664137	10.0062753	10.7726890	17
44	9.2280481	9.9937030	9.2343451	10.7656549	10.0062970	10.7719519	16
45	9.2287839	9.9936813	9.2351026	10.7648974	10.0063187	10.7712161	15
46	9.2295185	9.9936596	9.2358589	10.7641411	10.0063404	10.7704815	14
47	9.2302518	9.9936378	9.2366139	10.7633861	10.0063622	10.7697482	13
48	9.2309838	9.9936160	9.2373678	10.7626322	10.0063840	10.7690162	12
49	9.2317145	9.9935942	9.2381203	10.7618797	10.0064058	10.7682855	11
50	9.2324440	9.9935723	9.2388717	10.7611283	10.0064277	10.7675560	10
51	9.2331722	9.9935504	9.2396218	10.7603782	10.0064496	10.7668278	9
52	9.2338992	9.9935285	9.2403708	10.7596292	10.0064715	10.7661008	8
53	9.2346249	9.9935065	9.2411185	10.7588815	10.0064935	10.7653751	7
54	9.2353494	9.9934844	9.2418650	10.7581350	10.0065156	10.7646506	6
55	9.2360726	9.9934624	9.2426103	10.7573897	10.0065376	10.7639274	5
56	9.2367946	9.9934403	9.2433543	10.7566457	10.0065597	10.7632054	4
57	9.2375153	9.9934181	9.2440972	10.7559028	10.0065819	10.7624847	3
58	9.2382349	9.9933959	9.2448389	10.7551611	10.0066041	10.7617651	2
59	9.2389532	9.9933737	9.2455794	10.7544206	10.0066263	10.7610468	1
60	9.2396702	9.9933515	9.2463188	10.7536812	10.0066485	10.7603298	0
	Sine.		Tang.		Secant.		M

80 Degrees.

Hhh

10 Degrees.

M	Sine.		Tang.		Secant.		
0	9.2396700	9.9933515	9.2463188	10.7536812	10.0066487	10.7603298	60
1	9.2403861	9.9933292	9.2470569	10.7529431	10.0066708	10.7596139	59
2	9.2411007	9.9933068	9.2477939	10.7522061	10.0066932	10.7588993	58
3	9.2418141	9.9932845	9.2485297	10.7514703	10.0067155	10.7581859	57
4	9.2425264	9.9932621	9.2492643	10.7507357	10.0067379	10.7574736	56
5	9.2432374	9.9932396	9.2499978	10.7500022	10.0067604	10.7567626	55
6	9.2439472	9.9932171	9.2507301	10.7492699	10.0067829	10.7560528	54
7	9.2446558	9.9931946	9.2514612	10.7485388	10.0068054	10.7553442	53
8	9.2453632	9.9931720	9.2521912	10.7478088	10.0068280	10.7546368	52
9	9.2460695	9.9931494	9.2529200	10.7470800	10.0068506	10.7539305	51
10	9.2467746	9.9931268	9.2536477	10.7463523	10.0068732	10.7532254	50
11	9.2474784	9.9931041	9.2543743	10.7456257	10.0068959	10.7525216	49
12	9.2481811	9.9930814	9.2550997	10.7449003	10.0069186	10.7518189	48
13	9.2488827	9.9930587	9.2558240	10.7441760	10.0069413	10.7511173	47
14	9.2495830	9.9930359	9.2565472	10.7434528	10.0069641	10.7504170	46
15	9.2502822	9.9930131	9.2572692	10.7427308	10.0069869	10.7497178	45
16	9.2509802	9.9929902	9.2579901	10.7420099	10.0070098	10.7490197	44
17	9.2515772	9.9929673	9.2587099	10.7412901	10.0070327	10.7483228	43
18	9.2523729	9.9929444	9.2594285	10.7405715	10.0070556	10.7476271	42
19	9.2530675	9.9929214	9.2601461	10.7398539	10.0070786	10.7469325	41
20	9.2537609	9.9928984	9.2608625	10.7391375	10.0071016	10.7462391	40
21	9.2544532	9.9928753	9.2615779	10.7384221	10.0071247	10.7455468	39
22	9.2551444	9.9928522	9.2622921	10.7377079	10.0071478	10.7448556	38
23	9.2558344	9.9928291	9.2630053	10.7369947	10.0071709	10.7441656	37
24	9.2565233	9.9928059	9.2637173	10.7362827	10.0071941	10.7434767	36
25	9.2572110	9.9927827	9.2644283	10.7355717	10.0072173	10.7427890	35
26	9.2578977	9.9927595	9.2651382	10.7348618	10.0072405	10.7421023	34
27	9.2585832	9.9927362	9.2658470	10.7341530	10.0072638	10.7414168	33
28	9.2592676	9.9927129	9.2665547	10.7334453	10.0072871	10.7407324	32
29	9.2599509	9.9926895	9.2672613	10.7327387	10.0073105	10.7400491	31
30	9.2606330	9.9926661	9.2679669	10.7320331	10.0073339	10.7393670	30
	Sine.		Tang.		Secant		M

79 Degrees.

10 *Degrees.*

M	Sine.		Tang.		Secant.		
30	9.2606330	9.9926661	9.2679669	10.7320331	10.0073339	10.7393670	30
31	9.2613141	9.9926427	9.2686714	10.7313286	10.0073573	10.7386859	29
32	9.2619941	9.9926192	9.2693749	10.7306251	10.0073808	10.7380059	28
33	9.2626729	9.9925957	9.2700772	10.7299228	10.0074043	10.7373271	27
34	9.2633507	9.9925722	9.2707786	10.7292214	10.0074278	10.7366493	26
35	9.2640274	9.9925486	9.2714788	10.7285212	10.0074514	10.7359726	25
36	9.2647030	9.9925250	9.2721780	10.7278220	10.0074750	10.7352970	24
37	9.2653775	9.9925013	9.2728762	10.7271238	10.0074987	10.7346225	23
38	9.2660509	9.9924776	9.2735733	10.7264267	10.0075224	10.7339491	22
39	9.2667232	9.9924539	9.2742694	10.7257306	10.0075461	10.7332768	21
40	9.2673945	9.9924301	9.2749644	10.7250356	10.0075699	10.7326055	20
41	9.2680647	9.9924063	9.2756584	10.7243416	10.0075937	10.7319353	19
42	9.2687338	9.9923824	9.2763514	10.7236486	10.0076176	10.7312662	18
43	9.2694019	9.9923585	9.2770434	10.7229566	10.0076415	10.7305981	17
44	9.2700689	9.9923346	9.2777343	10.7222657	10.0076654	10.7299311	16
45	9.2707348	9.9923106	9.2784242	10.7215758	10.0076894	10.7292652	15
46	9.2713997	9.9922866	9.2791131	10.7208869	10.0077134	10.7286003	14
47	9.2720635	9.9922626	9.2798009	10.7201991	10.0077374	10.7279365	13
48	9.2727263	9.9922385	9.2804878	10.7195122	10.0077615	10.7272737	12
49	9.2733880	9.9922144	9.2811736	10.7188264	10.0077856	10.7266120	11
50	9.2740487	9.9921902	9.2818585	10.7181415	10.0078098	10.7259513	10
51	9.2747083	9.9921660	9.2825423	10.7174577	10.0078340	10.7252917	9
52	9.2753669	9.9921418	9.2832251	10.7167749	10.0078582	10.7246331	8
53	9.2760245	9.9921175	9.2839070	10.7160930	10.0078825	10.7239755	7
54	9.2766811	9.9920932	9.2845878	10.7154122	10.0079068	10.7233189	6
55	9.2773366	9.9920689	9.2852677	10.7147323	10.0079311	10.7226634	5
56	9.2779911	9.9920445	9.2859466	10.7140534	10.0079555	10.7220089	4
57	9.2786445	9.9920201	9.2866245	10.7133755	10.0079799	10.7213555	3
58	9.2792970	9.9919956	9.2873014	10.7126986	10.0080044	10.7207030	2
59	9.2799484	9.9919711	9.2879773	10.7120227	10.0080289	10.7200516	1
60	9.2805988	9.9919466	9.2886523	10.7113477	10.0080534	10.7194012	0
	Sine.		Tang.		Secant.		M

79 *Degrees.*

11 Degrees.

M	Sine.		Tang.		Secant.		
0	9.2805986	9.9919466	9.2886523	10.7113477	10.0080534	10.7194012	60
1	9.2812433	9.9919220	9.2893263	10.7106737	10.0080780	10.7187517	59
2	9.2818967	9.9918974	9.2899593	10.7100007	10.0081026	10.7181033	58
3	9.2825441	9.9918727	9.2906713	10.7093287	10.0081273	10.7174559	57
4	9.2831905	9.9918480	9.2913424	10.7086576	10.0081520	10.7168095	56
5	9.2838359	9.9918233	9.2920126	10.7079874	10.0081767	10.7161641	55
6	9.2844803	9.9917986	9.2926817	10.7073183	10.0082014	10.7155197	54
7	9.2851237	9.9917737	9.2933500	10.7066500	10.0082263	10.7148763	53
8	9.2857661	9.9917489	9.2940172	10.7059828	10.0082511	10.7142339	52
9	9.2864075	9.9917240	9.2946836	10.7053164	10.0082760	10.7135924	51
10	9.2870480	9.9916991	9.2953489	10.7046511	10.0083009	10.7129520	50
11	9.2876875	9.9916741	9.2960134	10.7039866	10.0083259	10.7123125	49
12	9.2883260	9.9916492	9.2966769	10.7033231	10.0083508	10.7116740	48
13	9.2889636	9.9916241	9.2973395	10.7026605	10.0083759	10.7110364	47
14	9.2896001	9.9915990	9.2980011	10.7019989	10.0084010	10.7103999	46
15	9.2902357	9.9915739	9.2986618	10.7013382	10.0084261	10.7097643	45
16	9.2908704	9.9915488	9.2993216	10.7006784	10.0084512	10.7091296	44
17	9.2915040	9.9915236	9.2999804	10.7000196	10.0084764	10.7084960	43
18	9.2921367	9.9914984	9.3006383	10.6993617	10.0085016	10.7078633	42
19	9.2927685	9.9914731	9.3012954	10.6987046	10.0085269	10.7072315	41
20	9.2933993	9.9914478	9.3019514	10.6980486	10.0085522	10.7066007	40
21	9.2940291	9.9914225	9.3026066	10.6973934	10.0085775	10.7059709	39
22	9.2946580	9.9913971	9.3032609	10.6967391	10.0086029	10.7053420	38
23	9.2952859	9.9913717	9.3039143	10.6960857	10.0086283	10.7047141	37
24	9.2959129	9.9913462	9.3045667	10.6954333	10.0086538	10.7040871	36
25	9.2965390	9.9913207	9.3052183	10.6947817	10.0086793	10.7034610	35
26	9.2971641	9.9912952	9.3058689	10.6941311	10.0087048	10.7028359	34
27	9.2977883	9.9912695	9.3065187	10.6934813	10.0087304	10.7022117	33
28	9.2984116	9.9912440	9.3071675	10.6928325	10.0087560	10.7015884	32
29	9.2990339	9.9912184	9.3078155	10.6921845	10.0087816	10.7009661	31
30	9.2996553	9.9911927	9.3084626	10.6915374	10.0088073	10.7003447	30
	Sine.		Tang.		Secant.		M

78 Degrees.

11 *Degrees.*

M	Sine.		Tang.		Secant.		
30	9.2996553	9.9911927	9.3084626	10.6915374	10.0088073	10.7003447	30
31	9.3002758	9.9911670	9.3091088	10.6908912	10.0088330	10.6997242	29
32	9.3008953	9.9911412	9.3097541	10.6902459	10.0088588	10.6991047	28
33	9.3015140	9.9911154	9.3103985	10.6896015	10.0088846	10.6984860	27
34	9.3021317	9.9910896	9.3110421	10.6889579	10.0089104	10.6978683	26
35	9.3027485	9.9910637	9.3116848	10.6883152	10.0089363	10.6972515	25
36	9.3033644	9.9910378	9.3123266	10.6876734	10.0089622	10.6966356	24
37	9.3039794	9.9910119	9.3129675	10.6870325	10.0089881	10.6960206	23
38	9.3045934	9.9909859	9.3136076	10.6863924	10.0090141	10.6954066	22
39	9.3052066	9.9909598	9.3142468	10.6857532	10.0090402	10.6947934	21
40	9.3058189	9.9909338	9.3148851	10.6851149	10.0090662	10.6941811	20
41	9.3064303	9.9909077	9.3155226	10.6844774	10.0090923	10.6935697	19
42	9.3070407	9.9908815	9.3161592	10.6838408	10.0091185	10.6929593	18
43	9.3076503	9.9908553	9.3167950	10.6832250	10.0091447	10.6923497	17
44	9.3082590	9.9908291	9.3174299	10.6825701	10.0091709	10.6917410	16
45	9.3088668	9.9908029	9.3180640	10.6819360	10.0091971	10.6911332	15
46	9.3094737	9.9907766	9.3186972	10.6813028	10.0092234	10.6905263	14
47	9.3100798	9.9907502	9.3193295	10.6806705	10.0092498	10.6899202	13
48	9.3106849	9.9907239	9.3199611	10.6800389	10.0092761	10.6893151	12
49	9.3112892	9.9906974	9.3205918	10.6794082	10.0093026	10.6887108	11
50	9.3118926	9.9906710	9.3212216	10.6787784	10.0093290	10.6881074	10
51	9.3124951	9.9906445	9.3218576	10.6781494	10.0093555	10.6875049	9
52	9.3130968	9.9906180	9.3224788	10.6775212	10.0093820	10.6869032	8
53	9.3136976	9.9905914	9.3231061	10.6768939	10.0094086	10.6863024	7
54	9.3142975	9.9905648	9.3237327	10.6762673	10.0094352	10.6857025	6
55	9.3148965	9.9905382	9.3243584	10.6756416	10.0094618	10.6851035	5
56	9.3154947	9.9905115	9.3249832	10.6750168	10.0094885	10.6845053	4
57	9.3160921	9.9904848	9.3256073	10.6743927	10.0095152	10.6839079	3
58	9.3166885	9.9904580	9.3262305	10.6737695	10.0095420	10.6833115	2
59	9.3172841	9.9904312	9.3268529	10.6731471	10.0095688	10.6827159	1
60	9.3178789	9.9904044	9.3274745	10.6725255	10.0095956	10.6821211	0
	Sine.		Tang.		Secant.		M

78 *Degrees.*

12 Degrees.

M	Sine.		Tang.		Secant.		
0	9.3175785	9.9974542	9.3274745	10.6725255	10.0095956	10.6821211	60
1	9.3184725	9.9903775	9.3289953	10.6719047	10.0096225	10.6815272	59
2	9.3190555	9.9903535	9.3287153	10.671284	10.0096494	10.6809341	58
3	9.3195551	9.9903257	9.3293345	10.6706655	10.0096763	10.6803419	57
4	9.3202495	9.9902977	9.3299528	10.670047	10.0097033	10.6797505	56
5	9.3208400	9.9902697	9.3305704	10.6694296	10.0097303	10.6791600	55
6	9.3214297	9.9902426	9.3311872	10.6688128	10.0097574	10.6785703	54
7	9.3220186	9.9902155	9.3318031	10.6681969	10.0097845	10.6779814	53
8	9.3226060	9.9901883	9.3324183	10.6675817	10.0098117	10.6773934	52
9	9.3231935	9.9901612	9.3330327	10.6669673	10.0098388	10.6768062	51
10	9.3237805	9.9901339	9.3336463	10.6663537	10.0098661	10.6762198	50
11	9.3243657	9.9901067	9.3342591	10.6657409	10.0098933	10.6756343	49
12	9.3249503	9.9900794	9.3348711	10.6651289	10.0099206	10.6750495	48
13	9.3255341	9.9900521	9.3354823	10.6645177	10.0099479	10.6744656	47
14	9.3261171	9.9900247	9.3360927	10.6639073	10.0099753	10.6738826	46
15	9.3266993	9.9899973	9.3367024	10.6632976	10.0100027	10.6733003	45
16	9.3272811	9.9899698	9.3373113	10.6626887	10.0100302	10.6727189	44
17	9.3278517	9.9899425	9.3379194	10.6620806	10.0100577	10.6721383	43
18	9.3284416	9.9899145	9.3385267	10.6614733	10.0100852	10.6715584	42
19	9.3290206	9.9898873	9.3391333	10.6608667	10.0101127	10.6709794	41
20	9.3295985	9.9898597	9.3397391	10.6602609	10.0101403	10.6704012	40
21	9.3301761	9.9898320	9.3403441	10.6596559	10.0101680	10.6698239	39
22	9.3307527	9.9898043	9.3409484	10.6590516	10.0101957	10.6692473	38
23	9.3313285	9.9897766	9.3415519	10.6584481	10.0102234	10.6686715	37
24	9.3319035	9.9897459	9.3421549	10.6578454	10.0102511	10.6680965	36
25	9.3324777	9.9897211	9.3427566	10.6572434	10.0102789	10.6675223	35
26	9.3330511	9.9896932	9.3433578	10.6566422	10.0103068	10.6669489	34
27	9.3336237	9.9896654	9.3439583	10.6560417	10.0103346	10.6663763	33
28	9.3341955	9.9896374	9.3445580	10.6554420	10.0103626	10.6658045	32
29	9.3347665	9.9896095	9.3451570	10.6548430	10.0103905	10.6652335	31
30	9.3353368	9.9895815	9.3457552	10.6542448	10.0104185	10.6646632	30
	Sine.		Tang.		Secant.		M

77 Degrees.

12 *Degrees.*

M	Sine.		Tang.		Secant.		
30	9.3353368	9.9895819	9.3457552	10.6542448	10.0104185	10.6646632	30
31	9.3359062	9.9895535	9.3463527	10.6536473	10.0104465	10.6647938	29
32	9.3364749	9.9895254	9.3469494	10.6530506	10.0104746	10.6635251	28
33	9.3370428	9.9894972	9.3475454	10.6524546	10.0105027	10.6629572	27
34	9.3376099	9.9894692	9.3481407	10.6518593	10.0105308	10.6623901	26
35	9.3381762	9.9894410	9.3487352	10.6512648	10.0105590	10.6618235	25
36	9.3387418	9.9894128	9.3493290	10.6506710	10.0105872	10.6612582	24
37	9.3393065	9.9893845	9.3499220	10.6500780	10.0106155	10.6606935	23
38	9.3398706	9.9893562	9.3505143	10.6494857	10.0106438	10.6601294	22
39	9.3404338	9.9893279	9.3511059	10.6488941	10.0106721	10.6595662	21
40	9.3409963	9.9892995	9.3516968	10.6483032	10.0107005	10.6590037	20
41	9.3415580	9.9892711	9.3522869	10.6477131	10.0107289	10.6584420	19
42	9.3421190	9.9892427	9.3528763	10.6471237	10.0107573	10.6578810	18
43	9.3426792	9.9892142	9.3534651	10.6465349	10.0107858	10.6573208	17
44	9.3432386	9.9891856	9.3540530	10.6459470	10.0108144	10.6567614	16
45	9.3437973	9.9891571	9.3546402	10.6453598	10.0108429	10.6562027	15
46	9.3443552	9.9891284	9.3552267	10.6447733	10.0108716	10.6556448	14
47	9.3449124	9.9890998	9.3558126	10.6441874	10.0109002	10.6550876	13
48	9.3454688	9.9890711	9.3563977	10.6436023	10.0109289	10.6545312	12
49	9.3460245	9.9890424	9.3569821	10.6430179	10.0109576	10.6539755	11
50	9.3465794	9.9890137	9.3575658	10.6424342	10.0109863	10.6534206	10
51	9.3471336	9.9889849	9.3581487	10.6418513	10.0110151	10.6528664	9
52	9.3476870	9.9889560	9.3587310	10.6412690	10.0110440	10.6523130	8
53	9.3482397	9.9889271	9.3593126	10.6406874	10.0110729	10.6517603	7
54	9.3487917	9.9888982	9.3598935	10.6401065	10.0111018	10.6512083	6
55	9.3493429	9.9888693	9.3604736	10.6395264	10.0111307	10.6506571	5
56	9.3498934	9.9888403	9.3610531	10.6389469	10.0111597	10.6501066	4
57	9.3504432	9.9888112	9.3616319	10.6383681	10.0111887	10.6495568	3
58	9.3509922	9.9887822	9.3622100	10.6377900	10.0112178	10.6490078	2
59	9.3515405	9.9887531	9.3627874	10.6372126	10.0112469	10.6484595	1
60	9.3520880	9.9887239	9.3633641	10.6366359	10.0112761	10.6479120	0
	Sine.		Tang.		Secant.		M

77 *Degrees.*

13 Degrees.

M	Sine.		Tang.		Secant.		
	9.3520985	9.9587239	9.3633641	10.6366359	10.0112761	10.6479120	60
1	9.3525047	9.9586947	9.3639401	10.6360599	10.0113051	10.6473651	59
2	9.3531010	9.9586655	9.3645155	10.6354845	10.0113346	10.6468190	58
3	9.3537264	9.9586366	9.3650908	10.6349092	10.0113637	10.6462736	57
4	9.3542710	9.9586070	9.3656641	10.6343359	10.0113937	10.6457290	56
5	9.3548150	9.9585776	9.3662374	10.6337626	10.0114224	10.6451850	55
6	9.3553582	9.9585452	9.3668100	10.6331900	10.0114518	10.6446418	54
7	9.3559007	9.9585188	9.3673819	10.6326181	10.0114812	10.6440993	53
8	9.3564426	9.9584891	9.3679532	10.6320468	10.0115106	10.6435574	52
9	9.3569836	9.9584593	9.3685238	10.6314762	10.0115401	10.6430164	51
10	9.3575240	9.9584303	9.3690937	10.6309063	10.0115697	10.6424760	50
11	9.3580637	9.9584008	9.3696629	10.6303371	10.0115992	10.6419363	49
12	9.3586027	9.9583712	9.3702315	10.6297685	10.0116288	10.6413973	48
13	9.3591409	9.9583415	9.3707994	10.6292006	10.0116585	10.6408591	47
14	9.3596755	9.9583118	9.3713667	10.6286333	10.0116882	10.6403215	46
15	9.3602154	9.9582821	9.3719333	10.6280667	10.0117179	10.6397846	45
16	9.3607515	9.9582523	9.3724992	10.6275008	10.0117477	10.6392485	44
17	9.3612870	9.9582225	9.3730645	10.6269355	10.0117775	10.6387130	43
18	9.3618211	9.9581927	9.3736291	10.6263709	10.0118073	10.6381783	42
19	9.3623558	9.9581628	9.3741930	10.6258070	10.0118372	10.6376442	41
20	9.3628892	9.9581329	9.3747563	10.6252437	10.0118671	10.6371108	40
21	9.3634216	9.9581029	9.3753190	10.6246810	10.0118971	10.6365781	39
22	9.3639539	9.9580729	9.3758810	10.6241190	10.0119271	10.6360461	38
23	9.3644854	9.9580429	9.3764423	10.6235577	10.0119571	10.6355148	37
24	9.3650155	9.9580128	9.3770030	10.6229970	10.0119872	10.6349842	36
25	9.3655458	9.9579827	9.3775631	10.6224369	10.0120173	10.6344542	35
26	9.3660750	9.9579525	9.3781225	10.6218775	10.0120475	10.6339250	34
27	9.3666036	9.9579223	9.3786813	10.6213187	10.0120777	10.6333964	33
28	9.3671315	9.9578921	9.3792394	10.6207606	10.0121079	10.6328685	32
29	9.3676587	9.9578618	9.3797969	10.6202031	10.0121382	10.6323413	31
30	9.3681852	9.9578315	9.3803537	10.6196463	10.0121685	10.6318147	30
	Sine.		Tang.		Secant.		M

76 Degrees.

13 Degrees.

M	Sine.		Tang.		Secant.		
30	9.3681853	9.9878315	9.3803537	10.6196463	10.0121685	10.6318147	30
31	9.3687111	9.9878012	9.3809100	10.6190900	10.0121988	10.6312889	29
32	9.3692363	9.9877708	9.3814655	10.6185345	10.0122292	10.6307637	28
33	9.3697608	9.9877404	9.3820205	10.6179795	10.0122596	10.6302392	27
34	9.3702847	9.9877095	9.3825748	10.6174252	10.0122901	10.6297153	26
35	9.3708079	9.9876794	9.3831285	10.6168715	10.0123206	10.6291921	25
36	9.3713304	9.9876488	9.3836815	10.6163184	10.0123512	10.6286696	24
37	9.3718523	9.9876183	9.3842340	10.6157660	10.0123817	10.6281477	23
38	9.3723735	9.9875876	9.3847858	10.6152142	10.0124124	10.6276265	22
39	9.3728940	9.9875570	9.3853370	10.6146630	10.0124430	10.6271060	21
40	9.3734139	9.9875263	9.3858876	10.6141124	10.0124737	10.6265861	20
41	9.3739331	9.9874955	9.3864376	10.6135624	10.0125045	10.6260669	19
42	9.3744517	9.9874648	9.3869869	10.6130131	10.0125352	10.6255483	18
43	9.3749696	9.9874339	9.3875356	10.6124644	10.0125661	10.6250304	17
44	9.3754868	9.9874031	9.3880837	10.6119163	10.0125969	10.6245132	16
45	9.3760034	9.9873722	9.3886312	10.6113688	10.0126278	10.6239966	15
46	9.3765194	9.9873413	9.3891781	10.6108219	10.0126587	10.6234806	14
47	9.3770347	9.9873103	9.3897244	10.6102756	10.0126897	10.6229653	13
48	9.3775493	9.9872793	9.3902700	10.6097300	10.0127207	10.6224507	12
49	9.3780633	9.9872482	9.3908151	10.6091849	10.0127518	10.6219367	11
50	9.3785767	9.9872171	9.3913595	10.6086405	10.0127829	10.621423	10
51	9.3790894	9.9871860	9.3919034	10.6080966	10.0128140	10.6209106	9
52	9.3796015	9.9871548	9.3924466	10.6075534	10.0128451	10.6203985	8
53	9.3801129	9.9871236	9.3929893	10.6070107	10.0128764	10.6198871	7
54	9.3806237	9.9870924	9.3935313	10.6064687	10.0129076	10.6193763	6
55	9.3811339	9.9870611	9.3940727	10.6059273	10.0129389	10.6188661	5
56	9.3816434	9.9870298	9.3946136	10.6053864	10.0129702	10.6183566	4
57	9.3821523	9.9869984	9.3951538	10.6048462	10.0130716	10.6178477	3
58	9.3826605	9.9869670	9.3956935	10.6043065	10.0130332	10.6173395	2
59	9.3831682	9.9869356	9.3962326	10.6037674	10.0130644	10.6168318	1
60	9.3836752	9.9869041	9.3967711	10.6032289	10.0130959	10.6163248	0
	Sine.		Tang.		Secant.		M

76 Degrees.

14 Degrees.

M	Sine.		Tang.		Secant.		
0	9.3836752	9.9865041	9.3967711	10.6032289	10.0130959	10.6163248	60
1	9.3841816	9.9868726	9.3973089	10.6026911	10.0131274	10.6158185	59
2	9.3845875	9.9868410	9.3978463	10.6021537	10.0131590	10.6153127	58
3	9.3851924	9.9868094	9.3983830	10.6016170	10.0131906	10.6148076	57
4	9.3856967	9.9867778	9.3989191	10.6010809	10.0132222	10.6143031	56
5	9.3862005	9.9867461	9.3994547	10.6005453	10.0132539	10.6137995	55
6	9.3867040	9.9867145	9.3999896	10.6000104	10.0132856	10.6132960	54
7	9.3872067	9.9866827	9.4005240	10.5994760	10.0133173	10.6127933	53
8	9.3877087	9.9866509	9.4010578	10.5989422	10.0133491	10.6122913	52
9	9.3882101	9.9866191	9.4015910	10.5984090	10.0133809	10.6117899	51
10	9.3887110	9.9865872	9.4021237	10.5978763	10.0134128	10.6112891	50
11	9.3892111	9.9865553	9.4026558	10.5973442	10.0134447	10.6107889	49
12	9.3897106	9.9865233	9.4031873	10.5968127	10.0134767	10.6102894	48
13	9.3902096	9.9864913	9.4037182	10.5962818	10.0135087	10.6097904	47
14	9.3907079	9.9864593	9.4042486	10.5957514	10.0135407	10.6092921	46
15	9.3912057	9.9864273	9.4047784	10.5952216	10.0135727	10.6087943	45
16	9.3917028	9.9863952	9.4053076	10.5946924	10.0136048	10.6082972	44
17	9.3921993	9.9863630	9.4058363	10.5941637	10.0136370	10.6078007	43
18	9.3926952	9.9863308	9.4063644	10.5936356	10.0136692	10.6073048	42
19	9.3931905	9.9862986	9.4068919	10.5931081	10.0137014	10.6068095	41
20	9.3936852	9.9862663	9.4074189	10.5925811	10.0137337	10.6063148	40
21	9.3941794	9.9862340	9.4079453	10.5920547	10.0137660	10.6058206	39
22	9.3946729	9.9862017	9.4084712	10.5915288	10.0137983	10.6053271	38
23	9.3951658	9.9861693	9.4089965	10.5910035	10.0138307	10.6048342	37
24	9.3956581	9.9861369	9.4095212	10.5904788	10.0138631	10.6043419	36
25	9.3961499	9.9861045	9.4100454	10.5899546	10.0138955	10.6038501	35
26	9.3966410	9.9860720	9.4105690	10.5894310	10.0139280	10.6033590	34
27	9.3971315	9.9860394	9.4110921	10.5889079	10.0139606	10.6028685	33
28	9.3976215	9.9860069	9.4116146	10.5883854	10.0139931	10.6023785	32
29	9.3981109	9.9859742	9.4121366	10.5878634	10.0140258	10.6018891	31
30	9.3985996	9.9859416	9.4126581	10.5873419	10.0140584	10.6014004	30
	Sine.		Tang.		Secant.		M

75 Degrees.

14 Degrees.

M	Sine.		Tang.		Secant.		
30	9.3985996	9.9859416	9.4126581	10.5873419	10.0140584	10.6014006	30
31	9.3990878	9.9859085	9.4131789	10.5868211	10.0140911	10.600912	29
32	9.3995754	9.9858762	9.4136993	10.5863007	10.0141238	10.6004246	28
33	9.4000625	9.9858434	9.4142191	10.5857809	10.0141566	10.5999375	27
34	9.4005489	9.9858106	9.4147383	10.5852617	10.0141894	10.5994511	26
35	9.4010348	9.9857777	9.4152570	10.5847430	10.0142223	10.5989265	25
36	9.4015201	9.9857449	9.4157752	10.5842248	10.0142551	10.5984799	24
37	9.4020048	9.9857119	9.4162928	10.5837072	10.0142881	10.5979952	23
38	9.4024889	9.9856790	9.4168099	10.5831901	10.0143210	10.5975111	22
39	9.4029724	9.9856460	9.4173265	10.5826735	10.0143540	10.5970276	21
40	9.4034554	9.9856129	9.4178425	10.5821575	10.0143871	10.5965446	20
41	9.4039378	9.9855798	9.4183580	10.5816420	10.0144202	10.5960622	19
42	9.4044196	9.9855467	9.4188729	10.5811271	10.0144533	10.5955804	18
43	9.4049009	9.9855135	9.4193874	10.5806126	10.0144865	10.5950991	17
44	9.4053816	9.9854803	9.4199013	10.5800987	10.0145197	10.5946184	16
45	9.4058617	9.9854471	9.4204148	10.5795854	10.0145529	10.5941383	15
46	9.4063413	9.9854138	9.4209275	10.5790725	10.0145862	10.5936587	14
47	9.4068203	9.9853805	9.4214398	10.5785602	10.0146195	10.5931797	13
48	9.4072987	9.9853471	9.4219515	10.5780485	10.0146529	10.5927013	12
49	9.4077766	9.9853138	9.4224628	10.5775372	10.0146862	10.5922234	11
50	9.4082539	9.9852803	9.4229735	10.5770265	10.0147197	10.5917461	10
51	9.4087306	9.9852468	9.4234838	10.5765162	10.0147532	10.5912694	9
52	9.4092068	9.9852133	9.4239935	10.5760065	10.0147867	10.5907932	8
53	9.4096824	9.9851798	9.4245026	10.5754974	10.0148202	10.5903176	7
54	9.4101575	9.9851462	9.4250113	10.5749887	10.0148538	10.5898429	6
55	9.4106320	9.9851125	9.4255194	10.5744806	10.0148875	10.5893680	5
56	9.4111059	9.9850789	9.4260271	10.5739729	10.0149211	10.5888941	4
57	9.4115793	9.9850452	9.4265342	10.5734658	10.0149548	10.5884207	3
58	9.4120522	9.9850114	9.4270408	10.5729592	10.0149886	10.5879478	2
59	9.4125245	9.9849776	9.4275469	10.5724531	10.0150224	10.5874755	1
60	9.4129962	9.9849438	9.4280525	10.5719475	10.0150562	10.5870038	0
	Sine.		Tang.		Secant.		M

75 Degrees.

15 Degrees.

M	Sine.		Tang.		Secant.		
0	9.4129962	9.9849435	9.4280525	10.5719475	10.0150562	10.5870038	60
1	9.4131674	9.9849099	9.4285575	10.5714425	10.0150901	10.5865326	59
2	9.4139381	9.9848760	9.4290621	10.5709379	10.0151240	10.5860619	58
3	9.4144082	9.9848420	9.4295661	10.5704339	10.0151580	10.5855918	57
4	9.4148778	9.9848081	9.4300697	10.5699303	10.0151919	10.5851222	56
5	9.4153468	9.9847740	9.4305727	10.5694273	10.0152260	10.5846532	55
6	9.4158152	9.9847400	9.4310753	10.5689247	10.0152600	10.5841848	54
7	9.4162832	9.9847059	9.4315773	10.5684227	10.0152941	10.5837168	53
8	9.4167506	9.9846717	9.4320789	10.5679211	10.0153283	10.5832494	52
9	9.4172174	9.9846375	9.4325799	10.5674201	10.0153625	10.5827826	51
10	9.4176837	9.9846033	9.4330804	10.5669196	10.0153957	10.5823163	50
11	9.4181495	9.9845690	9.4335805	10.5664195	10.0154310	10.5818505	49
12	9.4186148	9.9845347	9.4340800	10.5659200	10.0154653	10.5813852	48
13	9.4190795	9.9845004	9.4345791	10.5654209	10.0154996	10.5809205	47
14	9.4195436	9.9844660	9.4350776	10.5649224	10.0155340	10.5804564	46
15	9.4200073	9.9844316	9.4355757	10.5644243	10.0155684	10.5799927	45
16	9.4204704	9.9843971	9.4360733	10.5639267	10.0156029	10.5795296	44
17	9.4209330	9.9843626	9.4365704	10.5634296	10.0156374	10.5790670	43
18	9.4213950	9.9843281	9.4370670	10.5629330	10.0156719	10.5786050	42
19	9.4218566	9.9842935	9.4375631	10.5624369	10.0157065	10.5781434	41
20	9.4223176	9.9842589	9.4380587	10.5619413	10.0157411	10.5776824	40
21	9.4227780	9.9842242	9.4385538	10.5614462	10.0157758	10.5772220	39
22	9.4232380	9.9841895	9.4390485	10.5609515	10.0158105	10.5767620	38
23	9.4236974	9.9841548	9.4395426	10.5604574	10.0158452	10.5763026	37
24	9.4241563	9.9841200	9.4400363	10.5599637	10.0158800	10.5758437	36
25	9.4246147	9.9840852	9.4405295	10.5594705	10.0159148	10.5753853	35
26	9.4250726	9.9840503	9.4410222	10.5589778	10.0159497	10.5749274	34
27	9.4255299	9.9840154	9.4415145	10.5584855	10.0159846	10.5744701	33
28	9.4259867	9.9839805	9.4420062	10.5579938	10.0160195	10.5740133	32
29	9.4264430	9.9839455	9.4424975	10.5575025	10.0160545	10.5735570	31
30	9.4268988	9.9839105	9.4429883	10.5570117	10.0160895	10.5731012	30
	Sine,		Tang.		Secant		M

74 Degrees.

15 Degrees.

M	Sine.		Tang.		Secant.		
30	9.4268988	9.9839105	9.4429883	10.5570117	10.0160895	10.5731012	30
31	9.4273541	9.9838755	9.4434786	10.5565214	10.0161245	10.5726459	29
32	9.4278089	9.9838404	9.4439685	10.5560315	10.0161596	10.5721911	28
33	9.4282631	9.9838052	9.4444579	10.5555421	10.0161948	10.5717369	27
34	9.4287169	9.9837701	9.4449468	10.5550532	10.0162299	10.5712831	26
35	9.4291701	9.9837348	9.4454352	10.5545648	10.0162652	10.5708299	25
36	9.4296228	9.9836996	9.4459232	10.5540768	10.0163004	10.5703772	24
37	9.4300750	9.9836643	9.4464107	10.5535893	10.0163357	10.5699250	23
38	9.4305267	9.9836290	9.4468978	10.5531022	10.0163710	10.5694733	22
39	9.4309779	9.9835936	9.4473843	10.5526157	10.0164064	10.5690221	21
40	9.4314286	9.9835582	9.4478704	10.5521296	10.0164418	10.5685714	20
41	9.4318788	9.9835227	9.4483561	10.5516439	10.0164773	10.5681212	19
42	9.4323285	9.9834872	9.4488413	10.5511587	10.0165128	10.5676715	18
43	9.4327777	9.9834517	9.4493260	10.5506740	10.0165483	10.5672223	17
44	9.4332264	9.9834161	9.4498102	10.5501898	10.0165839	10.5667736	16
45	9.4336746	9.9833805	9.4502940	10.5497060	10.0166195	10.5663254	15
46	9.4341223	9.9833449	9.4507774	10.5492226	10.0166551	10.5658777	14
47	9.4345694	9.9833092	9.4512602	10.5487398	10.0166908	10.5654306	13
48	9.4350161	9.9832735	9.4517427	10.5482573	10.0167265	10.5649839	12
49	9.4354623	9.9832377	9.4522246	10.5477754	10.0167623	10.5645377	11
50	9.4359080	9.9832019	9.4527061	10.5472939	10.0167981	10.5640920	10
51	9.4363532	9.9831661	9.4531872	10.5468128	10.0168339	10.5636468	9
52	9.4367980	9.9831302	9.4536678	10.5463322	10.0168698	10.5632020	8
53	9.4372422	9.9830942	9.4541479	10.5458521	10.0169058	10.5627578	7
54	9.4376859	9.9830583	9.4546276	10.5453724	10.0169417	10.5623141	6
55	9.4381292	9.9830223	9.4551069	10.5448931	10.0169777	10.5618708	5
56	9.4385719	9.9829862	9.4555857	10.5444143	10.0170138	10.5614281	4
57	9.4390142	9.9829501	9.4560641	10.5439359	10.0170499	10.5609858	3
58	9.4394560	9.9829140	9.4565420	10.5434580	10.0170860	10.5605440	2
59	9.4398973	9.9828778	9.4570194	10.5429806	10.0171222	10.5601027	1
60	9.4403381	9.9828416	9.4574964	10.5425036	10.0171584	10.5596619	0
	Sine.		Tang.		Secant.		

74 Degrees.

16 Degrees.

M	Sine.		Tang.		Secant.		
0	9.440338	9.9828416	9.4574964	10.542503	10.0171584	10.5596619	60
1	9.4407784	9.9828054	9.4579730	10.5420270	10.0171946	10.5592216	59
2	9.4412182	9.9827691	9.4584491	10.5415509	10.0172309	10.5587818	58
3	9.4416576	9.9827328	9.4589248	10.5410752	10.0172672	10.5583424	57
4	9.4420966	9.9826964	9.4594001	10.5405999	10.0173036	10.5579035	56
5	9.4425349	9.9826600	9.4598749	10.5401251	10.0173400	10.5574651	55
6	9.4429728	9.9826236	9.4603492	10.5396508	10.0173764	10.5570272	54
7	9.4434102	9.9825871	9.4608232	10.5391768	10.0174129	10.5565897	53
8	9.4438472	9.9825506	9.4612967	10.5387033	10.0174494	10.5561528	52
9	9.4442837	9.9825140	9.4617697	10.5382303	10.0174860	10.5557163	51
10	9.4447197	9.9824774	9.4622423	10.5377577	10.0175226	10.5552803	50
11	9.4451553	9.9824408	9.4627145	10.5372855	10.0175592	10.5548447	49
12	9.4455904	9.9824041	9.4631863	10.5368137	10.0175959	10.5544096	48
13	9.4460250	9.9823674	9.4636576	10.5363424	10.0176326	10.5539750	47
14	9.4464591	9.9823306	9.4641285	10.5358715	10.0176694	10.5535409	46
15	9.4468927	9.9822939	9.4645990	10.5354010	10.0177062	10.5531073	45
16	9.4473259	9.9822569	9.4650690	10.5349310	10.0177431	10.5526741	44
17	9.4477586	9.9822201	9.4655386	10.5344614	10.0177799	10.5522414	43
18	9.4481909	9.9821831	9.4660078	10.5339922	10.0178169	10.5518091	42
19	9.4486227	9.9821462	9.4664765	10.5335235	10.0178538	10.5513773	41
20	9.4490540	9.9821092	9.4669448	10.5330552	10.0178908	10.5509460	40
21	9.4494849	9.9820721	9.4674127	10.5325873	10.0179279	10.5505151	39
22	9.4499153	9.9820351	9.4678802	10.5321198	10.0179649	10.5500847	38
23	9.4503452	9.9819979	9.4683473	10.5316527	10.0180021	10.5496548	37
24	9.4507747	9.9819608	9.4688139	10.5311861	10.0180392	10.5492253	36
25	9.4512037	9.9819236	9.4692801	10.5307199	10.0180764	10.5487963	35
26	9.4516322	9.9818863	9.4697459	10.5302541	10.0181137	10.5483678	34
27	9.4520603	9.9818490	9.4702112	10.5297888	10.0181510	10.5479397	33
28	9.4524879	9.9818117	9.4706762	10.5293238	10.0181883	10.5475121	32
29	9.4529151	9.9817744	9.4711407	10.5288593	10.0182256	10.5470849	31
30	9.4533418	9.9817370	9.4716048	10.5283952	10.0182630	10.5466582	30
	Sine.		Tang.		Secant.		M

73 Degrees.

16 Degrees.

M	Sine.		Tang.		Secant.		
30	9.4533418	9.9817370	9.4716048	10.5283952	10.0182630	10.5466582	30
31	9.4537681	9.9816995	9.4720685	10.5279315	10.0183005	10.5462319	29
32	9.4541939	9.9816620	9.4725318	10.5274682	10.0183380	10.5458061	28
33	9.4545192	9.9816245	9.4729947	10.5270053	10.0183755	10.5453808	27
34	9.4550441	9.9815870	9.4734572	10.5265428	10.0184130	10.5449559	26
35	9.4554686	9.9815494	9.4739192	10.5260808	10.0184506	10.5445314	25
36	9.4558926	9.9815117	9.4743808	10.5256192	10.0184883	10.5441074	24
37	9.4563161	9.9814740	9.4748421	10.5251579	10.0185260	10.5436839	23
38	9.4567392	9.9814363	9.4753029	10.5246971	10.0185637	10.5432608	22
39	9.4571618	9.9813986	9.4757633	10.5242367	10.0186014	10.5428382	21
40	9.4575840	9.9813608	9.4762233	10.5237767	10.0186392	10.5424160	20
41	9.4580058	9.9813229	9.4766829	10.5233171	10.0186771	10.5419942	19
42	9.4584271	9.9812850	9.4771421	10.5228579	10.0187150	10.5415729	18
43	9.4588480	9.9812471	9.4776009	10.5223991	10.0187529	10.5411520	17
44	9.4592684	9.9812091	9.4780592	10.5219408	10.0187909	10.5407315	16
45	9.4596884	9.9811711	9.4785172	10.5214828	10.0188289	10.5403116	15
46	9.4601079	9.9811331	9.4789748	10.5210252	10.0188669	10.5398921	14
47	9.4605270	9.9810950	9.4794319	10.5205681	10.0189050	10.5394730	13
48	9.4609456	9.9810569	9.4798887	10.5201113	10.0189431	10.5390544	12
49	9.4613638	9.9810187	9.4803451	10.5196549	10.0189813	10.5386362	11
50	9.4617816	9.9809805	9.4808011	10.5191989	10.0190195	10.5382184	10
51	9.4621989	9.9809423	9.4812566	10.5187434	10.0190577	10.5378011	9
52	9.4626158	9.9809040	9.4817118	10.5182882	10.0190960	10.5373842	8
53	9.4630323	9.9808657	9.4821666	10.5178334	10.0191343	10.5369677	7
54	9.4634483	9.9808273	9.4826210	10.5173790	10.0191727	10.5365517	6
55	9.4638639	9.9807889	9.4830750	10.5169250	10.0192111	10.5361361	5
56	9.4642790	9.9807505	9.4835286	10.5164714	10.0192495	10.5357210	4
57	9.4646938	9.9807120	9.4839818	10.5160182	10.0192880	10.5353062	3
58	9.4651081	9.9806735	9.4844346	10.5155654	10.0193265	10.5348919	2
59	9.4655219	9.9806349	9.4848870	10.5151130	10.0193651	10.5344781	1
60	9.4659352	9.9805963	9.4853390	10.5146610	10.0194037	10.5340647	0
	Sine.		Tang.		Secant.		M

73 Degrees.

17 Degrees.

M	Sine.		Tang.		Secant.		
0	9.459353	9.980596	9.485339	10.514661	10.019403	10.534064	60
1	9.466348	9.980577	9.485790	10.514209	10.019442	10.533651	59
2	9.465760	9.980519	9.486241	10.513758	10.019481	10.533239	58
3	9.467173	9.980330	9.486692	10.513307	10.019519	10.532827	57
4	9.467584	9.980441	9.487143	10.512856	10.019558	10.532415	56
5	9.467996	9.980402	9.487593	10.512406	10.019597	10.532004	55
6	9.468406	9.980363	9.488043	10.511957	10.019636	10.531593	54
7	9.468817	9.980325	9.488492	10.511507	10.019675	10.531182	53
8	9.469227	9.980286	9.488941	10.511058	10.019714	10.530772	52
9	9.469636	9.980247	9.489389	10.510610	10.019752	10.530363	51
10	9.470045	9.980208	9.489838	10.510162	10.019791	10.529953	50
11	9.470454	9.980169	9.490288	10.509714	10.019831	10.529545	49
12	9.470863	9.980129	9.490733	10.509266	10.019870	10.529136	48
13	9.471271	9.980090	9.491180	10.508819	10.019909	10.528729	47
14	9.471678	9.980051	9.491626	10.508373	10.019948	10.528321	46
15	9.472085	9.980012	9.492073	10.507926	10.019987	10.527914	45
16	9.472492	9.979973	9.492519	10.507481	10.020026	10.527507	44
17	9.472898	9.979933	9.492964	10.507035	10.020066	10.527101	43
18	9.473304	9.979894	9.493409	10.506590	10.020105	10.526695	42
19	9.473709	9.979855	9.493855	10.506145	10.020144	10.526290	41
20	9.474114	9.979815	9.494298	10.505701	10.020184	10.525885	40
21	9.474519	9.979776	9.494742	10.505257	10.020223	10.525480	39
22	9.474923	9.979736	9.495186	10.504813	10.020263	10.525076	38
23	9.475327	9.979697	9.495629	10.504370	10.020302	10.524672	37
24	9.475730	9.979557	9.496072	10.503927	10.020342	10.524269	36
25	9.476132	9.979618	9.496515	10.503484	10.020381	10.523866	35
26	9.476535	9.979578	9.496957	10.503042	10.020421	10.523464	34
27	9.476937	9.979538	9.497399	10.502600	10.020461	10.523062	33
28	9.477339	9.979499	9.497840	10.502159	10.020500	10.522660	32
29	9.477740	9.979459	9.498281	10.501718	10.020540	10.522259	31
30	9.478141	9.979419	9.498722	10.501277	10.020580	10.521858	0
	Sine.		Tang.		Secant.		M

72 Degrees.

17 *Degrees.*

M	Sine.		Tang.		Secant.		
30	9.4781418	9.9794195	9.4987223	10.5012777	10.0205805	10.5218582	30
31	9.4785423	9.9793796	9.4991626	10.5008374	10.0206294	10.5214577	29
32	9.4789423	9.9793398	9.4996026	10.5003974	10.0206602	10.5210577	28
33	9.4793420	9.9792998	9.5000422	10.4999578	10.0207002	10.5206580	27
34	9.4797412	9.9792598	9.5004814	10.4995186	10.0207402	10.5202588	26
35	9.4801401	9.9792198	9.5009203	10.4990797	10.0207802	10.5198599	25
36	9.4805385	9.9791798	9.5013588	10.4986412	10.0208202	10.5194615	24
37	9.4809366	9.9791397	9.5017969	10.4982031	10.0208603	10.5190634	23
38	9.4813342	9.9790995	9.5022347	10.4977653	10.0209004	10.5186658	22
39	9.4817315	9.9790594	9.5026721	10.4973279	10.0209406	10.5182685	21
40	9.4821283	9.9790192	9.5031092	10.4968908	10.0209808	10.5178717	20
41	9.4825248	9.9789789	9.5035459	10.4964541	10.0210211	10.5174752	19
42	9.4829208	9.9789386	9.5039822	10.4960178	10.0210614	10.5170792	18
43	9.4833165	9.9788983	9.5044182	10.4955818	10.0211017	10.5166835	17
44	9.4837117	9.9788579	9.5048538	10.4951462	10.0211421	10.5162883	16
45	9.4841066	9.9788175	9.5052891	10.4947109	10.0211825	10.5158934	15
46	9.4845010	9.9787770	9.5057240	10.4942760	10.0212230	10.5154990	14
47	9.4848951	9.9787365	9.5061586	10.4938414	10.0212635	10.5151049	13
48	9.4852888	9.9786960	9.5065928	10.4934072	10.0213040	10.5147112	12
49	9.4856820	9.9786554	9.5070267	10.4929733	10.0213446	10.5143180	11
50	9.4860749	9.9786148	9.5074602	10.4925398	10.0213852	10.5139251	10
51	9.4864674	9.9785741	9.5078933	10.4921067	10.0214259	10.5135326	9
52	9.4868595	9.9785334	9.5083261	10.4916739	10.0214666	10.5131405	8
53	9.4872512	9.9784927	9.5087586	10.4912414	10.0215073	10.5127488	7
54	9.4876426	9.9784519	9.5091907	10.4908093	10.0215481	10.5123574	6
55	9.4880335	9.9784111	9.5096224	10.4903776	10.0215889	10.5119665	5
56	9.4884240	9.9783702	9.5100539	10.4899461	10.0216298	10.5115760	4
57	9.4888142	9.9783293	9.5104849	10.4895151	10.0216707	10.5111858	3
58	9.4892040	9.9782883	9.5109156	10.4890844	10.0217117	10.5107960	2
59	9.4895934	9.9782474	9.5113460	10.4886540	10.0217526	10.5104066	1
60	9.4899824	9.9782063	9.5117760	10.4882240	10.0217937	10.5100176	0
	Sine.		Tang.		Secant.		M

72 *Degrees.*

18 *Degrees.*

M	Sine.		Tang.		Secant.		
0	9.4899824	9.9782063	9.5117760	10.4882240	10.0217937	10.5100176	00
1	9.4903719	9.9781653	9.5122297	10.4877943	10.0218347	10.5096290	59
2	9.4907592	9.9781241	9.5125351	10.4873649	10.0218759	10.5092408	58
3	9.4911171	9.9780833	9.5130641	10.4869353	10.0219170	10.5088520	57
4	9.4915345	9.9780418	9.5134927	10.4865073	10.0219582	10.5084655	56
5	9.4915216	9.9780006	9.5139210	10.4860790	10.0219994	10.5080784	55
6	9.4923053	9.9779593	9.5143490	10.4856510	10.0220407	10.5076917	54
7	9.4926946	9.9779130	9.5147766	10.4852234	10.0220820	10.5073054	53
8	9.4930505	9.9778766	9.5152039	10.4847961	10.0221234	10.5069194	52
9	9.4934661	9.9778353	9.5156309	10.4843691	10.0221647	10.5065339	51
10	9.4938513	9.9777938	9.5160575	10.4839425	10.0222062	10.5061487	50
11	9.4942361	9.9777523	9.5164838	10.4835162	10.0222477	10.5057639	49
12	9.4946205	9.9777108	9.5169097	10.4830903	10.0222892	10.5053795	48
13	9.4950046	9.9776693	9.5173353	10.4826647	10.0223307	10.5049954	47
14	9.4953883	9.9776277	9.5177606	10.4822394	10.0223723	10.5046117	46
15	9.4957717	9.9775861	9.5181855	10.4818145	10.0224140	10.5042284	45
16	9.4961545	9.9775444	9.5186101	10.4813899	10.0224556	10.5038455	44
17	9.4965370	9.9775026	9.5190344	10.4809656	10.0224974	10.5034630	43
18	9.4969192	9.9774609	9.5194583	10.4805417	10.0225391	10.5030808	42
19	9.4973010	9.9774191	9.5198819	10.4801181	10.0225809	10.5026990	41
20	9.4976824	9.9773772	9.5203052	10.4796948	10.0226228	10.5023176	40
21	9.4980635	9.9773354	9.5207282	10.4792718	10.0226646	10.5019365	39
22	9.4984112	9.9772934	9.5211508	10.4788492	10.0227066	10.5015558	38
23	9.4988245	9.9772515	9.5215730	10.4784270	10.0227485	10.5011755	37
24	9.4992045	9.9772095	9.5219950	10.4780050	10.0227905	10.5007955	36
25	9.4995840	9.9771674	9.5224166	10.4775834	10.0228326	10.5004160	35
26	9.4999633	9.9771253	9.5228379	10.4771621	10.0228747	10.5000367	34
27	9.5003421	9.9770832	9.5232589	10.4767411	10.0229168	10.4996579	33
28	9.5007206	9.9770410	9.5236795	10.4763205	10.0229590	10.4992794	32
29	9.5010987	9.9769988	9.5240999	10.4759001	10.0230012	10.4989013	31
30	9.5014764	9.9769566	9.5245199	10.4754801	10.0230434	10.4985236	30
	Sine.		Tang.		Secant.		M

71 *Degrees.*

18 *Degrees.*

M	Sine.		Tang.		Secant.		
30	9.5014764	9.9769566	9.5245199	10.4754801	10.0230434	10.4985236	30
31	9.5018538	9.9769143	9.5249395	10.4750605	10.0230857	10.4981462	29
32	9.5022308	9.9768720	9.5253589	10.4746411	10.0231280	10.4977692	28
33	9.5026075	9.9768296	9.5257779	10.4742221	10.0231704	10.4973925	27
34	9.5029838	9.9767872	9.5261966	10.4738034	10.0232128	10.4970162	26
35	9.5033597	9.9767447	9.5266150	10.4733850	10.0232553	10.4966403	25
36	9.5037353	9.9767022	9.5270331	10.4729669	10.0232978	10.4962647	24
37	9.5041105	9.9766597	9.5274508	10.4725492	10.0233403	10.4958895	23
38	9.5044853	9.9766171	9.5278682	10.4721318	10.0233829	10.4955147	22
39	9.5048598	9.9765745	9.5282853	10.4717147	10.0234255	10.4951402	21
40	9.5052339	9.9765318	9.5287021	10.4712979	10.0234682	10.4947661	20
41	9.5056077	9.9764891	9.5291186	10.4708814	10.0235109	10.4943923	19
42	9.5059811	9.9764464	9.5295347	10.4704653	10.0235536	10.4940189	18
43	9.5063542	9.9764036	9.5299505	10.4700495	10.0235964	10.4936458	17
44	9.5067269	9.9763608	9.5303661	10.4696339	10.0236392	10.4932731	16
45	9.5070992	9.9763179	9.5307813	10.4692187	10.0236821	10.4929008	15
46	9.5074712	9.9762750	9.5311961	10.4688039	10.0237250	10.4925288	14
47	9.5078428	9.9762321	9.5316107	10.4683893	10.0237679	10.4921572	13
48	9.5082141	9.9761891	9.5320250	10.4679750	10.0238109	10.4917859	12
49	9.5085850	9.9761461	9.5324389	10.4675611	10.0238539	10.4914150	11
50	9.5089556	9.9761030	9.5328526	10.4671474	10.0238970	10.4910444	10
51	9.5093258	9.9760599	9.5332659	10.4667341	10.0239401	10.4906742	9
52	9.5096956	9.9760167	9.5336789	10.4663211	10.0239833	10.4903044	8
53	9.5100651	9.9759736	9.5340916	10.4659084	10.0240264	10.4899349	7
54	9.5104343	9.9759303	9.5345040	10.4654960	10.0240697	10.4895657	6
55	9.5108031	9.9758870	9.5349161	10.4650839	10.0241130	10.4891969	5
56	9.5111716	9.9758437	9.5353278	10.4646722	10.0241563	10.4888284	4
57	9.5115397	9.9758004	9.5357393	10.4642607	10.0241996	10.4884603	3
58	9.5119074	9.9757570	9.5361505	10.4638495	10.0242430	10.4880926	2
59	9.5122749	9.9757135	9.5365613	10.4634387	10.0242865	10.4877251	1
60	9.5126419	9.9756701	9.5369719	10.4630281	10.0243299	10.4873581	0
	Sine.		Tang.		Secant.		M

71 *Degrees.*

Kkk 2

19 Degrees.

M	Sine.		Tang.		Secant.		
0	9.5126419	9.9756701	9.5369719	10.4630281	10.0243299	10.4873581	57
1	9.5130086	9.9756265	9.5373821	10.4626179	10.0243735	10.4869914	59
2	9.5133750	9.9755830	9.5377920	10.4622080	10.0244170	10.4866250	58
3	9.5137410	9.9755394	9.5382017	10.4617983	10.0244606	10.4862590	57
4	9.5141067	9.9754957	9.5386110	10.4613890	10.0245403	10.4858933	56
5	9.5144721	9.9754521	9.5390200	10.4609800	10.0245479	10.4855279	55
6	9.5148371	9.9754083	9.5394287	10.4605713	10.0245917	10.4851629	54
7	9.5152011	9.9753646	9.5398371	10.4601629	10.0246354	10.4847983	53
8	9.5155669	9.9753208	9.5402453	10.4597547	10.0246792	10.4844340	52
9	9.5159300	9.9752769	9.5406531	10.4593469	10.0247231	10.4840700	51
10	9.5162936	9.9752330	9.5410606	10.4589394	10.0247670	10.4837064	50
11	9.5166565	9.9751891	9.5414678	10.4585322	10.0248109	10.4833431	49
12	9.5170198	9.9751451	9.5418747	10.4581253	10.0248549	10.4829802	48
13	9.5173824	9.9751011	9.5422813	10.4577187	10.0248989	10.4826176	47
14	9.5177447	9.9750570	9.5426877	10.4573123	10.0249430	10.4822553	46
15	9.5181066	9.9750129	9.5430937	10.4569063	10.0249871	10.4818934	45
16	9.5184682	9.9749688	9.5434994	10.4565006	10.0250312	10.4815318	44
17	9.5188295	9.9749246	9.5439048	10.4560952	10.0250754	10.4811705	43
18	9.5191904	9.9748804	9.5443100	10.4556900	10.0251196	10.4808096	42
19	9.5195510	9.9748361	9.5447148	10.4552852	10.0251639	10.4804490	41
20	9.5199112	9.9747918	9.5451193	10.4548807	10.0252082	10.4800888	40
21	9.5202711	9.9747475	9.5455236	10.4544764	10.0252525	10.4797289	39
22	9.5206307	9.9747031	9.5459276	10.4540724	10.0252969	10.4793693	38
23	9.5209899	9.9746587	9.5463312	10.4536688	10.0253413	10.4790101	37
24	9.5213488	9.9746142	9.5467346	10.4532654	10.0253858	10.4786512	36
25	9.5217074	9.9745697	9.5471377	10.4528623	10.0254303	10.4782926	35
26	9.5220656	9.9745252	9.5475405	10.4524595	10.0254748	10.4779344	34
27	9.5224235	9.9744806	9.5479430	10.4520570	10.0255194	10.4775765	33
28	9.5227811	9.9744359	9.5483452	10.4516548	10.0255641	10.4772189	32
29	9.5231383	9.9743913	9.5487471	10.4512529	10.0256608	10.4768617	31
30	9.5234952	9.9743466	9.5491487	10.4508513	10.0256534	10.4765047	30
	Sine.		Tang.		Secant.		M

70 Degrees.

19 Degrees.

M	Sine.		Tang.		Secant.		
30	9.5234953	9.9743466	9.5491487	10.4508513	10.0256534	10.4765247	30
31	9.5238518	9.9743018	9.5495500	10.4504500	10.0256982	10.476148.	29
32	9.5242081	9.9742570	9.5499511	10.4500489	10.0257430	10.475791;	28
33	9.5245640	9.9742122	9.5503519	10.4496481	10.0257878	10.4754360	27
34	9.5249196	9.9741673	9.5507523	10.4492477	10.0258327	10.4750804	26
35	9.5252749	9.9741224	9.5511525	10.4488475	10.0258776	10.4747251	25
36	9.5256298	9.9740774	9.5515524	10.4484476	10.0259226	10.4743702	24
37	9.5259844	9.9740324	9.5519521	10.4480479	10.0259676	10.4740156	23
38	9.5263387	9.9739873	9.5523514	10.4476486	10.0260127	10.4736613	22
39	9.5266927	9.9739422	9.5527504	10.4472496	10.0260578	10.4733073	21
40	9.5270463	9.9738971	9.5531492	10.4468508	10.0261029	10.4729537	20
41	9.5273997	9.9738519	9.5535477	10.4464523	10.0261481	10.4726003	19
42	9.5277526	9.9738067	9.5539459	10.4460541	10.0261933	10.4722474	18
43	9.5281053	9.9737615	9.5543438	10.4456562	10.0262385	10.4718947	17
44	9.5284577	9.9737162	9.5547415	10.4452585	10.0262838	10.4715423	16
45	9.5288097	9.9736709	9.5551388	10.4448612	10.0263291	10.4711903	15
46	9.5291614	9.9736255	9.5555359	10.4444641	10.0263745	10.4708386	14
47	9.5295128	9.9735801	9.5559327	10.4440673	10.0264199	10.4704872	13
48	9.5298638	9.9735346	9.5563292	10.4436708	10.0264654	10.4701362	12
49	9.5302146	9.9734891	9.5567255	10.4432745	10.0265109	10.4697854	11
50	9.5305650	9.9734435	9.5571214	10.4428786	10.0265565	10.4694350	10
51	9.5309151	9.9733980	9.5575171	10.4424829	10.0266020	10.4690849	9
52	9.5312649	9.9733523	9.5579125	10.4420875	10.0266477	10.4687351	8
53	9.5316143	9.9733067	9.5583077	10.4416923	10.0266933	10.4683857	7
54	9.5319635	9.9732610	9.5587025	10.4412975	10.0267390	10.4680365	6
55	9.5323123	9.9732152	9.5590971	10.4409029	10.0267848	10.4676877	5
56	9.5326608	9.9731694	9.5594914	10.4405086	10.0268306	10.4673392	4
57	9.5330090	9.9731236	9.5598854	10.4401146	10.0268764	10.4669910	3
58	9.5333569	9.9730777	9.5602792	10.4397208	10.0269223	10.4666431	2
59	9.5337044	9.9730318	9.5606727	10.4393273	10.0269682	10.4662956	1
60	9.5340517	9.9729858	9.5610659	10.4389341	10.0270142	10.4659483	0
	Sine.		Tang.		Secant.		M

70 Degrees.

20 Degrees.

M	Sine.		Tang.		Secant.		
0	9.5340517	9.9729358	9.5610659	10.4389341	10.0270142	10.4659483	60
1	9.5343586	9.9729395	9.5614588	10.4385412	10.0270602	10.4656014	59
2	9.5347452	9.9728938	9.5618515	10.4381485	10.0271062	10.4652548	58
3	9.5350915	9.9728477	9.5622439	10.4377561	10.0271523	10.4649085	57
4	9.5354375	9.9728016	9.5626360	10.4373640	10.0271984	10.4645625	56
5	9.5357532	9.9727554	9.5630278	10.4369722	10.0272446	10.4642168	55
6	9.5361286	9.9727092	9.5634194	10.4365806	10.0272908	10.4638714	54
7	9.5364737	9.9726629	9.5638107	10.4361893	10.0273371	10.4635263	53
8	9.5368184	9.9726166	9.5642018	10.4357982	10.0273834	10.4631816	52
9	9.5371623	9.9725703	9.5645925	10.4354075	10.0274297	10.4628372	51
10	9.5375070	9.9725239	9.5649831	10.4350169	10.0274761	10.4624930	50
11	9.5378505	9.9724775	9.5653733	10.4346267	10.0275225	10.4621492	49
12	9.5381943	9.9724310	9.5657633	10.4342367	10.0275690	10.4618057	48
13	9.5385375	9.9723845	9.5661530	10.4338470	10.0276155	10.4614625	47
14	9.5388805	9.9723380	9.5665424	10.4334576	10.0276620	10.4611196	46
15	9.5392230	9.9722914	9.5669316	10.4330684	10.0277086	10.4607770	45
16	9.5395653	9.9722448	9.5673205	10.4326795	10.0277552	10.4604347	44
17	9.5399073	9.9721981	9.5677091	10.4322909	10.0278019	10.4600927	43
18	9.5402489	9.9721514	9.5680975	10.4319025	10.0278486	10.4597511	42
19	9.5405903	9.9721047	9.5684856	10.4315144	10.0278953	10.4594097	41
20	9.5409314	9.9720579	9.5688735	10.4311265	10.0279421	10.4590686	40
21	9.5412721	9.9720110	9.5692611	10.4307389	10.0279890	10.4587279	39
22	9.5416126	9.9719642	9.5696484	10.4303516	10.0280358	10.4583874	38
23	9.5419527	9.9719172	9.5700355	10.4299645	10.0280828	10.4580473	37
24	9.5422926	9.9718703	9.5704223	10.4295777	10.0281297	10.4577074	36
25	9.5426321	9.9718233	9.5708088	10.4291912	10.0281767	10.4573679	35
26	9.5429713	9.9717762	9.5711951	10.4288049	10.0282238	10.4570287	34
27	9.5433103	9.9717291	9.5715811	10.4284189	10.0282709	10.4566897	33
28	9.5436489	9.9716820	9.5719669	10.4280331	10.0283180	10.4563511	32
29	9.5439873	9.9716348	9.5723524	10.4276476	10.0283652	10.4560127	31
30	9.5443253	9.9715876	9.5727377	10.4272623	10.0284124	10.4556747	30
	Sine.		Tang.		Secant.		M

69 Degrees.

20 *Degrees.*

M	Sine.		Tang.		Secant.		
30	9.544325	9.971587	9.5727377	10.427262	10.0284124	10.4556747	30
31	9.544663	9.971540	9.5731227	10.426877	10.0284594	10.455337	29
32	9.545000	9.9714931	9.5735074	10.4249492	10.0235069	10.454999	28
33	9.5453376	9.9714457	9.5738919	10.4261081	10.0285543	10.4546242	27
34	9.5456749	9.9713984	9.5742761	10.4257239	10.0286016	10.4543255	26
35	9.5460110	9.9713509	9.5746601	10.4253399	10.0286491	10.4539850	25
36	9.5463472	9.9713035	9.5750438	10.424956	10.0286965	10.4536528	24
37	9.5466832	9.9712560	9.5754272	10.4245728	10.0287440	10.4533168	23
38	9.5470189	9.9712084	9.5758104	10.4241896	10.0287916	10.4529811	22
39	9.5473542	9.9711608	9.5761934	10.4238066	10.0288392	10.4526458	21
40	9.5476893	9.9711132	9.5765761	10.4234239	10.0288868	10.4523107	20
41	9.5480240	9.9710655	9.5769585	10.4230415	10.0289345	10.4519760	19
42	9.5483585	9.9710178	9.5773407	10.4226593	10.0289822	10.4516415	18
43	9.5486927	9.9709701	9.5777226	10.4222774	10.0290299	10.4513073	17
44	9.5490267	9.9709223	9.5781043	10.4218957	10.0290777	10.4509733	16
45	9.5493602	9.9708744	9.5784858	10.4215142	10.0291256	10.4506398	15
46	9.5496935	9.9708265	9.5788669	10.4211331	10.0291735	10.4503065	14
47	9.5500265	9.9707786	9.5792479	10.4207521	10.0292214	10.4499735	13
48	9.5503592	9.9707306	9.5796286	10.4203714	10.0292694	10.4496408	12
49	9.5506916	9.9706826	9.5800090	10.4199910	10.0293174	10.4493084	11
50	9.5510237	9.9706346	9.5803892	10.4196108	10.0293654	10.4489763	10
51	9.5513556	9.9705865	9.5807691	10.4192309	10.0294135	10.4486444	9
52	9.5516871	9.9705383	9.5811488	10.4188512	10.0294617	10.4483129	8
53	9.5520184	9.9704902	9.5815282	10.4184718	10.0295098	10.4479816	7
54	9.5523494	9.9704415	9.5819074	10.4180926	10.0295581	10.4476506	6
55	9.5526801	9.9703937	9.5822864	10.4177136	10.0296063	10.4473199	5
56	9.5530105	9.9703454	9.5826651	10.4173349	10.0296546	10.4469895	4
57	9.5533406	9.9702971	9.5830435	10.4169565	10.0297030	10.4466594	3
58	9.5536704	9.9702486	9.5834217	10.4165783	10.0297514	10.4463296	2
59	9.5539999	9.9702002	9.5837997	10.4162003	10.0297998	10.4460001	1
60	9.5543292	9.9701517	9.5841774	10.4158226	10.0298483	10.4456708	0
	Sine.		Tang.		Secant.		

69 *Degrees.*

21 Degrees.

M	Sine.		Tang.		Secant.		
0	9.554329	9.9701517	9.5841774	10.4158226	10.0298483	10.4456708	60
1	9.554658	9.9701032	9.5845549	10.4154451	10.0298968	10.4453415	59
2	9.554986	9.9700547	9.5849321	10.4150679	10.0299453	10.4450132	58
3	9.555314	9.9700061	9.5853091	10.4146909	10.0299939	10.4446848	57
4	9.555643	9.9699574	9.5856859	10.4143141	10.0300426	10.4443567	56
5	9.555971	9.9699087	9.5860624	10.4139376	10.0300913	10.4440289	55
6	9.556298	9.9698600	9.5864386	10.4135614	10.0301400	10.4437013	54
7	9.556625	9.9698112	9.5868147	10.4131853	10.0301888	10.4433741	53
8	9.556952	9.9697624	9.5871904	10.4128096	10.0302376	10.4430471	52
9	9.557279	9.9697136	9.5875660	10.4124340	10.0302864	10.4427204	51
10	9.557606	9.9696647	9.5879413	10.4120587	10.0303353	10.4423940	50
11	9.557932	9.9696158	9.5883163	10.4116837	10.0303842	10.4420679	49
12	9.558257	9.9695668	9.5886912	10.4113088	10.0304332	10.4417421	48
13	9.558583	9.9695177	9.5890657	10.4109343	10.0304823	10.4414165	47
14	9.558908	9.9694687	9.5894401	10.4105599	10.0305313	10.4410912	46
15	9.559233	9.9694196	9.5898142	10.4101858	10.0305804	10.4407662	45
16	9.559558	9.9693704	9.5901881	10.4098119	10.0306296	10.4404415	44
17	9.559882	9.9693212	9.5905617	10.4094383	10.0306788	10.4401171	43
18	9.560207	9.9692720	9.5909351	10.4090649	10.0307280	10.4397929	42
19	9.560531	9.9692227	9.5913082	10.4086918	10.0307773	10.4394690	41
20	9.560854	9.9691734	9.5916812	10.4083188	10.0308266	10.4391454	40
21	9.561177	9.9691241	9.5920539	10.4079461	10.0308759	10.4388221	39
22	9.561501	9.9690746	9.5924263	10.4075737	10.0309254	10.4384990	38
23	9.561823	9.9690252	9.5927985	10.4072015	10.0309748	10.4381762	37
24	9.562146	9.9689757	9.5931705	10.4068295	10.0310243	10.4378538	36
25	9.562468	9.9689262	9.5935423	10.4064577	10.0310738	10.4375315	35
26	9.562790	9.9688766	9.5939138	10.4060862	10.0311234	10.4372096	34
27	9.563112	9.9688270	9.5942851	10.4057149	10.0311730	10.4368879	33
28	9.563433	9.9687773	9.5946561	10.4053439	10.0312227	10.4365665	32
29	9.563754	9.9687276	9.5950269	10.4049731	10.0312724	10.4362454	31
30	9.564075	9.9686779	9.5953975	10.4046025	10.0313221	10.4359246	30
	Sine.		Tang.		Secant.		M

68 Degrees.

21 *Degrees.*

M	Sine.		Tang.		Secant.		
30	9.5640754	9.9686779	9.5953975	10.4046025	10.0313221	10.4359246	30
31	9.5643968	9.9686281	9.5957679	10.4042321	10.0313719	10.4356040	29
32	9.5647164	9.9685783	9.596138c	10.4038620	10.0314217	10.4352837	28
33	9.5650362	9.9685284	9.5965079	10.4034921	10.0314716	10.4349637	27
34	9.5653561	9.9684785	9.5958776	10.4031224	10.0315215	10.4346439	26
35	9.5656756	9.9684286	9.5972470	10.4027530	10.0315714	10.4343244	25
36	9.5659948	9.9683786	9.5976162	10.4023838	10.0316214	10.4340052	24
37	9.5663137	9.9683285	9.5979852	10.4020148	10.0316715	10.4336863	23
38	9.5666324	9.9682784	9.5983540	10.4016460	10.0317216	10.4333676	22
39	9.5669508	9.9682283	9.5987225	10.4012775	10.0317717	10.4330492	21
40	9.5672689	9.9681781	9.5990908	10.4009092	10.0318219	10.4327311	20
41	9.5675868	9.9681279	9.5994588	10.4005412	10.0318721	10.4324132	19
42	9.5679044	9.9680777	9.5998267	10.4001733	10.0319223	10.4320956	18
43	9.5682217	9.9680274	9.6001943	10.3998057	10.0319726	10.4317783	17
44	9.5685387	9.9679771	9.6005617	10.3994383	10.0320229	10.4314613	16
45	9.5688555	9.9679267	9.6009289	10.3990711	10.0320733	10.4311445	15
46	9.5691721	9.9678763	9.6012958	10.3987042	10.0321237	10.4308279	14
47	9.5694883	9.9678258	9.6016625	10.3983375	10.0321742	10.4305117	13
48	9.5698043	9.9677753	9.6020290	10.3979710	10.0322247	10.4301957	12
49	9.5701200	9.9677247	9.6023953	10.3976047	10.0322753	10.4298800	11
50	9.5704355	9.9676741	9.6027613	10.3972387	10.0323259	10.4295645	10
51	9.5707506	9.9676235	9.6031271	10.3968729	10.0323765	10.4292494	9
52	9.5710656	9.9675728	9.6034927	10.3965073	10.0324272	10.4289344	8
53	9.5713802	9.9675221	9.6038581	10.3961419	10.0324779	10.4286198	7
54	9.5716946	9.9674713	9.6042233	10.3957767	10.0325287	10.4283054	6
55	9.5720087	9.9674205	9.6045882	10.3954118	10.0325795	10.4279913	5
56	9.5723226	9.9673697	9.6049529	10.3950471	10.0326303	10.4276774	4
57	9.5726362	9.9673188	9.6053174	10.3946826	10.0326812	10.4273638	3
58	9.5729495	9.9672679	9.6056817	10.3943183	10.0327321	10.4270505	2
59	9.5732626	9.9672169	9.6060457	10.3939543	10.0327831	10.4267374	1
60	9.5735754	9.9671659	9.6064096	10.3935904	10.0328341	10.4264246	0
	Sine.		Tang.		Secant.		M

68 *Degrees.*

22 Degrees.

M	Sine.		Tang.		Secant.		M
0	9.5735754	9.9671659	9.6064096	10.3935904	10.0328341	10.4264246	60
1	9.5738880	9.9671645	9.6067732	10.3932268	10.0328852	10.4261120	59
2	9.5742003	9.9970537	9.6071366	10.3928634	10.0329363	10.4257997	58
3	9.5745123	9.9670125	9.6074997	10.3925003	10.0329875	10.4254877	57
4	9.5748243	9.9669514	9.6078627	10.3921373	10.0330386	10.4251750	56
5	9.5751355	9.9669101	9.6082254	10.3917746	10.0330899	10.4248644	55
6	9.5754465	9.9668595	9.6085880	10.3914120	10.0331412	10.4245532	54
7	9.5757573	9.9668075	9.6089503	10.3910497	10.0331925	10.4242422	53
8	9.5760680	9.9667552	9.6093124	10.3906876	10.0332438	10.4239315	52
9	9.5763790	9.9667048	9.6096742	10.3903258	10.0332952	10.4236210	51
10	9.5766892	9.9666533	9.6100359	10.3899641	10.0333467	10.4233108	50
11	9.5769991	9.9666015	9.6103973	10.3896027	10.0333982	10.4230009	49
12	9.5773088	9.9665503	9.6107586	10.3892414	10.0334497	10.4226912	48
13	9.5776181	9.9664987	9.6111196	10.3888804	10.0335013	10.4223817	47
14	9.5779275	9.9664471	9.6114804	10.3885196	10.0335529	10.4220725	46
15	9.5782364	9.9663954	9.6118409	10.3881591	10.0336046	10.4217636	45
16	9.5785454	9.9663437	9.6122013	10.3877987	10.0336563	10.4214550	44
17	9.5788535	9.9662920	9.6125615	10.3874385	10.0337080	10.4211465	43
18	9.5791616	9.9662402	9.6129214	10.3870786	10.0337598	10.4208384	42
19	9.5794695	9.9661884	9.6132812	10.3867188	10.0338116	10.4205305	41
20	9.5797772	9.9661365	9.6136407	10.3863593	10.0338635	10.4202228	40
21	9.5800846	9.9660846	9.6140000	10.3860000	10.0339154	10.4199155	39
22	9.5803917	9.9660326	9.6143591	10.3856409	10.0339674	10.4196083	38
23	9.5806984	9.9659806	9.6147180	10.3852820	10.0340194	10.4193016	37
24	9.5810052	9.9659285	9.6150766	10.3849234	10.0340715	10.4189948	36
25	9.5813116	9.9658764	9.6154351	10.3845649	10.0341236	10.4186884	35
26	9.5816177	9.9658243	9.6157934	10.3842066	10.0341757	10.4183823	34
27	9.5819236	9.9657721	9.6161514	10.3838486	10.0342279	10.4180764	33
28	9.5822292	9.9657199	9.6165093	10.3834907	10.0342801	10.4177708	32
29	9.5825345	9.9656677	9.6168669	10.3831331	10.0343323	10.4174655	31
30	9.5828397	9.9656153	9.6172243	10.3827757	10.0343847	10.4171603	30

| | Sine | | Tang. | | Secant. | | M |

67 Degrees.

22 *Degrees.*

M	Sine.		Tang.		Secant.		
30	9.5828397	9.9656155	9.6172243	10.3827757	10.0343847	10.0417160 3	30
31	9.5831445	9.9655630	9.6175815	10.3824185	10.0344370	10.4168555	29
32	9.5834491	9.9655100	9.6179385	10.3820615	10.0344894	10.4165509	28
33	9.5837535	9.965458	9.6182953	10.3817047	10.0345418	10.4162465	27
34	9.5840576	9.9654052	9.6186519	10.3813481	10.0345943	10.4159424	26
35	9.5843615	9.9653653	9.6190083	10.3809917	10.0346468	10.4156385	25
36	9.5846651	9.9653000	9.6193645	10.3806355	10.0346994	10.4153349	24
37	9.5849681	9.9652480	9.6197205	10.3802795	10.0347520	10.4150315	23
38	9.5852716	9.9651953	9.6200762	10.3799238	10.0348047	10.4147284	22
39	9.5855745	9.9651426	9.6204318	10.3795682	10.0348574	10.4144255	21
40	9.5858771	9.9650899	9.6207872	10.3792128	10.0349101	10.4141229	20
41	9.5861795	9.9650371	9.6211423	10.3788577	10.0349629	10.4138205	19
42	9.5864816	9.9649843	9.6214974	10.3785026	10.0350157	10.4135184	18
43	9.5867836	9.9649314	9.6218520	10.3781480	10.0350686	10.4132165	17
44	9.5870851	9.9648785	9.6222066	10.3777934	10.0351215	10.4129149	16
45	9.5873865	9.9648256	9.6225609	10.3774391	10.0351744	10.4126135	15
46	9.5876876	9.9647726	9.6229150	10.3770850	10.0352274	10.4123124	14
47	9.5879885	9.9647195	9.6232690	10.3767310	10.0352805	10.4120115	13
48	9.5882892	9.9646664	9.6236227	10.3763773	10.0353335	10.4117108	12
49	9.5885896	9.9646133	9.6239763	10.3760237	10.0353867	10.4114104	11
50	9.5888897	9.9645602	9.6243296	10.3756704	10.0354398	10.4111103	10
51	9.5891897	9.9645069	9.6246827	10.3753173	10.0354931	10.4108103	9
52	9.5894893	9.9644537	9.6250356	10.3749644	10.0355463	10.4105107	8
53	9.5897888	9.9644004	9.6253884	10.3746116	10.0355996	10.4102112	7
54	9.5900880	9.9643470	9.6257409	10.3742591	10.0356530	10.4099120	6
55	9.5903869	9.9642937	9.6260932	10.3739068	10.0357063	10.4096131	5
56	9.5906856	9.9642402	9.6264454	10.3735546	10.0357598	10.4093144	2
57	9.5909841	9.9641868	9.6267973	10.3732027	10.0358132	10.4090159	3
58	9.5912823	9.9641332	9.6271491	10.3728509	10.0358668	10.4087177	4
59	9.5915803	9.9640797	9.6275006	10.3724994	10.0359203	10.4084197	1
60	9.5918780	9.9640261	9.6278519	10.3721481	10.0359739	10.4081220	0
	Sine.		Tang.		Secant.		M

67 *Degrees.*

23 *Degrees.*

M	Sine.		Tang.		Secant.		
0	9.591878c	9.9640261	9.6278519	10.3721481	10.0359739	10.408122c	6c
1	9.5921755	9.9639724	9.6282031	10.3717969	10.0360276	10.4078245	59
2	9.5924728	9.9639187	9.628554c	10.3714460	10.0360813	10.4075272	58
3	9.5927698	9.9638650	9.6289045	10.3710952	10.036135c	10.40723 2	57
4	9.5930666	9.9638112	9.6292553	10.3707447	10.0361888	10.406933c	56
5	9.5933631	9.9637574	9.6296057	10.3703943	10.0362426	10.406636c	55
6	9.5936594	9.9637036	9.6299558	10.3700442	10.0362964	10.406340c	54
7	9.5939555	9.9636496	9.6303058	10.3696942	10.0363504	10.406044c	53
8	9.5942513	9.9635957	9.6306556	10.3693444	10.0364043	10.4057487	52
9	9.5945469	9.9635417	9.6310052	10.3689948	10.0364583	10.4054531	51
10	9.5948422	9.9634877	9.6313545	10.3686455	10.0365123	10.4051578	5c
11	9.5951373	9.9634336	9.6317037	10.3682963	10.0365664	10.4048627	49
12	9.5954322	9.9633795	9.6320527	10.3679473	10.0366205	10.4045678	48
13	9.5957268	9.9633253	9.6324015	10.3675985	10.0366747	10.4042732	47
14	9.5960212	9.9632711	9.6327501	10.3672499	10.0367289	10.403978t	46
15	9.5963154	9.9632168	7.6330985	10.3669015	1c.0367832	10.4036846	45
16	9.5966093	9.9631625	9.6334468	10.3665532	10.0368375	10.4033907	44
17	9.5969030	9.9631082	9.6337948	10.3662052	10.0368918	10.403097c	43
18	9.5971965	9.963053t	9.6341426	10.3658574	10.0369462	1c.4028035	42
19	9.5974897	9.9629994	9.6344903	10.3655097	10.0370006	10.4025103	41
20	9.5977827	9.9629449	9.6348378	10.3651622	10.0370551	10.4022173	40
21	9.5980754	9.9628904	9.6351850	10.3648150	10.0371096	10.4019246	39
22	9.5983679	9.962835t	9.6355321	10.3644679	10.0371642	10.4016321	38
23	9.5986602	9.9627812	9.6358790	10.3641210	10.0372188	10.4013398	37
24	9.5989523	9.9627266	9.6362257	10.3637743	1c.0372734	1c.4010477	36
25	9.5992441	9.9626719	9.6365722	10.3634278	10.0373281	10.4007559	35
26	9.5995357	9.9626172	9.6369185	10.3630815	10.0373828	10.4004643	34
27	9.5998270	9.9625624	9.6372646	10.3627354	10.0374376	10.4001730	33
28	9.6001181	9.9625076	9.6376106	10.3623894	10.0374924	10.3998819	32
29	9.6004090	9.9624527	9.6379563	10.3620437	10.0375473	10.3995910	31
30	9.6006997	9.9623978	9.6383019	10.3616981	10.0376022	10.3993003	3c
		Sine		Tang.		Secant.	M

66 *Degrees.*

23 Degrees.

M	Sine.		Tang.		Secant.		M
30	9.6006997	9.9623978	9.6383019	10.3616981	10.0376022	10.3993003	30
31	9.6009901	9.9623428	9.6386473	10.3613527	10.0376572	10.3990099	29
32	9.6012803	9.9622878	9.6389925	10.3610075	10.0377122	10.3987197	28
33	9.6015703	9.9622328	9.6393375	10.3606625	10.0377672	10.3984297	27
34	9.6018600	9.9621777	9.6396823	10.3603177	10.0378223	10.3981400	26
35	9.6021496	9.9621226	9.6400269	10.3599731	10.0378774	10.3978505	25
36	9.6024388	9.9620674	9.6403714	10.3596286	10.0379326	10.3975614	24
37	9.6027278	9.9620122	9.6407156	10.3592844	10.0379878	10.3972722	23
38	9.6030166	9.9619569	9.6410597	10.3589403	10.0380431	10.3969834	22
39	9.6033052	9.9619016	9.6414036	10.3585964	10.0380984	10.3966948	21
40	9.6035936	9.9618463	9.6417473	10.3582527	10.0381537	10.3964064	20
41	9.6038817	9.9617909	9.6420908	10.3579092	10.0382091	10.3961183	19
42	9.6041696	9.9617355	9.6424342	10.3575658	10.0382645	10.3958304	18
43	9.6044573	9.9616800	9.6427773	10.3572227	10.0383200	10.3955427	17
44	9.6047448	9.9616245	9.6431203	10.3568797	10.0383755	10.3952552	16
45	9.6050320	9.9615689	9.6434631	10.3565369	10.0384311	10.3949680	15
46	9.6053190	9.9615133	9.6438057	10.3561943	10.0384867	10.3946810	14
47	9.6056057	9.9614576	9.6441481	10.3558519	10.0385424	10.3943943	13
48	9.6058923	9.9614020	9.6444903	10.3555097	10.0385980	10.3941077	12
49	9.6061786	9.9613462	9.6448324	10.3551676	10.0386538	10.3938214	11
50	9.6064647	9.9612904	9.6451743	10.3548257	10.0387096	10.3935353	10
51	9.6067506	9.9612345	9.6455160	10.3544840	10.0387655	10.3932494	9
52	9.6070362	9.9611787	9.6458575	10.3541425	10.0388213	10.3929638	8
53	9.6073216	9.9611228	9.6461988	10.3538012	10.0388772	10.3926784	7
54	9.6076068	9.9610668	9.6465400	10.3534600	10.0389332	10.3923932	6
55	9.6078918	9.9610108	9.6468810	10.3531190	10.0389892	10.3921082	5
56	9.6081765	9.9609548	9.6472217	10.3527783	10.0390452	10.3918235	4
57	9.6084611	9.9608987	9.6475624	10.3524376	10.0391013	10.3915389	3
58	9.6087454	9.9608426	9.6479028	10.3520972	10.0391574	10.3912546	2
59	9.6090294	9.9607864	9.6482431	10.3517569	10.0392136	10.3909706	1
60	9.6093133	9.9607302	9.6485831	10.3514169	10.0392698	10.3906867	0
	Sine.		Tang.		Secant.		M

66 Degrees.

24 *Degrees.*

M	Sine.		Tang.		Secant.		
0	9.6093133	9.9607302	9.6485851	10.3514169	10.039269	10.390686	60
1	9.6095969	9.9606739	9.6489230	10.3510770	10.0393326	10.390403	59
2	9.6098803	9.9606176	9.6492626	10.3507372	10.0393824	10.390119	58
3	9.6101635	9.9605612	9.6496023	10.3503977	10.0394388	10.389836	57
4	9.6104465	9.9605048	9.6499741	10.3500583	10.0394952	10.389553	56
5	9.6107293	9.9604483	9.6502809	10.3497191	10.0395516	10.389270	55
6	9.6110118	9.9603919	9.6506199	10.3493801	10.0396081	10.388988	54
7	9.6112941	9.9603354	9.6509587	10.3490413	10.0396646	10.388705	53
8	9.6115762	9.9602788	9.6512974	10.3487026	10.0397212	10.388423	52
9	9.6118581	9.9602222	9.6516359	10.3483641	10.0397779	10.388142	51
10	9.6121397	9.9601655	9.6519744	10.3480256	10.0398345	10.387850	50
11	9.6124211	9.9601088	9.6523123	10.3476877	10.0398912	10.387578	49
12	9.6127023	9.9600520	9.6526503	10.3473497	10.0399480	10.387297	48
13	9.6129833	9.9599952	9.6529881	10.3470119	10.0400048	10.387016	47
14	9.6132641	9.9599384	9.6533257	10.3466743	10.0400616	10.386735	46
15	9.6135446	9.9598815	9.6536631	10.3463369	10.0401185	10.386455	45
16	9.6138250	9.9598246	9.6540004	10.3459996	10.0401754	10.386175	44
17	9.6141051	9.9597676	9.6543375	10.3456625	10.0402324	10.385894	43
18	9.6143850	9.9597106	9.6546744	10.3453256	10.0402894	10.385615	42
19	9.6146647	9.9596535	9.6550112	10.3449888	10.0403465	10.385335	41
20	9.6149441	9.9595964	9.6553477	10.3446523	10.0404036	10.385055	40
21	9.6152234	9.9595393	9.6556841	10.3443159	10.0404607	10.384776	39
22	9.6155024	9.9594821	9.6560204	10.3439796	10.0405179	10.384497	38
23	9.6157814	9.9594248	9.6563564	10.3436436	10.0405752	10.384218	37
24	9.6160599	9.9593675	9.6566923	10.3433077	10.0406325	10.383940	36
25	9.6163383	9.9593102	9.6570280	10.3429720	10.0406898	10.383651	35
26	9.6166164	9.9592528	9.6573636	10.3426364	10.0407472	10.383383	34
27	9.6168944	9.9591954	9.6576989	10.3423011	10.0408046	10.383105	33
28	9.6171721	9.9591380	9.6580341	10.3419659	10.0408520	10.382827	32
29	9.6174495	9.9590804	9.6583692	10.3416308	10.0409195	10.382550	31
30	9.6177270	9.9590229	9.6587041	10.3412955	10.0409771	10.382273	30
	Sine.		Tang.		Secant.		M

65 *Degrees.*

24 Degrees.

M	Sine.		Tang.		Secant.		M
30	9.6177270	9.9590229	9.6587041	10.3412959	10.0403771	10.3822730	30
31	9.6180041	9.9589653	9.6590387	10.3409613	10.0410347	10.3819955	29
32	9.6182809	9.9589077	9.6593733	10.3406257	10.0410923	10.3817191	28
33	9.6185576	9.9588502	9.6597076	10.3402924	10.0411500	10.3814424	27
34	9.6188341	9.9587923	9.6600418	10.3399582	10.0412077	10.3811659	26
35	9.6191103	9.9587345	9.6603758	10.3396242	10.0412655	10.3808897	25
36	9.6193864	9.9586767	9.6607097	10.3392903	10.0413233	10.3806136	24
37	9.6196622	9.9586188	9.6610434	10.3389566	10.0413812	10.3803378	23
38	9.6199378	9.9585609	9.6613769	10.3386231	10.0414391	10.3800622	22
39	9.6202132	9.9585030	9.6617103	10.3382897	10.0414970	10.3797868	21
40	9.6204884	9.9584450	9.6620434	10.3379566	10.0415550	10.3795116	20
41	9.6207634	9.9583869	9.6623765	10.3376235	10.0416131	10.3792366	19
42	9.6210382	9.9583288	9.6627093	10.3372907	10.0416712	10.3789618	18
43	9.6213127	9.9582707	9.6630420	10.3369580	10.0417293	10.3786873	17
44	9.6215871	9.9582125	9.6633745	10.3366255	10.0417875	10.3784129	16
45	9.6218612	9.9581543	9.6637069	10.3362931	10.0418457	10.3781388	15
46	9.6221351	9.9580961	9.6640391	10.3359609	10.0419039	10.3778649	14
47	9.6224088	9.9580378	9.6643711	10.3356289	10.0419622	10.3775912	13
48	9.6226824	9.9579794	9.6647030	10.3352970	10.0420206	10.3773176	12
49	9.6229557	9.9579210	9.6650346	10.3349654	10.0420790	10.3770443	11
50	9.6232287	9.9578626	9.6653662	10.3346338	10.0421374	10.3767713	10
51	9.6235016	9.9578041	9.6656975	10.3343025	10.0421959	10.3764984	9
52	9.6237743	9.9577456	9.6660288	10.3339712	10.0422544	10.3762257	8
53	9.6240468	9.9576870	9.6663598	10.3336402	10.0423130	10.3759532	7
54	9.6243190	9.9576284	9.6666907	10.3333093	10.0423716	10.3756810	6
55	9.6245911	9.9575697	9.6670214	10.3329786	10.0424303	10.3754089	5
56	9.6248629	9.9575110	9.6673519	10.3326481	10.0424890	10.3751371	4
57	9.6251346	9.9574522	9.6676822	10.3323177	10.0425478	10.3748654	3
58	9.6254060	9.9573934	9.6680126	10.3319874	10.0426066	10.3745940	2
59	9.6256772	9.9573346	9.6683426	10.3316574	10.0426654	10.3743228	1
60	9.6259483	9.9572757	9.6686725	10.3313275	10.0427242	10.3740517	0
	Sine.		Tang		Secant.		M

65 Degrees.

25 Degrees.

M	Sine.		Tang.		Secant.		
0	9.6259483	9.9572757	9.6686725	10.3313275	10.0427243	10.3740517	60
1	9.6262191	9.9572168	9.6690023	10.3309977	10.0427832	10.3737806	59
2	9.6264897	9.9571578	9.6693319	10.3306681	10.0428422	10.3735101	58
3	9.6267601	9.9570988	9.6696613	10.3303387	10.0429012	10.3732399	57
4	9.6270303	9.9570397	9.6699906	10.3300094	10.0429603	10.3729697	56
5	9.6273003	9.9569806	9.6703197	10.3296803	10.0430194	10.3726997	55
6	9.6275701	9.9569215	9.6706486	10.3293514	10.0430785	10.3724299	54
7	9.6278397	9.9568623	9.6709774	10.3290226	10.0431377	10.3721603	53
8	9.6281092	9.9568030	9.6713060	10.3286940	10.0431970	10.3718910	52
9	9.6283782	9.9567437	9.6716345	10.3283655	10.0432563	10.3716218	51
10	9.6286472	9.9566844	9.6719628	10.3280372	10.0433156	10.3713528	50
11	9.6289160	9.9566250	9.6722910	10.3277090	10.0433750	10.3710840	49
12	9.6291845	9.9565656	9.6726190	10.3273810	10.0434344	10.3708155	48
13	9.6294529	9.9565061	9.6729468	10.3270532	10.0434939	10.3705471	47
14	9.6297211	9.9564466	9.6732745	10.3267255	10.0435534	10.3702789	46
15	9.6299890	9.9563871	9.6736020	10.3263980	10.0436130	10.3700110	45
16	9.6302568	9.9563274	9.6739294	10.3260706	10.0436726	10.3697432	44
17	9.6305243	9.9562678	9.6742566	10.3257434	10.0437322	10.3694757	43
18	9.6307917	9.9562081	9.6745836	10.3254164	10.0437919	10.3692083	42
19	9.6310589	9.9561483	9.6749105	10.3250895	10.0438517	10.3689411	41
20	9.6313258	9.9560886	9.6752372	10.3247628	10.0439114	10.3686742	40
21	9.6315926	9.9560287	9.6755638	10.3244362	10.0439713	10.3684074	39
22	9.6318591	9.9559689	9.6758903	10.3241097	10.0440311	10.3681405	38
23	9.6321255	9.9559089	9.6762165	10.3237835	10.0440911	10.3678745	37
24	9.6323916	9.9558490	9.6765426	10.3234574	10.0441510	10.3676084	36
25	9.6326576	9.9557890	9.6768686	10.3231314	10.0442110	10.3673424	35
26	9.6329233	9.9557283	9.6771944	10.3228056	10.0442711	10.3670767	34
27	9.6331889	9.9556688	9.6775201	10.3224799	10.0443312	10.3668111	33
28	9.6334542	9.9556087	9.6778456	10.3221544	10.0444391	10.3665458	32
29	9.6337194	9.9555485	9.6781709	10.3218291	10.0444515	10.3662806	31
30	9.6339844	9.9554882	9.6784961	10.3215039	10.0445118	10.3660156	30
	Sine.		Tang.		Secant.		M

64 Degrees.

25 Degrees.

M	Sine.		Tang.		Secant.		
30	9.6339844	9.9554882	9.6789461	10.3215039	10.0445118	10.3660156	20
31	9.6342491	9.9554280	9.6788211	10.3211789	10.0445720	10.3657509	29
32	9.6345137	9.9553676	9.6791460	10.3208540	10.0446324	10.3654862	28
33	9.6347780	9.9553073	9.6794708	10.3205292	10.0446927	10.3652220	27
34	9.6350422	9.9552469	9.6797953	10.3202047	10.0447531	10.3649578	26
35	9.6353062	9.9551864	9.6801198	10.3198802	10.0448136	10.3646938	25
36	9.6355699	9.9551259	9.6804440	10.3195560	10.0448741	10.3644301	24
37	9.6358335	9.9550653	9.6807682	10.3192318	10.0449347	10.3641665	23
38	9.6360969	9.9550047	9.6810921	10.3189079	10.0449953	10.3639031	22
39	9.6363601	9.9549441	9.6814160	10.3185840	10.0450559	10.3636399	21
40	9.6366231	9.9548834	9.6817396	10.3182604	10.0451166	10.3633769	20
41	9.6368859	9.9548227	9.6820632	10.3179368	10.0451773	10.3631141	19
42	9.6371484	9.9547619	9.6823865	10.3176135	10.0452381	10.3628516	18
43	9.6374108	9.9547011	9.6827098	10.3172902	10.0452989	10.3625892	17
44	9.6376731	9.9546402	9.6830328	10.3169672	10.0453598	10.3623269	16
45	9.6379351	9.9545793	9.6833557	10.3166443	10.0454207	10.3620649	15
46	9.6381969	9.9545184	9.6836785	10.3163215	10.0454816	10.3618031	14
47	9.6384585	9.9544574	9.6840011	10.3159989	10.0455426	10.3615415	13
48	9.6387199	9.9543963	9.6843236	10.3156764	10.0456037	10.3612801	12
49	9.6389812	9.9543352	9.6846459	10.3153541	10.0456648	10.3610188	11
50	9.6392422	9.9542741	9.6849681	10.3150319	10.0457259	10.3607578	10
51	9.6395030	9.9542129	9.6852901	10.3147099	10.0457871	10.3604970	9
52	9.6397637	9.9541517	9.6856120	10.3143880	10.0458483	10.3602363	8
53	9.6400241	9.9540904	9.6859338	10.3140662	10.0459096	10.3599759	7
54	9.6402844	9.9540291	9.6862553	10.3137447	10.0459709	10.3597156	6
55	9.6405445	9.9539677	9.6865768	10.3134232	10.0460323	10.3594555	5
56	9.6408044	9.9539063	9.6868981	10.3131019	10.0460937	10.3591956	4
57	9.6410640	9.9538448	9.6872192	10.3127808	10.0461552	10.3589360	3
58	9.6413235	9.9537833	9.6875402	10.3124598	10.0462167	10.3586765	2
59	9.6415828	9.9537218	9.6878611	10.3121389	10.0462782	10.3584172	1
60	9.6418420	9.9536602	9.6881818	10.3118182	10.0463398	10.3581580	0
	Sine.		Tang.		Secant.		M

64 Degrees.

26 Degrees.

M	Sine.		Tang.		Secant.		
0	9.6418420	9.9536502	9.6881818	10.3118182	10.0463398	10.3581580	60
1	9.6421009	9.9535985	9.6885023	10.3114977	10.0464015	10.3578991	59
2	9.6423596	9.9535369	9.6888227	10.3111772	10.0464631	10.3576404	58
3	9.6426182	9.9534751	9.6891430	10.3108570	10.0465249	10.3573818	57
4	9.6428769	9.9534134	9.6894631	10.3105309	10.0465866	10.3571235	56
5	9.6431347	9.9533515	9.6897831	10.3102169	10.0466485	10.3568653	55
6	9.6433926	9.9532897	9.6901032	10.3098970	10.0467103	10.3566074	54
7	9.6436504	9.9532278	9.6904226	10.3095774	10.0467722	10.3563496	53
8	9.6439080	9.9531658	9.6907422	10.3092578	10.0468342	10.3560920	52
9	9.6441654	9.9531038	9.6910616	10.3089384	10.0468962	10.3558346	51
10	9.6444226	9.9530418	9.6913809	10.3086191	10.0469582	10.3555774	50
11	9.6446796	9.9529797	9.6917000	10.3083000	10.0470203	10.3553204	49
12	9.6449366	9.9529175	9.6920189	10.3079811	10.0470825	10.3550635	48
13	9.6451931	9.9528553	9.6923378	10.3076622	10.0471447	10.3548059	47
14	9.6454490	9.9527931	9.6926565	10.3073435	10.0472069	10.3545504	46
15	9.6457058	9.9527308	9.6929750	10.3070250	10.0472692	10.3542942	45
16	9.6459619	9.9526685	9.6932934	10.3067066	10.0473315	10.3540381	44
17	9.6462178	9.9526061	9.6936117	10.3063883	10.0473939	10.3537822	43
18	9.6464735	9.9525437	9.6939298	10.3060702	10.0474563	10.3535265	42
19	9.6467290	9.9524812	9.6942478	10.3057522	10.0475187	10.3532710	41
20	9.6469844	9.9524188	9.6945656	10.3054344	10.0475812	10.3530156	40
21	9.6472395	9.9523562	9.6948833	10.3051167	10.0476438	10.3527605	39
22	9.6474945	9.9522936	9.6952009	10.3047991	10.0477064	10.3525055	38
23	9.6477492	9.9522310	9.6955183	10.3044817	10.0477690	10.3522508	37
24	9.6480038	9.9521683	9.6958355	10.3041645	10.0478317	10.3519962	36
25	9.6482582	9.9521055	9.6961527	10.3038473	10.0478945	10.3517418	35
26	9.6485124	9.9520428	9.6964697	10.3035303	10.0479572	10.3514876	34
27	9.6487665	9.9519799	9.6967865	10.3032135	10.0480201	10.3512335	33
28	9.6490203	9.9519171	9.6971032	10.3028968	10.0480829	10.3509797	32
29	9.6492740	9.9518541	9.6974198	10.3025802	10.0481459	10.3507260	31
30	9.6495274	9.9517912	9.6977363	10.3022637	10.0482088	10.3504726	30
	Sine.		Tang.		Secant.		M

63 Degrees.

26 Degrees.

M	Sine.		Tang.		Secant.		
30	9.6495274	9.9517912	9.6977363	10.3022637	10.0482088	10.3504728	30
31	9.6497807	9.9517282	9.6980526	10.3019474	10.0482718	10.3502193	29
32	9.6500338	9.9516651	9.6983687	10.3016313	10.0483349	10.3499662	28
33	9.6502868	9.9516020	9.6986847	10.3013153	10.0483980	10.3497132	27
34	9.6505395	9.9515389	9.6990006	10.3009994	10.0484611	10.3494605	26
35	9.6507920	9.9514757	9.6993154	10.3006836	10.0485243	10.3492080	25
36	9.6510444	9.9514124	9.6996320	10.3003680	10.0485876	10.3489556	24
37	9.6512966	9.9513492	9.5999474	10.3000526	10.0486508	10.3487034	23
38	9.6515486	9.9512858	9.7002628	10.2997372	10.0487142	10.3484514	22
39	9.6518004	9.9512224	9.7005780	10.2994220	10.0487776	10.3481996	21
40	9.6520521	9.9511590	9.7008930	10.2991070	10.0488410	10.3479479	20
41	9.6523035	9.9510956	9.7012080	10.2987920	10.0489044	10.3476965	19
42	9.6525548	9.9510320	9.7015227	10.2984773	10.0489680	10.3474452	18
43	9.6528059	9.9509685	9.7018374	10.2981626	10.0490315	10.3471941	17
44	9.6530568	9.9509049	9.7021519	10.2978481	10.0490951	10.3469432	16
45	9.6533075	9.9508412	9.7024663	10.2975337	10.0491588	10.3466925	15
46	9.6535581	9.9507775	9.7027805	10.2972195	10.0492225	10.3464419	14
47	9.6538084	9.9507138	9.7030946	10.2969054	10.0492862	10.3461916	13
48	9.6540586	9.9506500	9.7034086	10.2965914	10.0493500	10.3459414	12
49	9.6543086	9.9505861	9.7037225	10.2962775	10.0494139	10.3456914	11
50	9.6545584	9.9505223	9.7040362	10.2959638	10.0494777	10.3454416	10
51	9.6548081	9.9504583	9.7043497	10.2956503	10.0495417	10.3451919	9
52	9.6550575	9.9503944	9.7046632	10.2953368	10.0496056	10.3449425	8
53	9.6553068	9.9503303	9.7049765	10.2950235	10.0496697	10.3446932	7
54	9.6555559	9.9502663	9.7052897	10.2947103	10.0497337	10.3444441	6
55	9.6558048	9.9502022	9.7056027	10.2943973	10.0497978	10.3441952	5
56	9.6560536	9.9501380	9.7059156	10.2940844	10.0498620	10.3439464	4
57	9.6563021	9.9500738	9.7062284	10.2937716	10.0499262	10.3436979	3
58	9.6565505	9.9500095	9.7065410	10.2934590	10.0499905	10.3434495	2
59	9.6567987	9.9499452	9.7068535	10.2931465	10.0500548	10.3432013	1
60	9.6570468	9.9498809	9.7071659	10.2928341	10.0501191	10.3429532	0
	Sine.		Tang.		Secant.		M

63 Degrees.

27 Degrees.

'	Sine.		Tang.		Secant.		
0	9.6570453	9.9498809	9.7071659	10.2928341	10.0501191	10.3429532	60
1	9.6572946	9.9498165	9.7074781	10.2925219	10.0501835	10.3427054	59
2	9.6575423	9.9497521	9.7077902	10.2922098	10.0502479	10.3424577	58
3	9.6577898	9.9496876	9.7081022	10.2918978	10.0503124	10.3422102	57
4	9.6580371	9.9496230	9.7084141	10.2915859	10.0503770	10.3419629	56
5	9.6582842	9.9495585	9.7087258	10.2912742	10.0504415	10.3417158	55
6	9.6585312	9.9494938	9.7090374	10.2909626	10.0505062	10.3414688	54
7	9.6587780	9.9494292	9.7093488	10.2906512	10.0505708	10.3412220	53
8	9.6590245	9.9493645	9.7096601	10.2903399	10.0506355	10.3409754	52
9	9.6592710	9.9492997	9.7099713	10.2900287	10.0507003	10.3407290	51
10	9.6595173	9.9492349	9.7102824	10.2897176	10.0507651	10.3404827	50
11	9.6597634	9.9491700	9.7105933	10.2894057	10.0508300	10.3402366	49
12	9.6600093	9.9491051	9.7109041	10.2890959	10.0508949	10.3399907	48
13	9.6602550	9.9490402	9.7112148	10.2887852	10.0509598	10.3397450	47
14	9.6605005	9.9489752	9.7115254	10.2884746	10.0510248	10.3394995	46
15	9.6607459	9.9489101	9.7118358	10.2881642	10.0510899	10.3392541	45
16	9.6609911	9.9488450	9.7121461	10.2878539	10.0511550	10.3390089	44
17	9.6612361	9.9487799	9.7124562	10.2875438	10.0512201	10.3387639	43
18	9.6614810	9.9487147	9.7127662	10.2872338	10.0512853	10.3385190	42
19	9.6617257	9.9486495	9.7130761	10.2869239	10.0513505	10.3382743	41
20	9.6619702	9.9485842	9.7133859	10.2866141	10.0514158	10.3380298	40
21	9.6622145	9.9485189	9.7136956	10.2863044	10.0514811	10.3377855	39
22	9.6624586	9.9484535	9.7140051	10.2859949	10.0515465	10.3375414	38
23	9.6627026	9.9483881	9.7143145	10.2856855	10.0516119	10.3372974	37
24	9.6629464	9.9483227	9.7146237	10.2853763	10.0516773	10.3370536	36
25	9.6631900	9.9482572	9.7149329	10.2850671	10.0517428	10.3368100	35
26	9.6634335	9.9481916	9.7152419	10.2847581	10.0518084	10.3365665	34
27	9.6636758	9.9481260	9.7155508	10.2844492	10.0518740	10.3363232	33
28	9.6639199	9.9480604	9.7158595	10.2841405	10.0519396	10.3360801	32
29	9.6641628	9.9479947	9.7161682	10.2838318	10.0520053	10.3358372	31
30	9.6644056	9.9479289	9.7164767	10.2835233	10.0520711	10.3355944	30
	Sine.		Tang.		Secant.		M

62 Degrees.

27 Degrees.

M	Sine.		Tang.		Secant.		
30	9.6640456	9.9479269	9.7164767	10.2835233	10.0520711	10.335594	30
31	9.6646482	9.9478631	9.7167851	10.2832149	10.0521369	10.335351	29
32	9.6648906	9.9477973	9.7170933	10.2829067	10.0522027	10.335109	28
33	9.6651329	9.9477314	9.7174014	10.2825986	10.0522686	10.334867	27
34	9.6653749	9.9476655	9.7177094	10.2822906	10.0523345	10.334625	26
35	9.6656168	9.9475995	9.7180173	10.2819827	10.0524005	10.334383	25
36	9.6658586	9.9475335	9.7183251	10.2816749	10.0524665	10.334141	24
37	9.6661001	9.9474674	9.7186327	10.2813673	10.0525326	10.333899	23
38	9.6663415	9.9474013	9.7189402	10.2810598	10.0525987	10.333658	22
39	9.6665828	9.9473352	9.7192476	10.2807524	10.0526648	10.333417	21
40	9.6668238	9.9472689	9.7195549	10.2804451	10.0527311	10.333176	20
41	9.6670647	9.9472027	9.7198620	10.2801380	10.0527973	10.332935	19
42	9.6673054	9.9471364	9.7201690	10.2798310	10.0528636	10.332694	18
43	9.6675459	9.9470700	9.7204759	10.2795241	10.0529300	10.332454	17
44	9.6677863	9.9470036	9.7207827	10.2792173	10.0529964	10.332137	16
45	9.6680265	9.9469372	9.7210893	10.2789107	10.0530628	10.331973	15
46	9.6682665	9.9468707	9.7213958	10.2786042	10.0531293	10.331733	14
47	9.6685064	9.9468042	9.7217022	10.2782978	10.0531958	10.331493	13
48	9.6687461	9.9467376	9.7220084	10.2779915	10.0532624	10.331253	12
49	9.6689856	9.9466710	9.7223147	10.2776853	10.0533290	10.331014	11
50	9.6692250	9.9466043	9.7226207	10.2773793	10.0533957	10.330775	10
51	9.6694642	9.9465376	9.7229266	10.2770734	10.0534624	10.330535	9
52	9.6697032	9.9464708	9.7232324	10.2767676	10.0535292	10.330296	8
53	9.6699420	9.9464040	9.7235381	10.2764619	10.0535960	10.330058	7
54	9.6701807	9.9463371	9.7238436	10.2761564	10.0536629	10.329819	6
55	9.6704192	9.9462702	9.7241490	10.2758510	10.0537298	10.329580	5
56	9.6706576	9.9462032	9.7244543	10.2755457	10.0537968	10.329342	4
57	9.6708958	9.9461352	9.7247595	10.2752405	10.0538638	10.329104	3
58	9.6711338	9.9460692	9.7250646	10.2749354	10.0539308	10.328866	2
59	9.6713716	9.9460021	9.7253695	10.2746305	10.0539979	10.328628	1
60	9.6716093	9.9459349	9.7256744	10.2743256	10.0540651	10.328390	0

Sine.		Tang.		Secant.	M

62 Degrees.

28 *Degrees.*

M	Sine.		Tang.		Secant.		
0	9.6716093	9.9459349	9.7256744	10.2743256	10.0540651	10.3283907	60
1	9.6718468	9.9458677	9.7259791	10.2740209	10.0541323	10.3281532	59
2	9.6720841	9.9458005	9.7262837	10.2737163	10.0541995	10.3279159	58
3	9.6723213	9.9457332	9.7265881	10.2734119	10.0542668	10.3276787	57
4	9.6725583	9.9456659	9.7268925	10.2731075	10.0543341	10.3274417	56
5	9.6727952	9.9455985	9.7271967	10.2728033	10.0544015	10.3272048	55
6	9.6730319	9.9455310	9.7275008	10.2724992	10.0544690	10.3269681	54
7	9.6732684	9.9454636	9.7278048	10.2721952	10.0545364	10.3267316	53
8	9.6735047	9.9453960	9.7281087	10.2718913	10.0546040	10.3264953	52
9	9.6737409	9.9453285	9.7284124	10.2715876	10.0546715	10.3262591	51
10	9.6739769	9.9452609	9.7287161	10.2712839	10.0547391	10.3260231	50
11	9.6742128	9.9451932	9.7290196	10.2709804	10.0548068	10.3257872	49
12	9.6744485	9.9451255	9.7293230	10.2706770	10.0548745	10.3255515	48
13	9.6746840	9.9450577	9.7296263	10.2703737	10.0549423	10.3253160	47
14	9.6749194	9.9449899	9.7299295	10.2700705	10.0550101	10.3250806	46
15	9.6751546	9.9449220	9.7302325	10.2697675	10.0550780	10.3248454	45
16	9.6753896	9.9448541	9.7305354	10.2694646	10.0551459	10.3246104	44
17	9.6756245	9.9447862	9.7308383	10.2691617	10.0552138	10.3243755	43
18	9.6758592	9.9447182	9.7311410	10.2688590	10.0552818	10.3241408	42
19	9.6760937	9.9446501	9.7314436	10.2685564	10.0553499	10.3239063	41
20	9.6763281	9.9445821	7.7317460	10.2682540	100.554179	10.3236719	40
21	9.6765623	9.9445139	97320484	10.2679516	10.0554861	10.3234377	39
22	9.6767963	9.9444457	9.7323506	10.2676494	10.0555543	10.3232037	38
23	9.6770302	9.9443775	9.7326527	10.2673473	10.0556225	10.3229698	37
24	9.6772640	9.9443092	9.7329547	10.2670453	10.0556908	10.3227360	36
25	9.6774975	9.9442409	9.7332566	10.2667434	10.0557591	10.3225025	35
26	9.6777309	9.9441725	9.7335584	10.2664416	10.0558275	10.3222691	34
27	9.6779642	9.9441041	9.7338601	10.2661399	10.0558959	10.3220358	33
28	9.6781972	9.9440356	9.7341616	10.2658384	10.0559644	10.3218028	32
29	9.6784301	9.9439671	9.7344631	10.2655369	10.0560329	10.3215699	31
30	9.6786629	9.9438985	9.7347644	10.2652356	10.0561015	10.3213371	30
	Sine.		Tang.		Secant.		M

61 *Degrees.*

28 Degrees.

M	Sine.		Tang.		Secant.		M
30	9.6786629	9.9438985	9.7347644	10.2652356	10.0561015	10.3213371	30
31	9.6788955	9.9438299	9.7350656	10.2649344	10.0561701	10.3211045	29
32	9.6791279	9.9437612	9.7353667	10.2646333	10.0562388	10.3208721	28
33	9.6793602	9.9436925	9.7356677	10.2643323	10.0563075	10.3206398	27
34	9.6795923	9.9436238	9.7359685	10.2640315	10.0563762	10.3204077	26
35	9.6798243	9.9435549	9.7362693	10.2637307	10.0564451	10.3201757	25
36	9.6800560	9.9434861	9.7365699	10.2634301	10.0565139	10.3199440	24
37	9.6802877	9.9434172	9.7368705	10.2631295	10.0565828	10.3197123	23
38	9.6805191	9.9433482	9.7371709	10.2628291	10.0566518	10.3194809	22
39	9.6807504	9.9432792	9.7374712	10.2625288	10.0567208	10.3192496	21
40	9.6809816	9.9432102	9.7377714	10.2622286	10.0567898	10.3190184	20
41	9.6812126	9.9431411	9.7380715	10.2619285	10.0568589	10.3187874	19
42	9.6814434	9.9430720	9.7383714	10.2616286	10.0569280	10.3185566	18
43	9.6816741	9.9430028	9.7386713	10.2613287	10.0569972	10.3183259	17
44	9.6819046	9.9429335	9.7389710	10.2610290	10.0570665	10.3180954	16
45	9.6821349	9.9428643	9.7392707	10.2607293	10.0571357	10.3178651	15
46	9.6823651	9.9427949	9.7395702	10.2604298	10.0572051	10.3176349	14
47	9.6825952	9.9427255	9.7398696	10.2601304	10.0572745	10.3174048	13
48	9.6828250	9.9426561	9.7401689	10.2598311	10.0573439	10.3171750	12
49	9.6830548	9.9425866	9.7404681	10.2595319	10.0574134	10.3169452	11
50	9.6832843	9.9425171	9.7407672	10.2592328	10.0574829	10.3167157	10
51	9.6835137	9.9424476	9.7410662	10.2589338	10.0575524	10.3164863	9
52	9.6837430	9.9423779	9.7413650	10.2586350	10.0576221	10.3162570	8
53	9.6839720	9.9423083	9.7416638	10.2583362	10.0576917	10.3160280	7
54	9.6842010	9.9422386	9.7419624	10.2580376	10.0577614	10.3157990	6
55	9.6844297	9.9421688	9.7422609	10.2577391	10.0578312	10.3155703	5
56	9.6846583	9.9420990	9.7425594	10.2574406	10.0579010	10.3153417	4
57	9.6848868	9.9420291	9.7428577	10.2571423	10.0579709	10.3151132	3
58	9.6851151	9.9419592	9.7431559	10.2568441	10.0580408	10.3148849	2
59	9.6853432	9.9418893	9.7434540	10.2565460	10.0581107	10.3146568	1
60	9.6855712	9.9418193	9.7437520	10.2562480	10.0581807	10.3144288	0
	Sine.		Tang.		Secant.		M

61 Degrees.

29 Degrees.

M	Sine.		Tang.		Secant.		
0	9.6855712	9.9413193	9.7137520	10.2562480	10.0581807	10.3144288	60
1	9.6856791	9.9417492	9.7440495	10.2559501	10.0582508	10.3142029	59
2	9.6860267	9.9416791	9.7443476	10.2556524	10.0583205	10.3139733	58
3	9.6862542	9.9416090	9.7446453	10.2553547	10.0583910	10.3137458	57
4	9.6864815	9.9415388	9.7449428	10.2550572	10.0584612	10.3135184	56
5	9.6867088	9.9414685	9.7452403	10.2547597	10.0585315	10.3132912	55
6	9.6869355	9.9413982	9.7455376	10.2544624	10.0586018	10.3130641	54
7	9.6871628	9.9413279	9.7458345	10.2541651	10.0586721	10.3128372	53
8	9.6873599	9.9412575	9.7461320	10.2538680	10.0587425	10.3126105	52
9	9.6876161	9.9411871	9.7464290	10.2535710	10.0588129	10.3123839	51
10	9.6878425	9.9411166	9.7467259	10.2532741	10.0588834	10.3121575	50
11	9.6880688	9.9410461	9.7470227	10.2529773	10.0589539	10.3119312	49
12	9.6882949	9.9409755	9.7473194	10.2526806	10.0590245	10.3117051	48
13	9.6885209	9.9409048	9.7476160	10.2523840	10.0590952	10.3114791	47
14	9.6887467	9.9408342	9.7479125	10.2520875	10.0591658	10.3112533	46
15	9.6889723	9.9407634	9.7482089	10.2517911	10.0592366	10.3110277	45
16	9.6891978	9.9406927	9.7485052	10.2514948	10.0593073	10.3108022	44
17	9.6894232	9.9406219	9.7488013	10.2511987	10.0593781	10.3105768	43
18	9.6896484	9.9405510	9.7490974	10.2509026	10.0594490	10.3103516	42
19	9.6898734	9.9404801	9.7493934	10.2506066	10.0595199	10.3101266	41
20	9.6900983	9.9404091	9.7496892	10.2503108	10.0595909	10.3099017	40
21	9.6903231	9.9403381	9.7499850	10.2500150	10.0596619	10.3096769	39
22	9.6905476	9.9402670	9.7502806	10.2497194	10.0597330	10.3094524	38
23	9.6907721	9.9401959	9.7505762	10.2494238	10.0598041	10.3092279	37
24	9.6909964	9.9401248	9.7508716	10.2491284	10.0598752	10.3090036	36
25	9.6912205	9.9400535	9.7511669	10.2488331	10.0599465	10.3087795	35
26	9.6914445	9.9399823	9.7514622	10.2485378	10.0600177	10.3085555	34
27	9.6916683	9.9399110	9.7517573	10.2482427	10.0600890	10.3083317	33
28	9.6918919	9.9398396	9.7520523	10.2479477	10.0601604	10.3081081	32
29	9.6921155	9.9397682	9.7523472	10.2476528	10.0602318	10.3078845	31
30	9.6923388	9.9396968	9.7526420	10.2473580	10.0603032	10.3076612	30

	Sine.		Tang.		Secant.	M

60 Degrees.

29 Degrees.

M	Sine.		Tang.		Secant.		
30	9.692338	9.9396968	9.7526420	10.2473580	10.060303	10.3076612	30
31	9.692562	9.9396253	9.7529368	10.2470632	10.060374	10.3074380	29
32	9.692785	9.9395537	9.7532314	10.2467686	10.060446	10.3072149	28
33	9.693008	9.9394821	9.7535259	10.2464741	10.060517	10.3069920	27
34	9.693230	9.9394105	9.7538203	10.2461797	10.060589	10.3067692	26
35	9.693453	9.9393388	9.7541146	10.2458854	10.060661	10.3065466	25
36	9.693675	9.9392671	9.7544088	10.2455912	10.060732	10.3063242	24
37	9.693898	9.9391953	9.7547029	10.2452971	10.060804	10.3061019	23
38	9.694120	9.9391234	9.7549969	10.2450031	10.060876	10.3058797	22
39	9.694342	9.9390515	9.7552908	10.2447092	10.060948	10.3056577	21
40	9.694564	9.9389796	9.7555846	10.2444154	10.061020	10.3054358	20
41	9.694785	9.9389076	9.7558783	10.2441217	10.061092	10.3052141	19
42	9.695007	9.9388356	9.7561718	10.2438282	10.061164	10.3049926	18
43	9.695228	9.9387635	9.7564653	10.2435347	10.061236	10.3047711	17
44	9.695450	9.9386914	9.7567587	10.2432413	10.061308	10.3045499	16
45	9.695671	9.9386192	9.7570527	10.2429480	10.061380	10.3043288	15
46	9.695892	9.9385470	9.7573452	10.2426548	10.061453	10.3041078	14
47	9.696113	9.9384747	9.7576383	10.2423617	10.061525	10.3038870	13
48	9.696333	9.9384024	9.7579313	10.2420587	10.061597	10.3036663	12
49	9.696554	9.9383300	9.7582242	10.2417755	10.061670	10.3034455	11
50	9.696774	9.9382576	9.7585170	10.2414830	10.061742	10.3032255	10
51	9.696994	9.9381851	9.7588096	10.2411904	10.061814	10.3030253	9
52	9.697214	9.9381126	9.7591022	10.2408978	10.061887	10.3027852	8
53	9.697434	9.9380400	9.7593947	10.2406053	10.0619500	10.3025653	7
54	9.697654	9.9379674	9.7596871	10.2403129	10.0620326	10.3023455	6
55	9.697874	9.9378947	9.7599794	10.2400206	10.0621053	10.3021259	5
56	9.698093	9.9378220	9.7602716	10.2397284	10.0621780	10.3019064	4
57	9.698312	9.9377492	9.7605637	10.2394363	10.0622508	10.3016871	3
58	9.698532	9.9376764	9.7608557	10.2391443	10.0623236	10.3014675	2
59	9.698751	9.9376035	9.7611476	10.2388524	10.0623965	10.3012485	1
60	9.698970	9.9375306	9.7614394	10.2385606	10.0624694	10.3010300	0
	Sine.		Tang.		Secant.		M

60 Degrees.

N n n

A Table of Artificial Sines,

30 Degrees.

	Sine.		Tang.		Secant.		
	9.6989700	9.9375306	9.7614394	10.2385606	10.0624694	10.3010300	60
	9.6991887	9.9374577	9.7617311	10.2382689	10.0625423	10.3008113	59
	9.6994073	9.9373847	9.7620227	10.2379773	10.0626153	10.3005927	58
	9.6996258	9.9373116	9.7623142	10.2376858	10.0626884	10.3003742	57
	9.6998441	9.9372385	9.7626056	10.2373944	10.0627616	10.3001559	56
	9.7000622	9.9371653	9.7628969	10.2371031	10.0628347	10.2999378	55
	9.7002802	9.9370921	9.7631881	10.2368119	10.0629079	10.2997198	54
	9.7004981	9.9370189	9.7634792	10.2365208	10.0629811	10.2995019	53
	9.7007158	9.9369456	9.7637702	10.2362298	10.0630544	10.2992842	52
	9.7009334	9.9368722	9.7640612	10.2359388	10.0631278	10.2990666	51
	9.7011508	9.9367988	9.7643520	10.2356480	10.0632012	10.2988492	50
	9.7013681	9.9367254	9.7646427	10.2353573	10.0632746	10.2986319	49
	9.7015852	9.9366519	9.7649334	10.2350666	10.0633481	10.2984148	48
	9.7018022	9.9365783	9.7652239	10.2347761	10.0634217	10.2981978	47
	9.7020190	9.9365047	9.7655143	10.2344857	10.0634953	10.2979816	46
	9.7022357	9.9364311	9.7658047	10.2341953	10.0635689	10.2977643	45
	9.7024523	9.9363574	9.7660949	10.2339051	10.0636426	10.2975477	44
	9.7026687	9.9362836	9.7663851	10.2336149	10.0637164	10.2973313	43
	9.7028849	9.9362098	9.7666751	10.2333249	10.0637902	10.2971151	42
	9.7031011	9.9361360	9.7669651	10.2330349	10.0638642	10.2968989	41
	9.7033170	9.9360621	7.7672550	10.2327450	10.0639379	10.2966830	40
	9.7035329	9.9359881	9.7675448	10.2324552	10.0640119	10.2964671	39
	9.7037486	9.9359141	9.7678344	10.2321656	10.0640859	10.2962514	38
	9.7039641	9.9358401	9.7681240	10.2318760	10.0641599	10.2960359	37
	9.7041795	9.9357660	9.7684135	10.2315865	10.0642340	10.2958205	36
	9.7043947	9.9356918	9.7687029	10.2312971	10.0643082	10.2956053	35
	9.7046099	9.9356177	9.7689922	10.2310078	10.0643823	10.2953901	34
	9.7048248	9.9355434	9.7692814	10.2307186	10.0644566	10.2951752	33
	9.7050397	9.9354691	9.7695706	10.2304295	10.0645309	10.2949603	32
	9.7052545	9.9353948	9.7698596	10.2301404	10.0646051	10.2947457	31
	9.7054689	9.9353204	9.7701489	10.2298515	10.0646796	10.2945311	30
	Sine.		Tang.		Secant.		M

59 Degrees.

30 Degrees.

M	Sine.		Tang.		Secant.		
30	9.7054689	9.9353204	9.7701485	10.2298515	10.0646796	10.2945311	30
31	9.7056833	9.9352459	9.7704373	10.2295627	10.064754	10.2943167	29
32	9.7058975	9.9351715	9.7707261	10.2292739	10.0648285	10.2941025	28
33	9.7061116	9.9350969	9.7710147	10.2289853	10.0649031	10.2938884	27
34	9.7063256	9.9350223	9.7713032	10.2286967	10.0649777	10.2936744	26
35	9.7065394	9.9349477	9.7715917	10.2284083	10.0650523	10.2934606	25
36	9.7067531	9.9348730	9.7718801	10.2281199	10.0651270	10.2932469	24
37	9.7069667	9.9347983	9.7721684	10.2278316	10.0652017	10.2930333	23
38	9.7071801	9.9347235	9.7724566	10.2275434	10.0652765	10.2928199	22
39	9.7073933	9.9346486	9.7727447	10.2272553	10.0653514	10.2926067	21
40	9.7076064	9.9345738	9.7730327	10.2269673	10.0654262	10.2923936	20
41	9.7078194	9.9344988	9.7733206	10.2266794	10.0655012	10.2921806	19
42	9.7080323	9.9344238	9.7736084	10.2263916	10.0655762	10.2919677	18
43	9.7082450	9.9343488	9.7738961	10.2261039	10.0656512	10.2917550	17
44	9.7084575	9.9342737	9.7741838	10.2258162	10.0657262	10.2915425	16
45	9.7086699	9.9341986	9.7744713	10.2255287	10.0658014	10.2913301	15
46	9.7088822	9.9341234	9.7747588	10.2252412	10.0658766	10.2911178	14
47	9.7090943	9.9340482	9.7750462	10.2249538	10.0659518	10.2909057	13
48	9.7093063	9.9339729	9.7753334	10.2246666	10.0660271	10.2906937	12
49	9.7095182	9.9338976	9.7756206	10.2243794	10.0661024	10.2904818	11
50	9.7097299	9.9338222	9.7759077	10.2240923	10.0661778	10.2902701	10
51	9.7099415	9.9337467	9.7761947	10.2238053	10.0662533	10.2900585	9
52	9.7101529	9.9336713	9.7764816	10.2235184	10.0663287	10.2898471	8
53	9.7103642	9.9335957	9.7767685	10.2232315	10.0664043	10.2896358	7
54	9.7105753	9.9335201	9.7770552	10.2229448	10.0664799	10.2894247	6
55	9.7107863	9.9334445	9.7773418	10.2226582	10.0665555	10.2892137	5
56	9.7109972	9.9333688	9.7776284	10.2223716	10.0666312	10.2890028	4
57	9.7112080	9.9332931	9.7779149	10.2220851	10.0667069	10.2887920	3
58	9.7114186	9.9332173	9.7782012	10.2217988	10.0667827	10.2885814	2
59	9.7116290	9.9331415	9.7784879	10.2215125	10.0668585	10.2883710	1
60	9.7118393	9.9330656	9.7787737	10.2212263	10.0669344	10.2881607	0
	Sine.		Tang.		Secant.		M

59 Degrees.

31 Degrees.

	Sine.		Tang.		Secant.		
0	9.7118393	9.9330656	9.7787757	10.2212263	10.0669344	10.2881607	60
1	9.7120495	9.9329897	9.7790599	10.2209401	10.0670103	10.2879505	59
2	9.7122596	9.9329137	9.7793459	10.2206541	10.0670863	10.2877404	58
3	9.7124695	9.9328376	9.7796318	10.2203682	10.0671624	10.2875305	57
4	9.7126792	9.9327616	9.7799177	10.2200823	10.0672384	10.2873208	56
5	9.7128889	9.9326854	9.7802034	10.2197966	10.0673146	10.2871111	55
6	9.7130984	9.9326092	9.7804891	10.2195109	10.0673908	10.2869017	54
7	9.7133077	9.9325330	9.7807747	10.2192253	10.0674570	10.2856923	53
8	9.7135169	9.9324567	9.7810602	10.2189398	10.0675433	10.2864831	52
9	9.7137260	9.9323804	9.7813456	10.2186544	10.0676196	10.2862740	51
10	9.7139349	9.9323040	9.7816309	10.2183691	10.0676960	10.2860651	50
11	9.7141437	9.9322276	9.7819162	10.2180838	10.0677724	10.2858563	49
12	9.7143524	9.9321511	9.7822013	10.2177987	10.0678489	10.2856476	48
13	9.7145609	9.9320746	9.7824864	10.2175136	10.0679254	10.2854391	47
14	9.7147693	9.9319981	9.7827713	10.2172287	10.0680020	10.2852307	46
15	9.7149776	9.9319213	9.7830562	10.2169438	10.0680787	10.2850224	45
16	9.7151857	9.9318447	9.7833410	10.2166590	10.0681553	10.2848143	44
17	9.7153937	9.9317679	9.7836258	10.2163742	10.0682321	10.2846063	43
18	9.7156015	9.9316911	9.7839104	10.2160896	10.0683089	10.2843985	42
19	9.7158092	9.9316143	9.7841949	10.2158051	10.0683857	10.2841908	41
20	9.7160168	9.9315374	9.7844794	10.2155206	10.0684626	10.2839832	40
21	9.7162243	9.9314605	9.7847638	10.2152362	10.0685395	10.2837757	39
22	9.7164316	9.9313835	9.7850481	10.2149519	10.0686165	10.2835684	38
23	9.7166387	9.9313065	9.7853323	10.2146677	10.0686935	10.2833613	37
24	9.7168458	9.9312294	9.7856164	10.2143836	10.0687706	10.2831542	36
25	9.7170526	9.9311522	9.7859004	10.2140996	10.0688478	10.2829474	35
26	9.7172594	9.9310750	9.7861844	10.2138156	10.0689250	10.2827406	34
27	9.7174660	9.9309978	9.7864682	10.2135318	10.0690022	10.2825340	33
28	9.7176725	9.9309205	9.7867520	10.2132480	10.0690795	10.2823275	32
29	9.7178789	9.9308432	9.7870357	10.2129643	10.0691568	10.2821211	31
30	9.7180851	9.9307658	9.7873193	10.2126807	10.0692342	10.2819149	30
	Sine.		Tang.		Secant.		M

58 Degrees.

31 Degrees.

M	Sine.		Tang.		Secant.		
30	9.7180851	9.9307658	9.7873193	10.2126807	10.0692342	10.2819149	30
31	9.7182912	9.9306883	9.7876028	10.2123972	10.0693117	10.2817088	29
32	9.7184971	9.9306109	9.7878863	10.2121137	10.0693891	10.2815029	28
33	9.7187030	9.9305333	9.7881696	10.2118304	10.0694667	10.2812970	27
34	9.7189086	9.9304557	9.7884529	10.2115471	10.0695443	10.2810914	26
35	9.7191142	9.9303781	9.7887361	10.2112639	10.0696219	10.2808858	25
36	9.7193196	9.9303004	9.7890192	10.2109808	10.0696996	10.2806804	24
37	9.7195249	9.9302226	9.7893023	10.2106977	10.0697774	10.2804751	23
38	9.7197300	9.9301448	9.7895852	10.2104148	10.0698552	10.2802700	22
39	9.7199350	9.9300670	9.7898681	10.2101319	10.0699330	10.2800650	21
40	9.7201399	9.9299891	9.7901508	10.2098492	10.0700109	10.2798601	20
41	9.7203447	9.9299112	9.7904335	10.2095665	10.0700888	10.2796553	19
42	9.7205493	9.9298332	9.7907161	10.2092839	10.0701668	10.2794507	18
43	9.7207538	9.9297551	9.7909987	10.2090013	10.0702449	10.2792462	17
44	9.7209581	9.9296770	9.7912811	10.2087189	10.0703230	10.2790419	16
45	9.7211623	9.9295989	9.7915635	10.2084365	10.0704011	10.2788377	15
46	9.7213664	9.9295207	9.7918458	10.2081542	10.0704793	10.2786336	14
47	9.7215704	9.9294424	9.7921280	10.2078720	10.0705576	10.2784296	13
48	9.7217742	9.9293641	9.7924101	10.2075899	10.0706359	10.2782258	12
49	9.7219779	9.9292857	9.7926921	10.2073079	10.0707143	10.2780221	11
50	9.7221814	9.9292073	9.7929741	10.2070259	10.0707927	10.2778186	10
51	9.7223848	9.9291289	9.7932560	10.2067440	10.0708711	10.2776152	9
52	9.7225881	9.9290504	9.7935378	10.2064622	10.0709496	10.2774119	8
53	9.7227913	9.9289718	9.7938195	10.2061805	10.0710282	10.2772087	7
54	9.7229943	9.9288932	9.7941011	10.2058989	10.0711068	10.2770057	6
55	9.7231972	9.9288145	9.7943827	10.2056173	10.0711855	10.2768028	5
56	9.7234000	9.9287358	9.7946641	10.2053359	10.0712642	10.2766000	4
57	9.7236026	9.9286571	9.7949455	10.2050545	10.0713429	10.2763974	3
58	9.7238051	9.9285783	9.7952268	10.2047732	10.0714217	10.2761949	2
59	9.7240075	9.9284994	9.7955081	10.2044919	10.0715006	10.2759925	1
60	9.7242097	9.9284205	9.7957892	10.2042108	10.0715795	10.2757903	0
	Sine.		Tang.		Secant.		M

58 Degrees.

32 Degrees.

M	Sine.		Tang.		Secant.		
0	9.7242097	9.9284205	9.7957892	10.2042108	10.071579	10.275790	
1	9.7244118	9.9283415	9.7960703	10.2039297	10.0716584	10.275588	59
2	9.7246138	9.9282625	9.7963513	10.2036487	10.0717374	10.275336	58
3	9.7248156	9.9281834	9.7966322	10.2033678	10.0718166	10.275184	57
4	9.7250174	9.9281043	9.7969130	10.2030870	10.0718957	10.274982	56
5	9.7252189	9.9280251	9.7971938	10.2028062	10.0719749	10.274781	55
6	9.7254204	9.9279459	9.7974745	10.2025255	10.0720541	10.274579	54
7	9.7256217	9.9278666	9.7977551	10.2022449	10.0721334	10.274378	53
8	9.7258229	9.9277873	9.7980356	10.2019644	10.0722127	10.274177	52
9	9.7260240	9.9277079	9.7983160	10.2016840	10.0722921	10.273976	51
10	9.7262249	9.9276285	9.7985964	10.2014036	10.0723715	10.273775	50
11	9.7264257	9.9275490	9.7988767	10.2011233	10.0724510	10.273574	49
12	9.7266264	9.9274695	9.7991569	10.2008431	10.0725309	10.273373	48
13	9.7268269	9.9273899	9.7994370	10.2005630	10.0726101	10.273173	47
14	9.7270273	9.9273103	9.7997172	10.2002830	10.0726897	10.272972	46
15	9.7272276	9.9272306	9.7999970	10.2000030	10.0727694	10.272772	45
16	9.7274278	9.9271509	9.8002769	10.1997231	10.0728491	10.272572	44
17	9.7276278	9.9270711	9.8005567	10.1994433	10.0729289	10.272372	43
18	9.7278277	9.9269913	9.8008365	10.1991635	10.0730087	10.272172	42
19	9.7280275	9.9269114	9.8011161	10.1988839	10.0730886	10.271972	41
20	9.7282271	9.9268314	9.8013957	10.1986043	10.0731686	10.271772	40
21	9.7284267	9.9267514	9.8016752	10.1983248	10.0732486	10.271573	39
22	9.7286260	9.9266714	9.8019546	10.1980454	10.0733286	10.271374	38
23	9.7288253	9.9265912	9.8022340	10.1977660	10.0734087	10.271174	37
24	9.7290244	9.9265112	9.8025133	10.1974867	10.0734888	10.270975	36
25	9.7292234	9.9264310	9.8027925	10.1972075	10.0735690	10.270776	35
26	9.7294223	9.9263507	9.8030716	10.1969284	10.0736493	10.270577	34
27	9.7296211	9.9262704	9.8033506	10.1966494	10.0737296	10.270378	33
28	9.7298197	9.9261901	9.8036296	10.1963724	10.0738099	10.270180	32
29	9.7300182	9.9261096	9.8039084	10.1960915	10.0738904	10.269981	31
30	9.7302165	9.9260292	9.8041873	10.1958127	10.0739708	10.269783	30
	Sine.		Tang.		Secant.		M

57 Degrees.

32 Degrees.

M	Sine.		Tang.		Secant.		
30	9.7302165	9.9260292	9.8041873	10.1958127	10.0739708	10.2697835	30
31	9.7304148	9.9259487	9.8044661	10.1955339	10.0740513	10.2695852	29
32	9.7306129	9.9258681	9.8047447	10.1952553	10.0741319	10.2693871	28
33	9.7308109	9.9257875	9.8050233	10.1949767	10.0742125	10.2691891	27
34	9.7310087	9.9257069	9.8053019	10.1946981	10.0742931	10.2689913	26
35	9.7312064	9.9256261	9.8055803	10.1944197	10.0743739	10.2687936	25
36	9.7314040	9.9255454	9.8058587	10.1941413	10.0744546	10.2685960	24
37	9.7316015	9.9254646	9.8061370	10.1938630	10.0745354	10.2683985	23
38	9.7317989	9.9253837	9.8064152	10.1935848	10.0746163	10.2682011	22
39	9.7319961	9.9253028	9.8066933	10.1933067	10.0746972	10.2680039	21
40	9.7321932	9.9252218	9.8069714	10.1930286	10.0747782	10.2678068	20
41	9.7323902	9.9251408	9.8072494	10.1927506	10.0748592	10.2676098	19
42	9.7325870	9.9250597	9.8075273	10.1924727	10.0749403	10.2674130	18
43	9.7327837	9.9249786	9.8078052	10.1921948	10.0750214	10.2672163	17
44	9.7329803	9.9248974	9.8080829	10.1919171	10.0751026	10.2670197	16
45	9.7331768	9.9248161	9.8083606	10.1916394	10.0751839	10.2668232	15
46	9.7333731	9.9247349	9.8086383	10.1913617	10.0752651	10.2666269	14
47	9.7335693	9.9246535	9.8089158	10.1910842	10.0753465	10.2664307	13
48	9.7337654	9.9245721	9.8091933	10.1908067	10.0754279	10.2662346	12
49	9.7339614	9.9244907	9.8094707	10.1905293	10.0755093	10.2660386	11
50	9.7341572	9.9244092	9.8097480	10.1902520	10.0755908	10.2658428	10
51	9.7343529	9.9243277	9.8100253	10.1899747	10.0756723	10.2656471	9
52	9.7345485	9.9242461	9.8103025	10.1896975	10.0757539	10.2654515	8
53	9.7347440	9.9241644	9.8105796	10.1894204	10.0758356	10.2652560	7
54	9.7349393	9.9240827	9.8108566	10.1891434	10.0759173	10.2650607	6
55	9.7351345	9.9240010	9.8111336	10.1888664	10.0759990	10.2648655	5
56	9.7353296	9.9239191	9.8114105	10.1885895	10.0760809	10.2646704	4
57	9.7355246	9.9238373	9.8116873	10.1883127	10.0761627	10.2644754	3
58	9.7357195	9.9237554	9.8119641	10.1880359	10.0762446	10.2642805	2
59	9.7359142	9.9236734	9.8122408	10.1877592	10.0763266	10.2640858	1
60	9.7361088	9.9235914	9.8125174	10.1874826	10.0764086	10.2638912	0
	Sine.		Tang.		Secant.		M

57 Degrees.

33 Degrees.

	Sine.		Tang.		Secant.		
0	9.7361285	9.9235914	9.8125174	10.1874826	10.0764086	10.2638912	60
1	9.7363502	9.9235093	9.8127939	10.1872061	10.0764900	10.2636968	59
2	9.7364376	9.9234274	9.8130704	10.1869296	10.0765728	10.2635024	58
3	9.7366918	9.9233450	9.8133468	10.1866532	10.0765550	10.2633082	57
4	9.7368855	9.9232628	9.8136231	10.1863769	10.0766737	10.2631141	56
5	9.7370799	9.9231805	9.8138993	10.1861007	10.0768195	10.2629201	55
6	9.7372737	9.9230982	9.8141755	10.1858245	10.0769015	10.2627263	54
7	9.7374675	9.9230155	9.8144516	10.1855484	10.0769842	10.2625325	53
8	9.7376611	9.9229334	9.8147277	10.1852723	10.0770666	10.2623389	52
9	9.7378545	9.9228509	9.8150036	10.1849964	10.0771491	10.2621454	51
10	9.7380479	9.9227684	9.8152795	10.1847205	10.0772316	10.2619521	50
11	9.7382412	9.9226859	9.8155554	10.1844446	10.0773142	10.2617588	49
12	9.7384343	9.9226032	9.8158311	10.1841689	10.0773968	10.2615657	48
13	9.7386273	9.9225205	9.8161068	10.1838932	10.0774795	10.2613727	47
14	9.7388201	9.9224377	9.8163824	10.1836176	10.0775623	10.2611799	46
15	9.7390129	9.9223549	9.8166580	10.1833420	10.0776451	10.2609871	45
16	9.7392055	9.9222721	9.8169335	10.1830665	10.0777279	10.2607945	44
17	9.7393980	9.9221891	9.8172089	10.1827911	10.0778109	10.2606020	43
18	9.7395904	9.9221062	9.8174842	10.1825158	10.0778938	10.2604096	42
19	9.7397827	9.9220232	9.8177595	10.1822405	10.0779768	10.2602173	41
20	9.7399748	9.9219401	9.8180347	10.1819653	10.0780599	10.2600252	40
21	9.7401668	9.9218570	9.8183098	10.1816902	10.0781430	10.2598332	39
22	9.7403587	9.9217738	9.8185849	10.1814151	10.0782262	10.2596413	38
23	9.7405505	9.9216905	9.8188599	10.1811401	10.0783094	10.2594495	37
24	9.7407421	9.9216072	9.8191348	10.1808652	10.0783927	10.2592579	36
25	9.7409337	9.9215240	9.8194096	10.1805904	10.0784760	10.2590663	35
26	9.7411251	9.9214406	9.8196844	10.1803156	10.0785594	10.2588749	34
27	9.7413164	9.9213572	9.8199592	10.1800408	10.0786428	10.2586836	33
28	9.7415075	9.9212737	9.8202338	10.1797662	10.0787263	10.2584925	32
29	9.7416986	9.9211902	9.8205084	10.1794916	10.0788098	10.2583014	31
30	9.7418895	9.9211066	9.8207829	10.1792171	10.0788934	10.2581105	30
	Sine.		Tang.		Secant.		M

56 Degrees.

33 Degrees.

M	Sine.		Tang.		Secant.		
30	9.7418895	9.9211066	9.8207829	10.1792171	10.0788934	10.2581105	30
31	9.7420803	9.9210229	9.8210574	10.1789426	10.0789771	10.2579197	29
32	9.7422710	9.9209393	9.8213317	10.1786683	10.0790607	10.2577290	28
33	9.7424616	9.9208555	9.8216060	10.1783940	10.0791445	10.2575384	27
34	9.7426520	9.9207717	9.8218803	10.1781197	10.0792283	10.2573480	26
35	9.7428423	9.9206878	9.8221545	10.1778455	10.0793122	10.2571577	25
36	9.7430325	9.9206039	9.8224286	10.1775714	10.0193961	10.2569675	24
37	9.7432226	9.9205200	9.8227026	10.1772974	10.0794800	10.2567774	23
38	9.7434126	9.9204360	9.8229766	10.1770234	10.0795640	10.2565874	22
39	9.7436024	9.9203519	9.8232505	10.1767495	10.0796481	10.2563976	21
40	9.7437921	9.9202678	9.8235244	10.1764756	10.0797322	10.2562079	20
41	9.7439817	9.9201836	9.8237981	10.1762019	10.0798164	10.2560183	19
42	9.7441712	9.9200994	9.8240719	10.1759281	10.0799006	10.2558288	18
43	9.7443606	9.9200151	9.8243455	10.1756545	10.0799849	10.2556394	17
44	9.7445498	9.9199308	9.8246191	10.1753809	10.0800692	10.2554502	16
45	9.7447390	9.9198464	9.8248926	10.1751074	10.0801536	10.2552610	15
46	9.7449280	9.9197619	9.8251660	10.1748340	10.0802381	10.2550720	14
47	9.7451169	9.9196775	9.8254394	10.1745606	10.0803225	10.2548831	13
48	9.7453056	9.9195929	9.8257127	10.1742873	10.0804071	10.2546944	12
49	9.7454943	9.9195083	9.8259860	10.1740140	10.0804917	10.2545057	11
50	9.7456828	9.9194237	9.8262592	10.1737408	10.0805763	10.2543172	10
51	9.7458712	9.9193390	9.8265323	10.1734677	10.0806610	10.2541288	9
52	9.7460595	9.9192542	9.8268053	10.1731947	10.0807458	10.2539405	8
53	9.7462477	9.9191694	9.8270783	10.1729217	10.0808306	10.2537523	7
54	9.7464358	9.9190845	9.8273513	10.1726487	10.0809155	10.2535642	6
55	9.7466237	9.9189996	9.8276241	10.1723759	10.0810004	10.2533763	5
56	9.7468115	9.9189146	9.8278969	10.1721031	10.0810854	10.2531885	4
57	9.7469992	9.9188296	9.8281696	10.1718304	10.0811704	10.2530008	3
58	9.7471868	9.9187445	9.8284423	10.1715577	10.0812555	10.2528132	2
59	9.7473743	9.9186594	9.8287149	10.1712851	10.0813406	10.2526256	1
60	9.7475617	9.9185742	9.8289874	10.1710126	10.0814258	10.2524381	0
	Sine.		Tang.		Secant.		M

56 Degrees.

O o o

34 *Degrees.*

M	Sine.		Tang.		Secant.		
0	9.7475617	9.9185742	9.8289374	10.1710126	10.0814258	10.2524383	60
1	9.7477487	9.9184893	9.8292599	10.1707401	10.0815110	10.2522511	59
2	9.7479360	9.9184037	9.8295323	10.1704677	10.0815963	10.2520640	58
3	9.7481230	9.9183183	9.8298047	10.1701953	10.0816817	10.2518770	57
4	9.7483039	9.9182329	9.8300769	10.1699231	10.0817671	10.2516901	56
5	9.7484967	9.9181475	9.8303492	10.1696508	10.0818525	10.2515033	55
6	9.7486833	9.9180620	9.8306215	10.1693787	10.0819380	10.2513167	54
7	9.7488698	9.9179764	9.8308934	10.1691066	10.0820236	10.2511302	53
8	9.7490562	9.9178908	9.8311654	10.1688346	10.0821092	10.2509438	52
9	9.7492125	9.9178051	9.8314374	10.1685626	10.0821949	10.2507575	51
10	9.7494257	9.9177194	9.8317093	10.1682907	10.0822806	10.2505713	50
11	9.7496148	9.9176336	9.8319811	10.1680189	10.0823664	10.2503852	49
12	9.7498007	9.9175478	9.8322529	10.1677471	10.0824522	10.2501993	48
13	9.7499866	9.9174619	9.8325246	10.1674754	10.0825381	10.2500134	47
14	9.7501723	9.9173760	9.8327963	10.1672037	10.0826240	10.2498277	46
15	9.7503579	9.9172900	9.8330679	10.1669321	10.0827100	10.2496421	45
16	9.7505434	9.9172040	9.8333394	10.1666606	10.0827960	10.2494566	44
17	9.7507287	9.9171179	9.8336109	10.1663891	10.0828821	10.2492713	43
18	9.7509140	9.9170317	9.8338823	10.1661177	10.0829583	10.2490860	42
19	9.7510991	9.9169455	9.8341536	10.1658464	10.0830545	10.2489009	41
20	9.7512842	9.9168593	9.8344249	10.1655751	10.0831407	10.2487158	40
21	9.7514691	9.9167737	9.8346961	10.1653039	10.0832270	10.2485309	39
22	9.7516538	9.9166866	9.8349673	10.1650327	10.0833134	10.2483462	38
23	9.7518385	9.9166002	9.8352384	10.1647616	10.0833998	10.2481615	37
24	9.7520231	9.9165137	9.8355094	10.1644906	10.0834862	10.2479769	36
25	9.7522075	9.9164272	9.8357804	10.1642196	10.0835728	10.2477925	35
26	9.7523919	9.9163406	9.8360513	10.1639487	10.0836594	10.2476081	34
27	9.7525761	9.9162539	9.8363221	10.1636779	10.0837461	10.2474239	33
28	9.7527602	9.9161673	9.8365929	10.1634071	10.0838327	10.2472398	32
29	9.7529442	9.9160805	9.8368636	10.1631364	10.0839195	10.2470558	31
30	9.7531280	9.9159937	9.8371343	10.1628657	10.0840063	10.2468720	30
	Sine.		Tang.		Secant.		M

55 *Degrees.*

34 Degrees.

M	Sine.		Tang.		Secant.		
30	9.7531280	9.9152937	9.8371343	10.1628657	10.0840063	10.2468720	30
31	9.7533118	9.9150069	9.8374049	10.1625951	10.0840931	10.2466882	29
32	9.7534954	9.9158200	9.8376755	10.1623245	10.0841800	10.2465046	28
33	9.7536790	9.9157330	9.8379460	10.1620540	10.0842670	10.2463210	27
34	9.7538624	9.9156460	9.8382164	10.1617836	10.0843540	10.2461376	26
35	9.7540457	9.9155589	9.8384867	10.1615133	10.0844411	10.2459543	25
36	9.7542288	9.9154718	9.8387571	10.1612429	10.0845282	10.2457712	24
37	9.7544119	9.9153846	9.8390273	10.1609727	10.0846154	10.2455881	23
38	9.7545949	9.9152974	9.8392975	10.1607025	10.0847026	10.2454051	22
39	9.7547777	9.9152101	9.8395676	10.1604324	10.0847899	10.2452223	21
40	9.7549604	9.9151228	9.8398377	10.1601623	10.0848772	10.2450396	20
41	9.7551431	9.9150354	9.8401077	10.1598923	10.0849646	10.2448569	19
42	9.7553256	9.9149479	9.8403776	10.1596224	10.0850521	10.2446744	18
43	9.7555080	9.9148604	9.8406475	10.1593525	10.0851396	10.2444920	17
44	9.7556902	9.9147729	9.8409174	10.1590826	10.0852271	10.2443098	16
45	9.7558724	9.9146852	9.8411871	10.1588129	10.0853148	10.2441276	15
46	9.7560544	9.9145976	9.8414569	10.1585431	10.0854024	10.2439456	14
47	9.7562364	9.9145099	9.8417265	10.1582735	10.0854901	10.2437636	13
48	9.7564182	9.9144221	9.8419961	10.1580039	10.0855779	10.2435818	12
49	9.7565999	9.9143342	9.8422657	10.1577343	10.0856658	10.2434001	11
50	9.7567815	9.9142464	9.8425351	10.1574649	10.0857536	10.2432185	10
51	9.7569630	9.9141584	9.8428046	10.1571954	10.0858416	10.2430370	9
52	9.7571444	9.9140704	9.8430739	10.1569261	10.0859296	10.2428556	8
53	9.7573256	9.9139824	9.8433432	10.1566568	10.0860176	10.2426744	7
54	9.7575068	9.9138943	9.8436125	10.1563875	10.0861057	10.2424937	6
55	9.7576878	9.9138061	9.8438817	10.1561183	10.0861939	10.2423122	5
56	9.7578687	9.9137179	9.8441508	10.1558492	10.0862821	10.2421313	4
57	9.7580495	9.9136296	9.8444199	10.1555801	10.0863704	10.2419505	3
58	9.7582302	9.9135413	9.8446889	10.1553111	10.0864587	10.2417695	2
59	9.7584108	9.9134529	9.8449579	10.1550421	10.0865471	10.2415892	1
60	9.7585913	9.9133645	9.8452268	10.1547732	10.0866355	10.2414087	0
	Sine.		Tang.		Secant.		

55 Degrees.

35 Degrees.

M	Sine.		Tang.		Secant.		
0	9.7585913	9.9133645	9.8452268	10.1547732	10.0866355	10.2414087	60
1	9.7587717	9.9132760	9.8454956	10.1545044	10.0867240	10.2412283	59
2	9.7589515	9.9131875	9.8457644	10.1542356	10.0868125	10.2410481	58
3	9.7591321	9.9130989	9.8460332	10.1539668	10.0869011	10.2408679	57
4	9.7593121	9.9130102	9.8463018	10.1536982	10.0869898	10.2406879	56
5	9.7594929	9.9129215	9.8465705	10.1534295	10.0870785	10.2405080	55
6	9.7596715	9.9128328	9.8468390	10.1531610	10.0871672	10.2403282	54
7	9.7598515	9.9127440	9.8471075	10.1528925	10.0872560	10.2401485	53
8	9.7600311	9.9126551	9.8473760	10.1526240	10.0873449	10.2399689	52
9	9.7602106	9.9125662	9.8476444	10.1523556	10.0874338	10.2397894	51
10	9.7603890	9.9124772	9.8479127	10.1520873	10.0875228	10.2396101	50
11	9.7605692	9.9123882	9.8481810	10.1518190	10.0876118	10.2394308	49
12	9.7607483	9.9122991	9.8484492	10.1515508	10.0877009	10.2392517	48
13	9.7609274	9.9122099	9.8487174	10.1512826	10.0877901	10.2390726	47
14	9.7611063	9.9121207	9.8489855	10.1510145	10.0878793	10.2388937	46
15	9.7612851	9.9120315	9.8492536	10.1507464	10.0879685	10.2387149	45
16	9.7614638	9.9119422	9.8495216	10.1504784	10.0880578	10.2385362	44
17	9.7616421	9.9118528	9.8497896	10.1502104	10.0881472	10.2383576	43
18	9.7618208	9.9117634	9.8500575	10.1499425	10.0882366	10.2381792	42
19	9.7619992	9.9116739	9.8503253	10.1496747	10.0883261	10.2380008	41
20	9.7621775	9.9115844	9.8505931	10.1494069	10.0884156	10.2378225	40
21	9.7623556	9.9114948	9.8508608	10.1491392	10.0885052	10.2376444	39
22	9.7625337	9.9114051	9.8511285	10.1488715	10.0885949	10.2374663	38
23	9.7627116	9.9113155	9.8513961	10.1486039	10.0886845	10.2372884	37
24	9.7628894	9.9112257	9.8516637	10.1483363	10.0887743	10.2371106	36
25	9.7630671	9.9111359	9.8519312	10.1480688	10.0888641	10.2369329	35
26	9.7632447	9.9110460	9.8521987	10.1478013	10.0889540	10.2367553	34
27	9.7634222	9.9109561	9.8524661	10.1475339	10.0890439	10.2365778	33
28	9.7635996	9.9108661	9.8527335	10.1472665	10.0891339	10.2364004	32
29	9.7637769	9.9107761	9.8530008	10.1469992	10.0892239	10.2362231	31
30	9.7639540	9.9106860	9.8532680	10.1467320	10.0893140	10.2360460	30

	Sine.		Tang.		Secant.	M

54 Degrees.

35 Degrees.

M	Sine.		Tang.		Secant.		
30	9.7639540	9.9106860	9.8532680	10.1467320	10.0893140	10.2360460	30
31	9.7641311	9.9105959	9.8535352	10.1464648	10.0894041	10.2358685	29
32	9.7643080	9.9105057	9.8538023	10.1461977	10.0894944	10.2356920	28
33	9.7644849	9.9104155	9.8540694	10.1459305	10.0895845	10.2355151	27
34	9.7646616	9.9103251	9.8543365	10.1456635	10.0896749	10.2353384	26
35	9.7648382	9.9102348	9.8546034	10.1453966	10.0897652	10.2351618	25
36	9.7650147	9.9101444	9.8548704	10.1451296	10.0898556	10.2349853	24
37	9.7651911	9.9100539	9.8551372	10.1448628	10.0899461	10.2348089	23
38	9.7653674	9.9099634	9.8554041	10.1445959	10.0900366	10.2346326	22
39	9.7655436	9.9098728	9.8556708	10.1443292	10.0901272	10.2344564	21
40	9.7657197	9.9097821	9.8559376	10.1440624	10.0902179	10.2342803	20
41	9.7658957	9.9096915	9.8562042	10.1437958	10.0903085	10.2341043	19
42	9.7660715	9.9096007	9.8564708	10.1435292	10.0903993	10.2339285	18
43	9.7662473	9.9095099	9.8567374	10.1432626	10.0904901	10.2337527	17
44	9.7664229	9.9094190	9.8570039	10.1429961	10.0905810	10.2335771	16
45	9.7665985	9.9093281	9.8572704	10.1427296	10.0906719	10.2334015	15
46	9.7667739	9.9092371	9.8575368	10.1424632	10.0907629	10.2332261	14
47	9.7669492	9.9091461	9.8578031	10.1421969	10.0908539	10.2330508	13
48	9.7671244	9.9090550	9.8580694	10.1419306	10.0909450	10.2328756	12
49	9.7672996	9.9089639	9.8583357	10.1416643	10.0910361	10.2327004	11
50	9.7674746	9.9088727	9.8586019	10.1413981	10.0911273	10.2325254	10
51	9.7676494	9.9087814	9.8588680	10.1411320	10.0912186	10.2323506	9
52	9.7678242	9.9086901	9.8591341	10.1408659	10.0913099	10.2321758	8
53	9.7679989	9.9085988	9.8594002	10.1405998	10.0914012	10.2320011	7
54	9.7681735	9.9085073	9.8596661	10.1403339	10.0914927	10.2318265	6
55	9.7683480	9.9084159	9.8599321	10.1400679	10.0915841	10.2316520	5
56	9.7685223	9.9083243	9.8601980	10.1398020	10.0916757	10.2314777	4
57	9.7686966	9.9082327	9.8604638	10.1395362	10.0917673	10.2313034	3
58	9.7688707	9.9081411	9.8607296	10.1392704	10.0918589	10.2311293	2
59	9.7690448	9.9080494	9.8609954	10.1390046	10.0919506	10.2309555	1
60	9.7692187	9.9079576	9.8612610	10.1387390	10.0920424	10.2307813	0
	Sine.		Tang.		Secant.		M

54 Degrees.

36 Degrees.

M	Sine.		Tang.		Secant.		
0	9.7592187	9.9070576	9.8612510	10.1387390	10.0920424	10.2307815	60
1	9.7593925	9.9078653	9.8615267	10.1384733	10.0921342	10.2306607	59
2	9.7595562	9.9077740	9.8617923	10.1382077	10.0922260	10.2304335	58
3	9.7697399	9.9076820	9.8620578	10.1379424	10.0923180	10.2302260	57
4	9.7599134	9.9075901	9.8623233	10.1376767	10.0924099	10.2300866	56
5	9.7700868	9.9074950	9.8625887	10.1374113	10.0925020	10.2299132	55
6	9.7702601	9.9074059	9.8628541	10.1371459	0.0925941	10.2297399	54
7	9.7704332	9.9073138	9.8631195	10.1368805	10.0926852	10.2295668	53
8	9.7706063	9.9072216	9.8633848	10.1366152	10.0927784	10.2293937	52
9	9.7707793	9.9071293	9.8636500	10.1363500	10.0928707	10.2292207	51
10	9.7709522	9.9070370	9.8639152	10.1360848	10.0929630	10.2290478	50
11	9.7711249	9.9069446	9.8641803	10.1358197	10.0930554	10.2288751	49
12	9.7712976	9.9068522	9.8644454	10.1355546	10.0931478	10.2287024	48
13	9.7714702	9.9067597	9.8647105	10.1352895	10.0932403	10.2285298	47
14	9.7716426	9.9066671	9.8649755	10.1350245	10.0933329	10.2283574	46
15	9.7718150	9.9065745	9.8652404	10.1347596	10.0934255	10.2281850	45
16	9.7719872	9.9064819	9.8655053	10.1344947	10.0935181	10.2280128	44
17	9.7721593	9.9063892	9.8657702	10.1342298	10.0936108	10.2278407	43
18	9.7723314	9.9062964	9.8660350	10.1339650	10.0937036	10.2276686	42
19	9.7725033	9.9062036	9.8662997	10.1337003	10.0937964	10.2274967	41
20	9.7726751	9.9061107	9.8665644	10.1334356	10.0938893	10.2273249	40
21	9.7728468	9.9060177	9.8668291	10.1331709	10.0939823	10.2271532	39
22	9.7730185	9.9059247	9.8670937	10.1329063	10.0940753	10.2269815	38
23	9.7731900	9.9058317	9.8673583	10.1326417	10.0941683	10.2268100	37
24	9.7733614	9.9057386	9.8676228	10.1323772	10.0942614	10.2266386	36
25	9.7735327	9.9056454	9.8678873	10.1321127	10.0943546	10.2264673	35
26	9.7737039	9.9055522	9.8681517	10.1318483	10.0944478	10.2262961	34
27	9.7738749	9.9054589	9.8684160	10.1315840	10.0945411	10.2261251	33
28	9.7740459	9.9053656	9.8686804	10.1313196	10.0946344	10.2259541	32
29	9.7742168	9.9052722	9.8689446	10.1310554	10.0947278	10.2257832	31
30	9.7743876	9.9051787	9.8692089	10.1307911	10.0948213	10.2256124	30

| | Sine. | | Tang. | | Secant. | | M |

53 Degrees.

36 Degrees.

M	Sine.		Tang.		Secant.		
30	9.7743876	9.9051787	9.8692089	10.1307911	10.0948213	10.2256124	30
31	9.7745583	9.9050852	9.8694731	10.1305269	10.0949148	10.2254417	29
32	9.7747288	9.9049916	9.8697372	10.1302628	10.0950084	10.2252712	28
33	9.7748993	9.9048980	9.8700013	10.1299987	10.0951020	10.2251007	27
34	9.7750697	9.9048043	9.8702653	10.1297347	10.0951957	10.2249303	26
35	9.7752399	9.9047106	9.8705293	10.1294707	10.0952894	10.2247601	25
36	9.7754101	9.9046168	9.8707933	10.1292067	10.0953832	10.2245899	24
37	9.7755801	9.9045230	9.8710572	10.1289428	10.0954770	10.2244199	23
38	9.7757501	9.9044291	9.8713210	10.1286790	10.0955709	10.2242499	22
39	9.7759199	9.9043351	9.8715848	10.1284152	10.0956649	10.2240801	21
40	9.7760897	9.9042411	9.8718486	10.1281514	10.0957589	10.2239103	20
41	9.7762593	9.9041470	9.8721123	10.1278877	10.0958530	10.2237407	19
42	9.7764289	9.9040529	9.8723760	10.1276240	10.0959471	10.2235711	18
43	9.7765983	9.9039587	9.8726396	10.1273604	10.0960413	10.2234017	17
44	9.7767676	9.9038644	9.8729032	10.1270968	10.0961356	10.2232324	16
45	9.7769369	9.9037701	9.8731668	10.1268332	10.0962299	10.2230631	15
46	9.7771060	9.9036757	9.8734302	10.1265698	10.0963243	10.2228940	14
47	9.7772750	9.9035813	9.8736937	10.1263063	10.0964187	10.2227250	13
48	9.7774439	9.9034868	9.8739571	10.1260429	10.0965132	10.2225561	12
49	9.7776128	9.9033923	9.8742204	10.1257796	10.0966077	10.2223872	11
50	9.7777815	9.9032977	9.8744838	10.1255162	10.0967023	10.2222185	10
51	9.7779501	9.9032031	9.8747470	10.1252530	10.0967969	10.2220499	9
52	9.7781186	9.9031084	9.8750102	10.1249898	10.0968916	10.2218814	8
53	9.7782870	9.9030136	9.8752734	10.1247266	10.0969864	10.2217130	7
54	9.7784553	9.9029188	9.8755365	10.1244635	10.0970812	10.2215447	6
55	9.7786235	9.9028239	9.8757996	10.1242004	10.0971761	10.2213765	5
56	9.7787916	9.9027289	9.8760627	10.1239373	10.0972711	10.2212084	4
57	9.7789596	9.9026339	9.8763257	10.1236743	10.0973661	10.2210404	3
58	9.7791275	9.9025389	9.8765886	10.1234114	10.0974611	10.2208725	2
59	9.7792953	9.9024438	9.8768515	10.1231485	10.0975562	10.2207047	1
60	9.7794630	9.9023486	9.8771144	10.1228856	10.0976514	10.2205370	0
	Sine.		Tang.		Secant.		M

53 Degrees.

37 Degrees.

M	Sine.		Tang.		Secant.		
0	9.779453-	9.9023456	9.8771144	10.1228856	10.0976514	10.2205370	60
1	9.7796326	9.902253-	9.8773772	10.1226228	10.0977460	10.2203694	59
2	9.7797581	9.9021581	9.8776400	10.1223600	10.0978415	10.2202019	58
3	9.7799655	9.9020628	9.8779027	10.122097	10.0979374	10.2200345	57
4	9.7801328	9.9019674	9.8781654	10.1218346	10.0980326	10.2198672	56
5	9.7803000	9.9018719	9.8784281	10.1215719	10.0981281	10.2197000	55
6	9.7804671	9.9017764	9.8786907	10.1213093	10.0982236	10.2195329	54
7	9.7806341	9.9016808	9.8789533	10.1210467	10.0983192	10.2193659	53
8	9.7808010	9.9015852	9.8792158	10.1207842	10.0984148	10.2191990	52
9	9.7809677	9.9014895	9.8794782	10.1205218	10.0985105	10.2190323	51
10	9.7811344	9.9013938	9.8797407	10.1202593	10.0986062	10.2188656	50
11	9.7813010	9.9012980	9.8800031	10.1199969	10.0987020	10.2186990	49
12	9.7814675	9.9012021	9.8802654	10.1197346	10.0987979	10.2185325	48
13	9.7816339	9.9011062	9.8805277	10.1194723	10.0988938	10.2183661	47
14	9.7818002	9.9010102	9.8807900	10.1192100	10.0989898	10.2181998	46
15	9.7819664	9.9009142	9.8810522	10.1189478	10.0990858	10.2180336	45
16	9.7821324	9.9008181	9.8813144	10.1186856	10.0991819	10.2178676	44
17	9.7822984	9.9007219	9.8815765	10.1184235	10.0992781	10.2177016	43
18	9.7824643	9.9006257	9.8818386	10.1181614	10.0993743	10.2175357	42
19	9.7826301	9.9005294	9.8821007	10.1178993	10.0994706	10.2173699	41
20	9.7827958	9.9004331	9.8823627	10.1176373	10.0995669	10.2172042	40
21	9.7829614	9.9003367	9.8826246	10.1173754	10.0996633	10.2170386	39
22	9.7831268	9.9002403	9.8828866	10.1171134	10.0997597	10.2168732	38
23	9.7832922	9.9001438	9.8831484	10.1168516	10.0998562	10.2167078	37
24	9.7834575	9.9000472	9.8834103	10.1165897	10.0999528	10.2165425	36
25	9.7836227	9.8999506	9.8836721	10.1163279	10.1000494	10.2163773	35
26	9.7837875	9.8998539	9.8839338	10.1160662	10.1001461	10.2162122	34
27	9.7839528	9.8997572	9.8841956	10.1158044	10.1002428	10.2160472	33
28	9.7841177	9.8996604	9.8844572	10.1155428	10.1003396	10.2158823	32
29	9.7842824	9.8995636	9.8847189	10.1152811	10.1004364	10.2157176	31
30	9.7844471	9.8994667	9.8849805	10.1150195	10.1005333	10.2155529	30

| | Sine. | | Tang. | | Secant. | | M |

52 Degrees.

37 Degrees.

M	Sine.		Tang.		Secant.		
30	9.7844471	9.8994667	9.8849805	10.1150195	10.1005333	10.2155529	30
31	9.7846117	9.8993697	9.8852420	10.1147580	10.1006303	10.2153883	29
32	9.7847764	9.8992727	9.8855035	10.1144965	10.1007274	10.2152236	28
33	9.7849406	9.8991756	9.8857650	10.1142350	10.1008244	10.2150594	27
34	9.7851049	9.8990284	9.8860264	10.1139736	10.1009216	10.2148951	26
35	9.7852691	9.8989812	9.8862878	10.1137122	10.1010188	10.2147309	25
36	9.7854332	9.8988840	9.8865492	10.1134508	10.1011160	10.2145668	24
37	9.7855972	9.8987867	9.8868105	10.1131895	10.1012133	10.2144028	23
38	9.7857611	9.8986893	9.8870718	10.1129282	10.1013107	10.2142389	22
39	9.7859249	9.8985919	9.8873330	10.1126670	10.1014081	10.2140751	21
40	9.7860886	9.8984944	9.8875942	10.1124058	10.1015056	10.2139114	20
41	9.7862522	9.8983968	9.8878554	10.1121446	10.1016032	10.2137478	19
42	9.7864157	9.8982992	9.8881165	10.1118835	10.1017008	10.2135843	18
43	9.7865791	9.8982015	9.8883775	10.1116225	10.1017985	10.2134209	17
44	9.7867424	9.8981038	9.8886386	10.1113614	10.1018962	10.2132576	16
45	9.7869056	9.8980060	9.8888996	10.1111004	10.1019940	10.2130944	15
46	9.7870687	9.8979082	9.8891605	10.1108395	10.1020918	10.2129313	14
47	9.7872317	9.8978103	9.8894214	10.1105786	10.1021897	10.2127683	13
48	9.7873946	9.8977123	9.8896823	10.1103177	10.1022877	10.2126054	12
49	9.7875574	9.8976143	9.8899432	10.1100568	10.1023857	10.2124426	11
50	9.7877202	9.8975162	9.8902040	10.1097960	10.1024838	10.2122798	10
51	9.7878828	9.8974181	9.8904647	10.1095353	10.1025819	10.2121172	9
54	9.7880453	9.8973199	9.8907254	10.1092746	10.1026801	10.2119547	8
53	9.7882077	9.8972216	9.8909861	10.1090139	10.1027784	10.2117923	7
54	9.7883701	9.8971233	9.8912468	10.1087532	10.1028767	10.2116299	6
55	9.7885323	9.8970249	9.8915074	10.1084926	10.1029751	10.2114677	5
56	9.7886944	9.8969265	9.8917679	10.1082321	10.1030735	10.2113056	4
57	9.7888565	9.8968280	9.8920285	10.1079715	10.1031720	10.2111435	3
58	9.7890184	9.8967294	9.8922890	10.1077110	10.1032706	10.2109816	2
59	9.7891802	9.8966308	9.8925494	10.1074506	10.1033692	10.2108198	1
60	9.7893420	9.8965321	9.8928098	10.1071902	10.1034679	10.2106580	0
	Sine.		Tang.		Secant.		M

52 Degrees.

38 Degrees.

M	Sine.		Tang.		Secant.		
0	9.7893420	9.8965321	9.8928098	10.1071902	10.1034679	10.2106580	60
1	9.7895031	9.8964334	9.8930702	10.1069298	10.1035666	10.2104964	59
2	9.7896655	9.8963346	9.8933306	10.1066694	10.1036654	10.2103348	58
3	9.7898265	9.8962358	9.8935909	10.1064091	10.1037642	10.2101734	57
4	9.7899885	9.8961369	9.8938511	10.1061489	10.1038631	10.2100120	56
5	9.7901490	9.8960379	9.8941114	10.1058886	10.1039621	10.2098507	55
6	9.7903104	9.8959389	9.8943715	10.1056285	10.1040611	10.2096896	54
7	9.7904715	9.8958395	9.8946317	10.1053683	10.1041602	10.2095285	53
8	9.7906325	9.8957406	9.8948918	10.1051082	10.1042594	10.2093675	52
9	9.7907933	9.8956414	9.8951519	10.1048481	10.1043586	10.2092067	51
10	9.7909541	9.8955422	9.8954119	10.1045881	10.1044578	10.2090459	50
11	9.7911148	9.8954428	9.8956719	10.1043281	10.1045572	10.2088852	49
12	9.7912753	9.8953435	9.8959319	10.1040681	10.1046565	10.2087246	48
13	9.7914359	9.8952440	9.8961918	10.1038082	10.1047560	10.2085641	47
14	9.7915963	9.8951445	9.8964517	10.1035483	10.1048555	10.2084037	46
15	9.7917566	9.8950450	9.8967116	10.1032884	10.1049550	10.2082434	45
16	9.7919169	9.8949453	9.8969714	10.1030286	10.1050547	10.2080832	44
17	9.7920769	9.8948457	9.8972312	10.1027688	10.1051543	10.2079231	43
18	9.7922369	9.8947459	9.8974910	10.1025090	10.1052541	10.2077631	42
19	9.7923969	9.8946461	9.8977507	10.1022493	10.1053539	10.2076032	41
20	9.7925566	9.8945463	9.8980104	10.1019896	10.1054537	10.2074434	40
21	9.7927163	9.8944463	9.8982700	10.1017300	10.1055537	10.2072837	39
22	9.7928760	9.8943464	9.8985296	10.1014704	10.1056536	10.2071240	38
23	9.7930355	9.8942463	9.8987892	10.1012108	10.1057537	10.2069645	37
24	9.7931949	9.8941462	9.8990487	10.1009513	10.1058538	10.2068051	36
25	9.7933543	9.8940461	9.8993082	10.1006918	10.1059539	10.2066457	35
25	9.7935135	9.8939458	9.8995677	10.1004323	10.1060542	10.2064865	34
27	9.7936727	9.8938456	9.8998271	10.1001729	10.1061544	10.2063273	33
28	9.7938317	9.8937452	9.9000865	10.0999135	10.1062548	10.2061683	32
29	9.7939907	9.8936448	9.9003459	10.0996541	10.1063552	10.2060093	31
30	9.7941496	9.8935444	9.9006052	10.0993948	10.1064556	10.2058504	30
	Sine.		Tang.		Secant.		M

51 Degrees.

38 Degrees.

M	Sine.		Tang.		Secant.		
30	9.7941496	9.8935444	9.9006057	10.0993948	10.1064556	10.2058504	30
31	9.7943083	9.8934439	9.9008644	10.0991355	10.1065561	10.2056917	29
32	9.7944670	9.8933433	9.9011237	10.0988763	10.1066567	10.2055330	28
33	9.7946256	9.8932426	9.9013830	10.0986170	10.1067574	10.2053744	27
34	9.7947841	9.8931419	9.9016422	10.0983578	10.1068581	10.2052159	26
35	9.7949425	9.8930412	9.9019013	10.0980987	10.1069588	10.2050575	25
36	9.7951008	9.8929404	9.9021604	10.0978396	10.1070596	10.2048992	24
37	9.7952590	9.8928395	9.9024195	10.0975805	10.1071605	10.2047410	23
38	9.7954171	9.8927385	9.9026786	10.0973214	10.1072615	10.2045829	22
39	9.7955751	9.8926375	9.9029376	10.0970624	10.1073625	10.2044249	21
40	9.7957330	9.8925365	9.9031966	10.0968034	10.1074635	10.2042670	20
41	9.7958909	9.8924354	9.9034555	10.0965445	10.1075646	10.2041091	19
42	9.7960486	9.8923342	9.9037144	10.0962856	10.1076658	10.2039514	18
43	9.7962062	9.8922329	9.9039733	10.0960267	10.1077671	10.2037938	17
44	9.7963638	9.8921316	9.9042321	10.0957679	10.1078684	10.2036362	16
45	9.7965212	9.8920303	9.9044910	10.0955090	10.1079697	10.2034788	15
46	9.7966786	9.8919289	9.9047497	10.0952503	10.1080711	10.2033214	14
47	9.7968359	9.8918274	9.9050085	10.0949915	10.1081726	10.2031641	13
48	9.7969930	9.8917258	9.9052672	10.0947328	10.1082742	10.2030070	12
49	9.7971501	9.8916242	9.9055259	10.0944741	10.1083758	10.2028499	11
50	9.7973071	9.8915226	9.9057845	10.0942155	10.1084774	10.2026929	10
51	9.7974640	9.8914208	9.9060431	10.0939569	10.1085792	10.2025360	9
52	9.7976208	9.8913191	9.9063017	10.0936983	10.1086809	10.2023792	8
53	9.7977775	9.8912172	9.9065603	10.0934397	10.1087828	10.2022225	7
54	9.7979241	9.8911153	9.9068188	10.0931812	10.1088847	10.2020659	6
55	9.7980906	9.8910133	9.9070773	10.0929227	10.1089867	10.2019094	5
56	9.7982470	9.8909113	9.9073357	10.0926643	10.1090887	10.2017530	4
57	9.7984034	9.8908092	9.9075941	10.0924059	10.1091908	10.2015966	3
58	9.7985590	9.8907071	9.9078525	10.0921475	10.1092929	10.2014404	2
59	9.7987158	9.8906049	9.9081109	10.0918891	10.1093951	10.2012842	1
60	9.7988718	9.8905026	9.9083692	10.0916308	10.1094974	10.2011282	0
	Sine.		Tang.		Secant.		M

51 Degrees.

A Table of Artificial Sines,

39 Degrees.

M	Sine.		Tang.		Secant.		
0	9.7988718	9.8905026	9.9083692	10.0916308	10.1094974	10.2011282	60
1	9.7990278	9.8904003	9.9086275	10.0913725	10.1095997	10.2009724	59
2	9.7991836	9.8902979	9.9088858	10.0911142	10.1097021	10.2008164	58
3	9.7993394	9.8901954	9.9091440	10.0908560	10.1098046	10.2006606	57
4	9.7994951	9.8900929	9.9094022	10.0905978	10.1099071	10.2005049	56
5	9.7996507	9.8899903	9.9096603	10.0903397	10.1100097	10.2003493	55
6	9.7998062	9.8898877	9.9099185	10.0900815	10.1101123	10.2001938	54
7	9.7999616	9.8897850	9.9101766	10.0898234	10.1102150	10.2000384	53
8	9.8001169	9.8896822	9.9104347	10.0895653	10.1103178	10.1998831	52
9	9.8002721	9.8895794	9.9106927	10.0893073	10.1104206	10.1997279	51
10	9.8004272	9.8894765	9.9109507	10.0890493	10.1105235	10.1995728	50
11	9.8005823	9.8893736	9.9112087	10.0887913	10.1106264	10.1994177	49
12	9.8007372	9.8892706	9.9114666	10.0885334	10.1107294	10.1992628	48
13	9.8008921	9.8891675	9.9117245	10.0882755	10.1108325	10.1991079	47
14	9.8010458	9.8890644	9.9119824	10.0880176	10.1109356	10.1989532	46
15	9.8012014	9.8889612	9.9122403	10.0877597	10.1110388	10.1987985	45
16	9.8013561	9.8888580	9.9124981	10.0875019	10.1111420	10.1986439	44
17	9.8015106	9.8887547	9.9127559	10.0872441	10.1112453	10.1984894	43
18	9.8016649	9.8886513	9.9130137	10.0869863	10.1113487	10.1983351	42
19	9.8018192	9.8885479	9.9132714	10.0867286	10.1114521	10.1981808	41
20	9.8019735	9.8884444	9.9135291	10.0864709	10.1115556	10.1980265	40
21	9.8021276	9.8883408	9.9137868	10.0862132	10.1116592	10.1978724	39
22	9.8022816	9.8882372	9.9140444	10.0859556	10.1117628	10.1977184	38
23	9.8024355	9.8881335	9.9143020	10.0856980	10.1118665	10.1975645	37
24	9.8025894	9.8880298	9.9145596	10.0854404	10.1119702	10.1974106	36
25	9.8027431	9.8879260	9.9148171	10.0851829	10.1120740	10.1972569	35
26	9.8028968	9.8878221	9.9150747	10.0849253	10.1121779	10.1971032	34
27	9.8030504	9.8877182	9.9153322	10.0846678	10.1122818	10.1969496	33
28	9.8032038	9.8876142	9.9155896	10.0844104	10.1123858	10.1967962	32
29	9.8033572	9.8875102	9.9158471	10.0841529	10.1124898	10.1966428	31
30	9.8035105	9.8874061	9.9161045	10.0838955	10.1125939	10.1964895	30
	Sine.		Tang.		Secant.		M

50 Degrees.

39 *Degrees.*

M	Sine.		Tang.		Secant.		
30	9.8035105	9.8874061	9.9161045	10.0838955	10.1125939	10.1964895	30
31	9.8036637	9.8873019	9.9163618	10.0836382	10.1126981	10.1963363	29
32	9.8038168	9.8871977	9.9166192	10.0833808	10.1128023	10.1961832	28
33	9.8039699	9.8870934	9.9168765	10.0831235	10.1129066	10.1960301	27
34	9.8041228	9.8869890	9.9171338	10.0828662	10.1130110	10.1958772	26
35	9.8042757	9.8868846	9.9173911	10.0826089	10.1131154	10.1957243	25
36	9.8044284	9.8867801	9.9176483	10.0823517	10.1132199	10.1955716	24
37	9.8045811	9.8866756	9.9179055	10.0820945	10.1133244	10.1954180	23
38	9.8047336	9.8865710	9.9181627	10.0818373	10.1134290	10.1952664	22
39	9.8048861	9.8864663	9.9184198	10.0815802	10.1135337	10.1951139	21
40	9.8050385	9.8863616	9.9186769	10.0813231	10.1136384	10.1949615	20
41	9.8051908	9.8862568	9.9189347	10.0810660	10.1137432	10.1948092	19
42	9.8053430	9.8861519	9.9191911	10.0808089	10.1138481	10.1946570	18
43	9.8054951	9.8860470	9.9194481	10.0805519	10.1139530	10.1945049	17
44	9.8056472	9.8859420	9.9197051	10.0802949	10.1140580	10.1943528	16
45	9.8057991	9.8858370	9.9199621	10.0800379	10.1141630	10.1942009	15
46	9.8059510	9.8857319	9.9202191	10.0797809	10.1142681	10.1940490	14
47	9.8061027	9.8856267	9.9204760	10.0795240	10.1143733	10.1938973	13
48	9.8062544	9.8855215	9.9207329	10.0792671	10.1144785	10.1937456	12
49	9.8064060	9.8854162	9.9209898	10.0790102	10.1145838	10.1935940	11
50	9.8065575	9.8853109	9.9212466	10.0787534	10.1146891	10.1934425	10
51	9.8067089	9.8852055	9.9215034	10.0784966	10.1147945	10.1932911	9
52	9.8068602	9.8851000	9.9217602	10.0782398	10.1149000	10.1931398	8
53	9.8070114	9.8849945	9.9220170	10.0779830	10.1150055	10.1929886	7
54	9.8071626	9.8848889	9.9222737	10.0777263	10.1151111	10.1928374	6
55	9.8073136	9.8847832	9.9225304	10.0774696	10.1152168	10.1926864	5
56	9.8074646	9.8846775	9.9227871	10.0772129	10.1153225	10.1925354	4
57	9.8076154	9.8845717	9.9230437	10.0769563	10.1154283	10.1923846	3
58	9.8077662	9.8844659	9.9233004	10.0766996	10.1155341	10.1922338	2
59	9.8079169	9.8843599	9.9235570	10.0764430	10.1156401	10.1920831	1
60	9.8080675	9.8842540	9.9238135	10.0761885	10.1157460	10.1919325	0
	Sine.		Tang.		Secant.		M

50 *Degrees.*

40 Degrees.

M	Sine.		Tang.		Secant.		
0	9.8080675	9.8842540	9.9238135	10.0751860	10.1157460	10.1919325	50
1	9.8082182	9.8841479	9.9240701	10.0759299	10.1158521	10.1917820	59
2	9.8083684	9.8840418	9.9243266	10.0756734	10.1159582	10.1916316	58
3	9.8085188	9.8839357	9.9245831	10.0754165	10.1160643	10.1914811	57
4	9.8086690	9.8838294	9.9248396	10.0751604	10.1161708	10.1913310	56
5	9.8088519	9.8837232	9.9250960	10.0749040	10.1162768	10.1911808	55
6	9.8089690	9.8836168	9.9253524	10.0746476	10.1163832	10.1910308	54
7	9.8091192	9.8835104	9.9256088	10.0743912	10.1164896	10.1908808	53
8	9.8092691	9.8834039	9.9258652	10.0741348	10.1165961	10.1907309	52
9	9.8094189	9.8832974	9.9261215	10.0738785	10.1167026	10.1905811	51
10	9.8095686	9.8831905	9.9263778	10.0736222	10.1168092	10.1904314	50
11	9.8097132	9.8830841	9.9266341	10.0733659	10.1169159	10.1902818	49
12	9.8098678	9.8829774	9.9268904	10.0731096	10.1170226	10.1901322	48
13	9.8100172	9.8828706	9.9271466	10.0728534	10.1171294	10.1899828	47
14	9.8101666	9.8827638	9.9274028	10.0725972	10.1172362	10.1898334	46
15	9.8103159	9.8826565	9.9276590	10.0723410	10.1173432	10.1896841	45
16	9.8104650	9.8825499	9.9279152	10.0720848	10.1174501	10.1895350	44
17	9.8106141	9.8824428	9.9281713	10.0718287	10.1175572	10.1893859	43
18	9.8107631	9.8823357	9.9284274	10.0715726	10.1176643	10.1892369	42
19	9.8109121	9.8822285	9.9286835	10.0713165	10.1177715	10.1890879	41
20	9.8110609	9.8821213	9.9289396	10.0710604	10.1178787	10.1889391	40
21	9.8112095	9.8820140	9.9291956	10.0708044	10.1179860	10.1887904	39
22	9.8113583	9.8819067	9.9294516	10.0705484	10.1180933	10.1886417	38
23	9.8115069	9.8817992	9.9297076	10.0702924	10.1182008	10.1884931	37
24	9.8116554	9.8816918	9.9299636	10.0700364	10.1183082	10.1883446	36
25	9.8118038	9.8815842	9.9302195	10.0697805	10.1184158	10.1881962	35
26	9.8119521	9.8814766	9.9304755	10.0695245	10.1185234	10.1880479	34
27	9.8121003	9.8813689	9.9307314	10.0692686	10.1186311	10.1878997	33
28	9.8122484	9.8812612	9.9309872	10.0690128	10.1187388	10.1877516	32
29	9.8123965	9.8811534	9.9312431	10.0687569	10.1188466	10.1876035	31
30	9.8125444	9.8810455	9.9314989	10.0685011	10.1189545	10.1874556	30
	Sine.		Tang.		Secant.		M

49 Degrees.

40 Degrees.

M	Sine.		Tang.		Secant.		M
30	9.8125444	9.8810455	9.9314989	10.0685011	10.1189545	10.1874556	30
31	9.8126923	9.8809376	9.9317547	10.0682453	10.1190624	10.1873077	29
32	9.8128401	9.8808296	9.9320105	10.0679895	10.1191704	10.1871599	28
33	9.8129878	9.8807215	9.9322662	10.0677338	10.1192785	10.1870122	27
34	9.8131354	9.8806134	9.9325220	10.0674780	10.1193866	10.1868646	26
35	9.8132829	9.8805052	9.9327777	10.0672223	10.1194948	10.1867171	25
36	9.8134303	9.8803970	9.9330334	10.0669566	10.1196030	10.1865697	24
37	9.8135777	9.8802887	9.9332890	10.0667110	10.1197113	10.1864223	23
38	9.8137250	9.8801803	9.9335446	10.0664554	10.1198197	10.1862750	22
39	9.8138721	9.8800719	9.9338003	10.0661997	10.1199281	10.1861279	21
40	9.8140192	9.8799634	9.9340559	10.0659441	10.1200366	10.1859808	20
41	9.8141662	9.8798548	9.9343114	10.0656886	10.1201452	10.1858338	19
42	9.8143131	9.8797462	9.9345670	10.0654330	10.1202538	10.1856869	18
43	9.8144600	9.8796375	9.9348225	10.0651775	10.1203625	10.1855400	17
44	9.8146067	9.8795287	9.9350780	10.0649220	10.1204713	10.1853933	16
45	9.8147534	9.8794199	9.9353335	10.0646665	10.1205801	10.1852466	15
46	9.8148999	9.8793110	9.9355889	10.0644111	10.1206890	10.1851001	14
47	9.8150464	9.8792021	9.9358444	10.0641556	10.1207979	10.1849536	13
48	9.8151928	9.8790930	9.9360998	10.0639002	10.1209070	10.1848072	12
49	9.8153391	9.8789840	9.9363552	10.0636448	10.1210160	10.1846609	11
50	9.8154854	9.8788748	9.9366105	10.0633895	10.1211252	10.1845146	10
51	9.8156315	9.8787656	9.9368659	10.0631341	10.1212344	10.1843685	9
52	9.8157776	9.8786563	9.9371212	10.0628788	10.1213437	10.1842224	8
53	9.8159235	9.8785470	9.9373765	10.0626235	10.1214530	10.1840765	7
54	9.8160694	9.8784376	9.9376318	10.0623682	10.1215624	10.1839306	6
55	9.8162152	9.8783281	9.9378871	10.0621129	10.1216719	10.1837848	5
56	9.8163609	9.8782186	9.9381423	10.0618577	10.1217814	10.1836391	4
57	9.8165066	9.8781090	9.9383975	10.0616025	10.1218910	10.1834934	3
58	9.8166521	9.8779994	9.9386527	10.0613473	10.1220006	10.1833479	2
59	9.8167975	9.8778896	9.9389079	10.0610921	10.1221104	10.1832025	1
60	9.8169429	9.8777799	9.9391631	10.0608369	10.1222201	10.1830571	0
	Sine.		Tang.		Secant.		M

49 Degrees.

41 Degrees.

M	Sine.		Tang.		Secant.		
0	9.8169429	9.8777799	9.9391631	10.0608369	10.122220	0.1830571	60
1	9.8170882	9.8776700	9.9394102	10.0605818	10.1223300	10.1829118	59
2	9.8172334	9.8775601	9.9396733	10.0603267	10.1224399	10.1827666	58
3	9.8173785	9.8774501	9.9399294	.0600716	10.1225491	10.1826215	57
4	9.8175235	9.8773401	9.9401833	10.0598166	10.1226599	10.1824765	56
5	9.8176685	9.8772300	9.9404385	10.0595615	10.1227700	10.1823315	55
6	9.8178133	9.8771198	9.9406936	10.0593064	10.1228802	10.1821867	54
7	9.8179581	9.8770096	9.9409486	10.0590514	10.1229909	10.1820419	53
8	9.8181028	9.8768993	9.9412036	10.0587964	10.1231007	10.1818972	52
9	9.8182474	9.8767889	9.9414585	10.0585415	10.1232111	10.1817526	51
10	9.8183919	9.8766785	9.9417135	10.0582865	10.1233215	10.1816081	50
11	9.8185364	9.8765680	9.9419684	10.0580316	10.1234320	10.1814636	49
12	9.8186807	9.8764574	9.9422233	10.0577767	10.1235426	10.1813193	48
13	9.8188250	9.8763468	9.9424782	10.0575218	10.1236532	10.1811750	47
14	9.8189692	9.8762361	9.9427331	10.0572669	10.1237639	10.1810308	46
15	9.8191133	9.8761253	9.9429879	10.0570121	10.1238747	10.1808867	45
16	9.8192573	9.8760145	9.9432428	10.0567572	10.1239855	10.1807427	44
17	9.8194012	9.8759036	9.9434975	10.0565024	10.1240964	10.1805988	43
18	9.8195450	9.8757927	9.9437524	10.0562476	10.1242073	10.1804550	42
19	9.8196888	9.8756816	9.9440072	10.0559928	10.1243184	10.1803112	41
20	9.8198325	9.8755706	9.9442619	10.0557381	10.1244294	10.1801675	40
21	9.8199761	9.8754594	9.9445166	10.0554834	10.1245406	10.1800239	39
22	9.8201196	9.8753482	9.9447714	10.0552286	10.1246518	10.1798804	38
23	9.8202630	9.8752359	9.9450261	10.0549739	10.1247631	10.1797370	37
24	9.8204063	9.8751256	9.9452807	10.0547193	10.1248744	10.1795937	36
25	9.8205496	9.8750142	9.9455354	10.0544646	10.1249858	10.1794504	35
26	9.8206927	9.8749027	9.9457900	10.0542100	10.1250973	10.1793073	34
27	9.8208358	9.8747912	9.9460447	10.0539553	10.1252088	10.1791642	33
28	9.8209788	9.8746795	9.9462993	10.0537007	10.1253205	10.1790212	32
29	9.8211217	9.8745679	9.9465539	10.0534461	10.1254321	10.1788783	31
30	9.8212646	9.8744561	9.9468084	10.0531916	10.1255439	10.1787354	30
	Sine.		Tang.		Secant.		M

48 Degrees.

Pamper, Pamper, Pamper, amper, Pamp

per, amper, Pamper, Pamper,

Pamper, Pamper, Pamper, Pamper,

amper, Pamper, Pamper, Pampe

amper, Pamper, Pamper, Pamper,

amper, Pamper, Pamper, Pamper,

amper, Pamper, Pamper, amper,

amper, Pamper, Pamper, Pam

amper, Pamper, Pamper, Pamper,

amper, Pamper, Pamper, Pamper, Pam

amper Pamper, Pamper, Pamper,

Pamper, Pamper, Pamper, Pamper,

Joshua Easton his Book. Jan

Quintus,

41 Degrees.

M	Sine.		Tang.		Secant.		M
30	9.8212646	9.8744561	9.9468084	10.0531916	10.1255439	10.1787354	30
31	9.8214073	9.8743443	9.9470630	10.052937c	10.1256557	10.1785927	29
32	9.8215500	9.8742325	9.9473175	10.0526825	10.1257675	10.178450c	28
33	9.8216926	9.8741205	9.9475720	10.0524280	10.1258795	10.1783074	27
34	9.8218351	9.8740085	9.9478265	10.0521735	10.1259915	10.1781649	26
35	9.8219775	9.8738965	9.9480810	10.0519190	10.1261035	10.1780225	25
36	9.9221198	9.8737844	9.9483355	10.0516645	10.1262156	10.1778802	24
37	9.8222621	9.8736722	9.9485899	10.0514101	10.1263278	10.1777379	23
38	9.8224042	9.8735599	9.9488443	10.0511557	10.1264401	10.1775958	22
39	9.8225463	9.8734476	9.9490987	10.0509013	10.1265524	10.1774537	21
40	9.8226883	9.8733352	9.9493531	10.0506469	10.1266648	10.1773117	20
41	9.8228302	9.8732227	9.9496075	10.0503925	10.126777?	10.1771698	19
42	9.8229721	9.8731102	9.9498619	10.0501381	10.1268898	10.1770279	18
43	9.8231138	9.8729976	9.9501162	10.0498838	10.1270024	10.1768862	17
44	9.8232555	9.8728849	9.9503705	10.0496295	10.1271151	10.1767445	16
45	9.8233971	9.8727722	9.9506248	10.0493752	10.1272278	10.1766029	15
46	9.8235386	9.8726594	9.9508791	10.0491209	10.1273406	10.1764614	14
47	9.8236800	9.8725466	9.9511334	10.0488666	10.1274534	10.176320?	13
48	9.8238213	9.8724337	9.9513876	10.0486124	10.1275663	10.1761787	12
49	9.8239626	9.8723207	9.9516419	10.0483581	10.1276793	10.1760374	11
50	9.8241037	9.8722076	9.9518961	10.0481039	10.1277924	10.1758963	10
51	9.8242448	9.8720945	9.9521503	10.0478497	10.1279055	10.1757552	9
52	9.8243858	9.8719813	9.9524245	10.0475955	10.1280187	10.1756142	8
53	9.8245267	9.8718681	9.9526587	10.0473413	10.1281319	10.1754733	7
54	9.8246676	9.8717548	9.9529128	10.0470872	10.1282452	10.1753324	6
55	9.8248083	9.8716414	9.953167c	10.0468330	10.1283586	10.1751917	5
56	9.8249490	9.8715279	9.9534211	10.0465789	10.1284721	10.1750510	4
57	9.8250896	9.8714144	9.9536752	10.0463248	10.1285856	10.1749104	3
58	9.8252301	9.8713008	9.9539293	10.0460707	10.1286992	10.1747699	2
59	9.8253705	9.8711872	9.9541834	10.0458166	10.1288128	10.1746295	1
60	9.8255109	9.8710735	9.9544374	10.0455626	10.1289265	10.1744891	0
	Sine.		Tang.		Secant.		M

48 Degrees.

42 Degrees.

M	Sine.		Tang.		Secant.		
0	9.8255109	9.8710735	9.9544374	10.0455626	10.1289265	10.1744891	60
1	9.8256512	9.8709597	9.9546915	10.0453085	10.1290403	10.1743488	59
2	9.8257915	9.8708458	9.9549455	10.0450545	10.1291542	10.1742087	58
3	9.8259314	9.8707319	9.9551935	10.0448000	10.1292681	10.1740686	57
4	9.8260715	9.8706179	9.9554535	10.0445465	10.1293821	10.1739285	56
5	9.8262114	9.8705039	9.9557075	10.0442925	10.1294961	10.1737886	55
6	9.8263512	9.8703898	9.9559615	10.0440385	10.1296102	10.1736488	54
7	9.8264910	9.8702756	9.9562154	10.0437846	10.1297244	10.1735090	53
8	9.8266307	9.8701613	9.9564694	10.0435306	10.1298387	10.1733693	52
9	9.8267703	9.8700470	9.9567233	10.0432767	10.1299530	10.1732297	51
10	9.8269098	9.8699326	9.9569772	10.0430228	10.1300674	10.1730902	50
11	9.8270473	9.8698182	9.9572311	10.0427689	10.1301818	10.1729507	49
12	9.8271887	9.8697037	9.9574850	10.0425150	10.1302963	10.1728113	48
13	9.8273279	9.8695891	9.9577389	10.0422611	10.1304109	10.1726721	47
14	9.8274671	9.8694744	9.9579927	10.0420073	10.1305256	10.1725329	46
15	9.8276062	9.8693597	9.9582465	10.0417535	10.1306403	10.1723937	45
16	9.8277452	9.8692449	9.9585004	10.0414996	10.1307551	10.1722547	44
17	9.8278842	9.8691301	9.9587542	10.0412458	10.1308699	10.1721157	43
18	9.8280231	9.8690152	9.9590080	10.0409920	10.1309848	10.1719769	42
19	9.8281619	9.8689002	9.9592618	10.0407382	10.1310998	10.1718381	41
20	9.8283006	9.8687851	9.9595155	10.0404845	10.1312149	10.1716994	40
21	9.8284393	9.8686700	9.9597693	10.0402307	10.1313300	10.1715607	39
22	9.8285778	9.8685548	9.9600230	10.0399770	10.1314452	10.1714222	38
23	9.8287163	9.8684396	9.9602767	10.0397233	10.1315604	10.1712837	37
24	9.8288547	9.8683242	9.9605305	10.0394695	10.1316758	10.1711453	36
25	9.8289930	9.8682088	9.9607842	10.0392158	10.1317912	10.1710070	35
26	9.8291312	9.8680934	9.9610378	10.0389622	10.1319066	10.1708688	34
27	9.8292694	9.8679779	9.9612915	10.0387085	10.1320221	10.1707306	33
28	9.8294075	9.8678623	9.9615452	10.0384548	10.1321377	10.1705925	32
29	9.8295454	9.8677466	9.9617988	10.0382012	10.1322534	10.1704546	31
30	9.8296833	9.8675309	9.9620525	10.0379475	10.1323691	10.1703167	30
	Sine.		Tang.		Secant.		M

47 Degrees.

42 *Degrees.*

M	Sine.		Tang.		Secant.		
30	9.8296833	9.8676305	9.9620525	10.0379475	10.1323691	1C.170316,	3C
31	9.8298212	9.8675151	9.9623061	1C.037693,	10.1324845	1C.170178,	29
32	9.8299586	9.8673992	9.9625597	10.0374403	10.1326008	1C.1700411	28
33	9.8300966	9.8672833	9.9628133	10.037186,	10.1327167	10.1699034	27
34	9.8302344	9.8671673	9.9630665	10.0369331	10.1328327	10.1697658	26
35	9.8303717	9.8670512	9.9633204	10.0366790	10.1329488	10.1696283	25
36	9.8305091	9.8669351	9.9635740	1C.0364260	10.1330649	1C.1694905	24
37	9.8306464	9.8668189	9.9638275	10.0361725	10.1331811	1C.1693530	23
38	9.8307837	9.8657026	9.9640811	10.0359189	10.1332974	10.1692163	22
39	9.8309209	9.8665863	9.9643346	10.0356654	10.1334137	10.1690791	21
4C	9.8310580	9.8664696	9.9645881	1C.0354119	10.1335301	10.1689420	2C
41	9.8311950	9.8663534	9.9648416	10.0351584	10.1336466	10.1688050	19
42	9.8313320	9.8662369	9.9650951	10.0349049	10.1337631	10.1686680	18
43	9.8314688	9.8661203	9.9653486	10.0346514	10.1338797	10.1685312	17
44	9.8316056	9.8660036	9.9656020	10.034398	10.1339964	10.1683944	16
45	9.8317423	9.8658868	9.9658555	10.0341445	10.1341132	10.1682577	15
46	9.8318789	9.8657700	9.9661089	1C.0338911	10.1342300	10.1681211	14
47	9.8320155	9.8656531	9.9663623	1C.0336377	10.1343469	10.1679845	13
48	9.8321519	9.8655362	9.9666157	10.0333843	10.1344638	10.1678481	12
49	9.8322883	9.8654192	9.9668692	10.0331308	10.1345808	10.1677117	11
5C	9.8324246	9.8653021	9.9671225	10.0328775	10.1346979	10.1675754	10
51	9.8325609	9.8651849	9.9673759	1C.0326241	10.1348151	10.1674391	9
52	9.8326970	9.8650677	9.9676293	10.0323707	10.1349323	10.1673030	8
53	9.8328331	9.8649504	9.9678827	10.0321173	10.1350496	10.1671669	7
54	9.8329691	9.8648331	9.9681360	10.0318640	10.1351669	10.1670309	6
55	9.8331050	9.8647156	9.9683893	1C.0316107	10.1352844	10.1668950	5
56	9.8332408	9.8645981	9.9686427	10.0313573	10.1354019	10.1667592	4
57	9.8333766	9.8644806	9.9688960	10.0311040	10.1355194	10.1666234	3
58	9.8335122	9.8643629	9.9691493	10.0308507	10.1356371	10.1664878	2
59	9.8336478	9.8642452	9.9694026	10.0305974	10.1357548	10.1663522	1
6C	9.8337833	9.8641275	9.9696555	10.0303441	10.1358725	10.1662167	0
	Sine.		Tang.		Secant.		M

47 *Degrees.*

43 Degrees.

M	Sine.		Tang.		Secant.		
0	9.8337833	9.8641275	9.9696559	10.0303441	10.1358725	10.1662167	60
1	9.8339188	9.8640096	9.9699091	10.0300909	10.1359904	10.1660812	59
2	9.8340541	9.8638917	9.9701624	10.0298376	10.1361083	10.1659459	58
3	9.8341894	9.8637737	9.9704157	10.0295843	10.1362263	10.1658106	57
4	9.8343246	9.8636557	9.9706689	10.0293311	10.1363443	10.1656754	56
5	9.8344597	9.8635376	9.9709221	10.0290779	10.1364524	10.1655402	55
6	9.8345948	9.8634194	9.9711754	10.0288246	10.1365806	10.1654052	54
7	9.8347297	9.8633011	9.9714286	10.0285714	10.1366989	10.1652703	53
8	9.8348646	9.8631928	9.9716818	10.0283182	10.1368172	10.1651354	52
9	9.8349991	9.8630644	9.9719350	10.0280650	10.1369356	10.1650006	51
10	9.8351341	9.8629460	9.9721882	10.0278118	10.1370540	10.1648659	50
11	9.8352688	9.8628274	9.9724413	10.0275587	10.1371726	10.1647312	49
12	9.8354033	9.8627088	9.9726945	10.0273055	10.1372912	10.1645967	48
13	9.8355378	9.8625902	9.9729477	10.0270523	10.1374098	10.1644622	47
14	9.8356722	9.8624714	9.9732008	10.0267992	10.1375286	10.1643278	46
15	9.8358066	9.8623526	9.9734539	10.0265461	10.1376474	10.1641934	45
16	9.8359408	9.8622338	9.9737071	10.0262929	10.1377662	10.1640592	44
17	9.8360750	9.8621148	9.9739602	10.0260398	10.1378852	10.1639250	43
18	9.8362091	9.8619958	9.9742133	10.0257867	10.1380042	10.1637909	42
19	9.8363431	9.8618767	9.9744664	10.0255336	10.1381233	10.1636569	41
20	9.8364771	9.8617576	9.9747195	10.0252805	10.1382424	10.1635229	40
21	9.8366109	9.8616383	9.9749726	10.0250274	10.1383617	10.1633891	39
22	9.8367447	9.8615190	9.9752257	10.0247743	10.1384810	10.1632553	38
23	9.8368784	9.8613997	9.9754787	10.0245213	10.1386003	10.1631216	37
24	9.8370121	9.8612803	9.9757318	10.0242682	10.1387197	10.1629879	36
25	9.8371456	9.8611608	9.9759849	10.0240151	10.1388392	10.1628544	35
26	9.8372791	9.8610412	9.9762379	10.0237621	10.1389588	10.1627209	34
27	9.8374125	9.8609215	9.9764909	10.0235091	10.1390785	10.1625875	33
28	9.8375458	9.8608018	9.9767440	10.0232560	10.1391982	10.1624542	32
29	9.8376790	9.8606821	9.9769970	10.0230030	10.1393179	10.1623210	31
30	9.8378122	9.8605622	9.9772500	10.0227500	10.1394378	10.1621878	30
	Sine.		Tang.			Secant.	M

46 Degrees.

43 *Degrees.*

M	Sine.		Tang.		Secant.		
30	9.8378122	9.8605622	9.9772500	10.0227500	10.1394378	10.1621878	30
31	9.8379453	9.8604423	9.9775030	10.0224970	10.1395577	10.1620547	29
32	9.8380783	9.8603223	9.9777560	10.0222440	10.1396777	10.1619217	28
33	9.8382112	9.8602022	9.9780090	10.0219910	10.1397978	10.1617882	27
34	9.8383441	9.8600821	9.9782620	10.0217380	10.1399179	10.1616559	26
35	9.8384769	9.8599619	9.9785149	10.0214851	10.1400381	10.1615231	25
36	9.8386096	9.8598416	9.9787679	10.0212321	10.1401584	10.1613904	24
37	9.8387422	9.8597213	9.9790209	10.0209791	10.1402787	10.1612578	23
38	9.8388747	9.8596009	9.9792738	10.0207262	10.1403991	10.1611253	22
39	9.8390072	9.8594804	9.9795268	10.0204732	10.1405196	10.1609928	21
40	9.8391396	9.8593599	9.9797797	10.0202203	10.1406401	10.1608604	20
41	9.8392719	9.8592393	9.9800326	10.0199674	10.1407607	10.1607281	19
42	9.8394041	9.8591186	9.9802856	10.0197144	10.1408814	10.1605959	18
43	9.8395363	9.8589978	9.9805385	10.0194615	10.1410022	10.1604637	17
44	9.8396684	9.8588770	9.9807914	10.0192086	10.1411230	10.1603316	16
45	9.8398004	9.8587561	9.9810443	10.0189557	10.1412439	10.1601996	15
46	9.8399323	9.8586351	9.9812972	10.0187028	10.1413649	10.1600677	14
47	9.8400642	9.8585141	9.9815501	10.0184499	10.1414859	10.1599358	13
48	9.8401959	9.8583929	9.9818030	10.0181970	10.1416071	10.1598041	12
49	9.8403276	9.8582718	9.9820559	10.0179441	10.1417282	10.1596724	11
50	9.8404593	9.8581505	9.9823087	10.0176913	10.1418495	10.1595407	10
51	9.8405908	9.8580292	9.9825616	10.0174384	10.1419708	10.1594092	9
52	9.8407223	9.8579078	9.9828145	10.0171855	10.1420922	10.1592777	8
53	9.8408537	9.8577863	9.9830673	10.0169327	10.1422137	10.1591463	7
54	9.8409850	9.8576648	9.9833202	10.0166798	10.1423352	10.1590150	6
55	9.8411162	9.8575432	9.9835730	10.0164270	10.1424568	10.1588838	5
56	9.8412474	9.8574215	9.9838259	10.0161741	10.1425785	10.1587526	4
57	9.8413785	9.8572998	9.9840787	10.0159213	10.1427002	10.1586215	3
58	9.8415095	9.8571779	9.9843315	10.0156685	10.1428221	10.1584905	2
59	9.8416404	9.8570561	9.9845844	10.0154156	10.1429439	10.1583596	1
60	9.8417713	9.8569341	9.9848372	10.0151628	10.1430659	10.1582287	0
	Sine.		Tang.		Secant.		M

46 *Degrees.*

44 Degrees.

M	Sine.		Tang.		Secant.		
0	9.8417713	9.8569241	9.9848372	10.0151628	10.1430659	10.1582287	60
1	9.8419021	9.8568121	9.9850900	10.0149100	10.1431879	10.1580975	59
2	9.8420328	9.8566990	9.9853428	10.0146572	10.1433100	10.1579672	58
3	9.8421634	9.8565678	9.9855956	10.0144044	10.1434322	10.1578360	57
4	9.8422939	9.8564456	9.9858484	10.0141516	10.1435545	10.1577061	56
5	9.8424244	9.8563234	9.9861012	10.0138988	10.1436768	10.1575756	55
6	9.8425548	9.8562002	9.9863540	10.0136460	10.1437992	10.1574452	54
7	9.8426851	9.8560784	9.9866068	10.0133934	10.1439216	10.1573149	53
8	9.8428154	9.8559555	9.9868596	10.0131404	10.1440442	10.1571846	52
9	9.8429456	9.8558333	9.9871123	10.0128877	10.1441668	10.1570544	51
10	9.8430757	9.8557100	9.9873651	10.0126349	10.1442894	10.1569243	50
11	9.8432057	9.8555879	9.9876179	10.0123821	10.1444122	10.1567943	49
12	9.8433357	9.8554650	9.9878706	10.0121294	10.1445350	10.1566644	48
13	9.8434655	9.8553421	9.9881234	10.0118766	10.1446579	10.1565345	47
14	9.8435953	9.8552194	9.9883761	10.0116239	10.1447808	10.1564047	46
15	9.8437250	9.8550961	9.9886289	10.0113711	10.1449039	10.1562750	45
16	9.8438547	9.8549730	9.9888816	10.0111184	10.1450270	10.1561453	44
17	9.8439842	9.8548499	9.9891344	10.0108656	10.1451501	10.1560158	43
18	9.8441137	9.8547266	9.9893871	10.0106129	10.1452734	10.1558863	42
19	9.8442432	9.8546033	9.9896399	10.0103601	10.1453967	10.1557568	41
20	9.8443725	9.8544799	9.9898926	10.0101074	10.1455201	10.1556275	40
21	9.8445018	9.8543564	9.9901453	10.0098547	10.1456436	10.1554982	39
22	9.8446310	9.8542329	9.9903981	10.0096019	10.1457671	10.1553690	38
23	9.8447601	9.8541093	9.9906508	10.0093492	10.1458907	10.1552399	37
24	9.8448891	9.8539856	9.9909035	10.0090965	10.1460144	10.1551109	36
25	9.8450181	9.8538619	9.9911562	10.0088438	10.1461381	10.1549819	35
26	9.8451470	9.8537381	9.9914089	10.0085911	10.1462619	10.1548530	34
27	9.8452758	9.8536142	9.9916616	10.0083384	10.1463858	10.1547242	33
28	9.8454045	9.8534902	9.9919143	10.0080857	10.1465098	10.1545955	32
29	9.8455332	9.8533662	9.9921670	10.0078330	10.1466338	10.1544668	31
30	9.8456018	9.8532421	9.9924197	10.0075803	10.1467579	10.1543382	30
	Sine.		Tang.		Secant.		M

45 Degrees.

44 Degrees.

M	Sine.		Tang.		Secant.		
30	9.8456618	9.8532421	9.9924197	10.0075803	10.1467579	10.1543382	30
31	9.8457903	9.8531179	9.9926724	10.0073276	10.1468821	10.1542097	29
32	9.8459188	9.8529936	9.9929251	10.0070749	10.1470064	10.1540812	28
33	9.8460471	9.8528693	9.9931778	10.0068222	10.1471307	10.1539529	27
34	9.8461754	9.8527449	9.9934305	10.0065695	10.1472551	10.1538246	26
35	9.8463036	9.8526204	9.9936832	10.0063168	10.1473795	10.1536964	25
36	9.8464318	9.8524959	9.9939359	10.0060641	10.1475041	10.1535682	24
37	9.8465599	9.8523713	9.9941886	10.0058114	10.1476287	10.1534401	23
38	9.8466879	9.8522466	9.9944413	10.0055587	10.1477534	10.1533121	22
39	9.8468158	9.8521218	9.9946940	10.0053060	10.1478782	10.1531842	21
40	9.8469436	9.8519970	9.9949466	10.0050534	10.1480030	10.1530564	20
41	9.8470714	9.8518721	9.9951993	10.0048007	10.1481279	10.1529286	19
42	9.8471991	9.8517471	9.9954520	10.0045480	10.1482529	10.1528009	18
43	9.8473267	9.8516220	9.9957047	10.0042953	10.1483780	10.1526733	17
44	9.8474543	9.8514969	9.9959573	10.0040427	10.1485031	10.1525457	16
45	9.8475817	9.8513717	9.9962100	10.0037900	10.1486283	10.1524183	15
46	9.8477091	9.8512465	9.9964627	10.0035373	10.1487535	10.1522909	14
47	9.8478365	9.8511211	9.9967154	10.0032846	10.1488789	10.1521635	13
48	9.8479637	9.8509957	9.9969680	10.0030320	10.1490043	10.1520363	12
49	9.8480909	9.8508702	9.9972207	10.0027793	10.1491298	10.1519091	11
50	9.8482180	9.8507446	9.9974734	10.0025266	10.1492554	10.1517820	10
51	9.8483450	9.8506190	9.9977260	10.0022740	10.1493810	10.1516550	9
52	9.8484720	9.8504933	9.9979787	10.0020213	10.1495067	10.1515280	8
53	9.8485989	9.8503675	9.9982314	10.0017686	10.1496325	10.1514011	7
54	9.8487257	9.8502417	9.9984840	10.0015160	10.1497583	10.1512743	6
55	9.8488524	9.8501157	9.9987367	10.0012633	10.1498843	10.1511476	5
56	9.8489791	9.8499897	9.9989893	10.0010107	10.1500103	10.1510209	4
57	9.8491057	9.8498637	9.9992420	10.0007580	10.1501363	10.1508943	3
58	9.8492322	9.8497375	9.9994947	10.0005053	10.1502625	10.1507678	2
59	9.8493586	9.8496113	9.9997473	10.0002527	10.1503887	10.1506414	1
60	9.8494850	9.8494850	10.0000000	10.0000000	10.1505150	10.1505150	0
	Sine.		Tang.		Secant.		M

45 Degrees.

A TABLE of the ANGLES, which every Rhomb (or Point of the Compass) maketh with the Meridian.

NORTH.	SOUTH	Points.	D.	M.	NORTH.	SOUTH.
		¼	02	49		
		½	05	37		
		¾	08	26		
North by East	South by East	1	11	15	N by W.	S. by W.
		1 ¼	14	04		
		1 ½	16	52		
		1 ¾	19	41		
N. N. E.	S. S. E.	2	22	30	N. N. W.	S. S. W.
		2 ¼	25	19		
		2 ½	28	07		
		2 ¾	30	56		
N. E. by N.	S. E. by S.	3	33	45	N. W. by N.	S. W. by S.
		3 ¼	36	34		
		3 ½	39	22		
		3 ¾	42	11		
North-East	South-East	4	45	00	North-West	South-West
		4 ¼	47	49		
		4 ½	50	37		
		4 ¾	53	26		
N. E. by E.	S. E. by E.	5	56	15	N. W. by W.	S. W. by W.
		5 ¼	59	04		
		5 ½	61	52		
		5 ¾	64	42		
E. N. E.	E. S. E.	6	67	30	W. N. W.	W. S. W.
		6 ¼	70	19		
		6 ½	73	07		
		6 ¾	75	56		
East by North	East by South	7	78	45	W. by N.	W. by S.
		7 ¼	81	34		
		7 ½	84	22		
		7 ¾	87	11		
East.	East.	8	90	00	West	West.

FINIS.

Lightning Source UK Ltd.
Milton Keynes UK
UKHW021827160223
417092UK00004B/349